Amin Abbasi
Negin Lohrasbi
Sara Arshadi
Faezeh Tejareh
Mohammad Hashemi
Hedayat Hosseini

Gluten-Targeted Dietary and Non-Dietary Therapeutic Approaches in Celiac Disease

nova
science publishers
www.novapublishers.com

DOI: https://doi.org/10.52305/VBCE6840

Library of Congress Cataloging-in-Publication Data
Library of Congress Control Number: 2025946043
ISBN: 979-8-89530-545-4 (Hardcover)
ISBN: 979-8-89530-845-5 (eBook)

Published by Nova Science Publishers, Inc. † New York

Dedication

This book is dedicated to all the individuals who have been affected by celiac disease, whose courage and resilience continue to inspire the medical and scientific communities.

We also dedicate this work to our families and colleagues for their unwavering support and encouragement throughout this journey.

May this book serve as a resource that advances the understanding and treatment of celiac disease, ultimately improving the lives of those living with it.

Contents

Foreword

Celiac Disease (CD) is a complex and increasingly recognized autoimmune disorder that affects millions worldwide. For decades, its understanding and treatment have evolved through research and clinical trials, but much remains to be explored. This book, Gluten-Targeted Dietary and Non-Dietary Therapeutic Approaches in Celiac Disease, represents a significant contribution to this ongoing scientific discourse, offering a detailed, multi-faceted examination of the condition from the perspectives of diet, pharmacological treatment, and immunology.

As we delve deeper into the realms of celiac disease, it becomes clear that the need for comprehensive and innovative approaches to its treatment is more pressing than ever. The authors, a distinguished group of researchers and clinicians, have assembled a wealth of knowledge that bridges gaps between the most current research findings and practical therapeutic strategies. This book's interdisciplinary approach - combining insights from gastroenterology, immunology, nutrition science, and even artificial intelligence - offers a holistic understanding of how both established and emerging therapies can improve patient outcomes.

One of the key strengths of this volume is its focus on non-dietary treatments, an area that has traditionally been overshadowed by the emphasis on gluten-free diets. While the gluten-free diet remains the cornerstone of managing celiac disease, this book highlights cutting-edge advances in pharmacology, including immunomodulation, probiotics, gluten vaccinations, and targeted therapies. The integration of these therapies could revolutionize the way we approach CD treatment, offering hope for patients who are non-responsive to conventional dietary interventions.

Moreover, the inclusion of chapters on diagnostic challenges, the role of the microbiome, and future directions in therapy underscores the depth and breadth of the research presented. This is not just a resource for clinicians and researchers, but a vital guide for anyone involved in the care of patients with celiac disease. It emphasizes the critical importance of interdisciplinary collaboration in addressing the diverse needs of these patients, whose lives are shaped by a condition that, though widely recognized, remains challenging to manage.

In reviewing the chapters, it is evident that the authors have painstakingly integrated evidence-based findings with clinical expertise, making this book an essential resource for understanding the complexities of celiac disease and the innovative therapeutic strategies that lie ahead. I commend the authors for their dedication to advancing the field of celiac disease research and for producing a work that is as informative as it is inspiring.

As our understanding of celiac disease continues to evolve, this book will undoubtedly play a pivotal role in shaping future research and treatment strategies. It is my sincere hope that it inspires further scientific inquiry and drives advancements that improve the lives of individuals affected by this chronic and often debilitating condition.

Dr. Leili Aghebati Maleki, PhD,
Head of the Medical Immunology Research Center
Tabriz University of Medical Sciences, Tabriz, Iran

Preface

Celiac disease (CD) represents a significant global health concern, with its intricate interplay of genetic, environmental, and immunological factors posing substantial challenges for researchers and clinicians alike. This book, *Gluten-Targeted Dietary and Non-Dietary Therapeutic Approaches in Celiac Disease*, seeks to provide a comprehensive exploration of the latest advancements in the understanding, diagnosis, and management of CD. Our intent is to serve as a valuable resource for a wide spectrum of readers, including healthcare professionals, researchers, students, and policy-makers, fostering an informed dialogue on this multifaceted condition.

The book is structured to encompass a thorough examination of CD's epidemiology, pathophysiology, and diagnostic methodologies, emphasizing both established practices and innovative techniques. It also delves deeply into the dietary and non-dietary therapeutic interventions that are shaping the future of CD management. From the critical role of gluten-free diets to groundbreaking pharmacological approaches, this text provides an integrative perspective that highlights the strides made in addressing both the symptomatic and underlying immunological aspects of the disease.

One of the unique strengths of this volume lies in its interdisciplinary approach, bridging insights from gastroenterology, immunology, nutrition science, and even artificial intelligence. The chapters offer a nuanced understanding of how evolving diagnostic tools and therapeutic strategies can be harmonized to improve patient outcomes. Furthermore, the inclusion of discussions on nutritional considerations, gluten-free food innovations, and the socioeconomic dimensions of CD management ensures a holistic coverage of the subject. In this book, we have strived to present evidence-based findings, supported by extensive clinical and preclinical research. The collaborative contributions from a distinguished group of authors underscore the collective effort to enhance the scientific community's understanding of CD and inspire further inquiry.

We recognize that scientific knowledge is ever-evolving and that the true potential of this work can only be realized through active engagement with our readers. We warmly invite feedback, critiques, and suggestions from our audience, as such interactions are invaluable in refining the understanding and application of the concepts presented here. Should you wish to share your thoughts, please feel free to contact us through the provided email addresses.

It is our sincere hope that this book not only enriches readers' knowledge of celiac disease but also inspires continued exploration and innovation in this vital field of study.

Dr. Amin Abbasi (abasi@tbzmed.ac.ir)
Negin Lohrasbi (negin.lohrasbi250@gmail.com)
Sara Arshadi (saraharshadii81@gmail.com)
Faezeh Tejareh (faezehtejareh135@gmail.com)
Dr. Mohammad Hashemi (mo_hashemi@hotmail.com)
Hedayat Hosseini (hedayat@sbmu.ac.ir)

Endorsements

The book provides a remarkable synthesis of immunological mechanisms and therapeutic interventions for celiac disease. The interdisciplinary approach is highly valuable for researchers and clinicians alike who are looking to advance their understanding of gluten-induced immune responses.

Dr. Hossein Samadi Kafil, PhD,
Head of Applied Pharmaceutical Research Center
Tabriz University of Medical Sciences, Tabriz, Iran

A comprehensive and accessible resource that bridges the gap between the latest research in celiac disease and practical dietary management. This book is essential for nutritionists and dieticians working with individuals affected by gluten intolerance and celiac disease.

Dr. Anahita Ghorbani Tajani, PhD,
University of Wyoming, Laramie, USA

This book is an essential addition to the growing body of literature on celiac disease. It comprehensively covers both dietary and non-dietary therapeutic approaches, providing valuable insights for anyone interested in the future of celiac disease management.

Dr. Sahar Sabahi, PhD,
Director of Nutrition Department
Ahvaz University of Medical Sciences, Ahvaz, Iran

This book offers an in-depth and up-to-date review of the diagnostic and therapeutic strategies for celiac disease. It provides a thorough understanding of both conventional and emerging approaches, making it an invaluable resource for clinicians in gastroenterology.

Dr. Kiana Ghafourian, MD,
Shahid Beheshti University of Medical Sciences, Tehran, Iran

Acknowledgments

We would like to express our deepest gratitude to all those who have contributed to the completion of this book.

First and foremost, we would like to thank the patients and their families living with celiac disease, whose resilience and experiences have been a constant source of inspiration for this work. It is their stories that drive us to continue seeking better therapeutic solutions.

We would also like to acknowledge our colleagues and experts in the fields of gastroenterology, immunology, and nutrition who have provided invaluable guidance and support. Their expertise has enriched the content of this book and ensured its scientific accuracy.

A special thanks goes to the research teams and clinical practitioners who are at the forefront of celiac disease diagnosis and treatment. Their dedication to advancing our understanding of this condition is truly commendable.

We are incredibly grateful to our families for their unwavering support, patience, and encouragement throughout the entire writing process. Without their love and understanding, this book would not have been possible.

Lastly, we extend our sincere thanks to the editorial and publishing teams at Nova Science Publishers for their professionalism and commitment in bringing this book to fruition.

Chapter 1

Introduction to Celiac Disease

Abstract

Celiac disease (CD) is a chronic immune-mediated disorder triggered by the ingestion of gluten in genetically predisposed individuals. This chapter introduces CD, tracing its historical development and the early recognition of its symptoms. It emphasizes the importance of understanding CD's impact on global health, as the disease poses challenges to clinicians and researchers. The chapter also highlights advancements in the diagnosis, treatment, and management of the condition, providing a foundational understanding for the rest of the book.

Introduction

Over the past few years, there has been significant discussion about celiac disease (CD) and non-celiac gluten sensitivity. However, historically, accounts of celiac disease are far from new. The earliest known description of the condition is attributed to the Greek physician Aretaeus, who noted that adult patients with the ailment experienced "a persistent impairment of digestive processes and malabsorption, resulting in a malnourished state, and whose symptoms are alleviated by fasting" (Dowd & Walker-Smith, 1974). In 1888, Samuel Jones Gee described what he referred to as the "Coeliac Affection," a chronic dyspepsia primarily affecting children, though it can occur in individuals of all ages. The condition is characterized by diarrhea and symptoms of malabsorption (Yan & Holt, 2009). Until the mid-20th century, the disease was often referred to as "Gee-Herter," named after both Gee in England and Christian Herter, who first characterized the disease in the USA. Dutch pediatrician Willem Dicke made the most significant and insightful historical observations regarding celiac disease in the 1930s and 1940s. At the time, the standard care for children with celiac disease consisted of a "banana diet" or "Fanconi diet," which included vegetables and fruits. The potential toxicity of wheat consumption, however, was not yet understood. Through careful observations, while advising families on various dietary approaches - including a wheat-free meal - and having them report back, Dicke proposed a wheat-free diet in 1941. Many of Dicke's patients saw clinical improvements during the "winter of famine" in the Netherlands during World War II. When bread was once again made available, the patients' conditions dramatically worsened. This experience led to a wider recognition of the harmful effects of wheat (Yan & Holt, 2009).

Definitions Regarding CD

There is no consensus on the terminology used to describe celiac disease and other illnesses related to gluten consumption. In the past, celiac disease has also been referred to by other names, including celiac sprue, gluten intolerance, sprue, and gluten-sensitive enteropathy. *Acta Paediatrica* published the first widely accepted terminology for celiac disease in 1970, nearly forty years ago. At that time, the term "celiac disease" was used to describe a chronic illness characterized by mucosal flattening and gluten sensitivity that (a) is cured on a gluten-free diet (GFD) and (b) reverts with the reintroduction of gluten (Weijers et al., 1970). With growing awareness of the broader range of illnesses linked to gluten consumption, a comprehensive literature evaluation led to the Oslo definitions, which were published in 2013 (Ludvigsson, Leffler, et al., 2013).

- *Celiac disease (CD)* is described as a chronic immune-mediated enteropathy of the intestine that develops in individuals with a genetic predisposition when they consume dietary gluten.
- The term *"classical CD"* refers to CD that exhibits malabsorption-related symptoms and signs. It must cause steatorrhea, diarrhea, weight loss, or growth failure.
- *Non-classical CD* refers to individuals who have the disease but lack any symptoms associated with malabsorption. These patients may experience constipation, abdominal discomfort, and other signs not typically associated with malabsorption.
- *Symptomatic CD* is defined by gastrointestinal and/or extraintestinal symptoms that are clinically apparent and linked to gluten consumption.

- The term *"gluten-related disorders"* encompasses all illnesses caused by gluten, including CD, non-celiac gluten sensitivity, dermatitis herpetiformis (DH), and gluten ataxia.

It was also advised against using the terms "gluten intolerance," "overt CD" (defined as dyspepsia, diarrhea, and bloating caused by gluten ingestion), and "silent CD," which is synonymous with "asymptomatic CD."

In the literature on celiac disease, other terminologies are often used, including:

- Several definitions exist for *latent CD.* The broadest definition applies to individuals with a positive CD serology, normal mucosa, no villous atrophy (VA), and no symptoms. The terms *potential CD* and *latent CD* have been used interchangeably. Family members of CD patients who test positive for the human leucocyte antigens (HLA) DQ2 and/or DQ8 are considered genetically at risk for CD. HLA and non-HLA genes, which account for about 65% of the genetic predisposition, contribute to the genetic risk for CD (Van Heel et al., 2007).

Epidemiology of CD

Incidence and Prevalence

Celiac disease is now recognized as a global condition, contrary to earlier beliefs that it primarily affected individuals in Western and Northern Europe. A comprehensive assessment of the global prevalence of celiac disease indicated a seroprevalence rate of 1.4%, with prevalence varying by continent: from 1.3% in South America (based on 11 studies) to 10.8% in Asia (based on 20 studies) (Sima et al., 2010; P. Singh et al., 2018). Given the poor sensitivity of celiac disease serologies, these figures may exaggerate the true frequency of the condition. This research also assessed the prevalence of celiac disease, which was found to be 0.7% overall, but varied by continent and region. Since not all individuals who are seropositive for celiac disease undergo thorough endoscopic evaluation, seroprevalence may be overstated, while biopsy-proven cases of celiac disease may be underestimated. The prevalence and incidence of CD have been rising over time, a trend observed across various geographical locations. In 33 studies that examined incidence at multiple time points and were subjected to systematic review and meta-analysis, substantial increases in diagnostic rates were reported in 24 (73%) of them over time (J. A. King et al., 2020). From 1950 to 2010, the diagnosis rate in Olmsted County, Minnesota, rose by 8.1% (Ludvigsson, Rubio-Tapia, et al., 2013). The development of serologic testing in the 1990s has been linked to significant increases in diagnosis rates, which have also been influenced by various incentives (Murray et al., 2003). For example, detection rates in Finland increased after a policy was implemented requiring individuals to have a doctor-confirmed diagnosis in order to be eligible for a government-funded gluten-free diet (Virta, Kaukinen, & Collin, 2009).

There is growing evidence that, in addition to increased awareness, the prevalence of celiac disease has risen, reflecting a true increase in its incidence. Cohort studies such as the Diabetes Autoimmunity Research in the Young study have shown this trend. In this study, celiac disease antibodies were assessed at 9, 15, and 24 months, as well as yearly, in 1,339 infants born at a hospital in Denver, Colorado, between 1993 and 2004 and possessing an HLA haplotype associated with celiac disease. Duodenal biopsy was offered to participants whose antibody levels were steadily rising. The prevalence of CD in the greater Denver region, by age 15 years, was projected to be 3.1%, based on data on population HLA distribution and the diagnosis of celiac disease in 66 children (4.9%) (E. Liu et al., 2017).

Celiac disease can manifest in individuals of any age, including the elderly (Zali, Sima, Hekmatdoost, Ghaziani, & Mashayekh, 2003). Such diagnoses may result from a de novo loss of gluten tolerance rather than the delayed detection of celiac disease. Studies using repeated blood samples have shown that adults can lose their ability to tolerate gluten. However, newer prospective cohort studies have revealed that celiac disease typically develops in individuals before the age of 10 (Jansson-Knodell et al., 2019). According to pooled research (J. A. King et al., 2020), women have a higher incidence of CD than men (17.0 vs. 7.8 per 100,000 person-years), although this difference may be attributed to higher rates of undiagnosed cases in men.

Female participants in screening trials exhibited somewhat higher seropositivity, according to a systematic review and meta-analysis (Jansson-Knodell et al., 2019), although other studies in adults have shown that men and women have similar seroprevalences (Katz et al., 2011). The lower frequency of duodenal biopsies performed on men during upper endoscopy for symptoms such as diarrhea and weight loss may contribute to an underdiagnosis in this population (Lebwohl et al., 2012).

The risk for celiac disease varies across nations. Despite the identical prevalence of the HLA-permissive haplotypes DQ2 and DQ8, the prevalence of celiac disease in India is higher in the Punjab region (1.2%) and other northern areas compared to the south (0.1%) (Ramakrishna et al., 2016). In that study, no difference in celiac disease prevalence was found between urban and rural areas or across different socioeconomic statuses. Similarly, a study of duodenal biopsy samples from upper endoscopies sent to pathology labs across the United States showed that individuals of Punjabi ancestry had the highest frequency of villous atrophy, significantly higher than those of Indian ancestry from other regions (Krigel et al., 2016).

The causes of these geographical and racial variations are unknown; however, they may be linked to the higher mean daily wheat intake in the Punjab region (Ramakrishna et al., 2016). Regional differences may also be explained by various environmental factors. Racial and ethnic disparities in the prevalence of CD persist even in screening studies, regardless of variations in testing rates. In the US, non-Hispanic Black and Hispanic individuals with celiac disease have a lower prevalence than white individuals. According to data from the National Health and Nutrition Examination Survey (NHANES), seroprevalence was 0.2% in non-Hispanic Black and 0.3% in Hispanic individuals, compared to 1.0% in white individuals (Ditah et al., 2015).

Similarly, despite being in close geographical proximity, the prevalence of CD can differ significantly between countries. A screening study found serological signs of CD in 1.4% of individuals in Finland, but only 0.6% in the nearby Russian Karelia, despite no discernible differences in compatible HLA haplotypes (Kondrashova et al., 2008). These variations have led researchers to explore environmental exposures as potential risk factors for the onset of celiac disease.

Chapter 2

Risk Factors and Prevention Strategies for Celiac Disease

Abstract

Celiac disease is primarily influenced by genetic and environmental factors, particularly the presence of HLA-DQ2/DQ8 alleles. This chapter investigates these risk factors and discusses their role in disease onset. Environmental triggers such as infections, microbiota imbalances, and dietary habits are explored. Additionally, it reviews prevention strategies, including the timing of gluten introduction in infants and the implications for at-risk populations. The chapter aims to provide insights into how modifiable factors may contribute to CD prevention and management.

Risk Factors

The presentation of deamidated gliadin peptide fragments by antigen-presenting cells through HLA proteins causes enteropathy associated with celiac disease. The major histocompatibility complex (MHC) region on chromosome 6 contains genes that encode for HLA proteins, which are found on the surface of antigen-presenting cells (N. K. Brown, Guandalini, Semrad, & Kupfer, 2019). Specific haplotypes produce proteins that bind to particular antigens. The DQ2 and DQ8 haplotypes enable antigen-presenting cells to display gluten antigens, which may trigger an immune response and the onset of celiac disease. While the expression of at least one of these haplotypes is required for the onset of celiac disease, it is not sufficient by itself. Approximately 35% of Americans carry a DQ2 or DQ8 haplotype, yet most of them never develop celiac disease (N. K. Brown et al., 2019). Additional, though minor, genetic risk factors for celiac disease have been identified through genome-wide association studies; however, DQ2 and DQ8 are the genetic traits most strongly linked to the onset of the condition (Romanos et al., 2014). In twin studies, only 49% to 83% of monozygotic twins had concordance rates, suggesting that environmental risk factors also play a role

(Kuja-Halkola et al., 2017). Moreover, the prevalence of celiac disease has increased recently in several countries. For example, the incidence of celiac disease serologies increased from 0.2% to 0.9% between blood samples collected in 1950 and 2006 from age-matched individuals at the Warren Air Force Base (Rubio–Tapia et al., 2009).

Similar research in Finland, where celiac disease is more prevalent overall, found an increase in prevalence from 1.05% in 1978 to 1.99% in 2000 (Lohi et al., 2007). This sudden rise in prevalence is likely due to environmental, rather than genetic, risk factors. Prevention strategies have mainly focused on infant feeding practices, particularly the timing of gluten introduction. Studies examining the sharp rise in CD incidence in Sweden during the 1980s led to the hypothesis that the epidemic was caused by early high-gluten introduction without concurrent breastfeeding (Ivarsson et al., 2000).

An analysis of the Diabetes Autoimmunity Research in the Young (DAISY) study found that celiac disease-associated antibodies were detected in a higher percentage of infants whose gluten exposure occurred either before age 3 months or after age 6 months (Norris et al., 2005). These observational studies prompted clinical trials to test methods for protecting children at higher risk of developing celiac disease, including those with a family history and a suitable HLA haplotype. In an Italian multicenter trial, 533 infants were randomized into two groups: one introduced gluten at 12 months, and the other at 6 months. Except for a slightly higher incidence of CD in the 12-month group, there were no significant differences in disease progression between the groups by the time the children reached 10 years of age (Lionetti et al., 2014).

In a multicenter randomized experiment, 944 infants were divided into groups at the age of 4 months and given either low doses of daily gluten or a placebo. Both groups were then introduced to full doses of gluten at 6 months. By the age of 5 years, 12.1% of participants had developed celiac disease, with no discernible difference between the groups (Vriezinga et al., 2014). The findings of these trials, based on observational research, disproved long-held theories that the timing of gluten intake increased the likelihood of developing celiac disease.

In response to these findings, the European Society for Pediatric Gastroenterology, Hepatology, and Nutrition revised their feeding recommendations, suggesting that gluten could be introduced at any time between 4 and 12 months of age (Szajewska et al., 2016). Despite these disappointing results, there is still considerable interest in how early gluten intake affects the likelihood of developing celiac disease. While it would be challenging to investigate this further due to the small number of reported outcomes, the therapies tested in this high-risk cohort likely had positive effects in lower-risk populations.

Gluten consumption has been found to be inversely correlated with the prevalence of celiac disease (Ramakrishna et al., 2016), suggesting that the quantity of gluten consumed, rather than the timing of its introduction, may influence the risk of developing the condition. This theory has gained further support from recent studies: three cohort studies found that children who consumed more gluten had a higher risk of developing celiac disease (Aronsson et al., 2019). These studies, which reported celiac disease frequencies ranging from 1.1% (Lund-Blix et al., 2019) to 7%, were conducted in several countries, including Norway (Lund-Blix et al., 2019), the United States (Mårild et al., 2019), and an international cohort that included Sweden, Germany, Finland, and the United States. Both clinically diagnosed and screen-detected cases of CD were included in these studies. The consistent findings, showing a gradient between early childhood gluten consumption and eventual celiac disease, suggest that the amount of gluten consumed should be evaluated in future intervention trials (Ludvigsson & Lebwohl, 2019). In addition to gluten consumption, other environmental risk factors for celiac disease have been identified. Small increases in the risk of celiac disease have been associated with perinatal factors such as elective (but not emergent) cesarean birth and being small for gestational age (Mårild, Stephansson, Montgomery, Murray, & Ludvigsson, 2012). However, the evidence regarding the effects of cesarean birth remains conflicting (Koletzko et al., 2018).

Prevention Strategies for CD

Celiac disease may be triggered by microbial infections such as *Campylobacter* species (Riddle, Murray, Cash, Pimentel, & Porter, 2013b), rotavirus (Inns, Fleming, Iturriza-Gomara, & Hungerford, 2021), or reovirus (Bouziat et al., 2017), and immunization against rotavirus may offer protection (K. M. Kemppainen et al., 2017). A subsequent diagnosis of celiac disease is more likely when certain features of the gastric environment are present, such as the absence of *Helicobacter pylori* survival and the use of proton pump inhibitors. However, these associations may be explained by protopathic bias and socioeconomic factors, respectively (Lebwohl, Spechler, Wang, Green, & Ludvigsson, 2014).

Although the exact mechanism behind these associations remains uncertain, factors such as a non-smoking lifestyle (Wijarnpreecha et al., 2018) and socioeconomic characteristics, including greater maternal education (Canova et al., 2014), have been linked to an increased risk of celiac disease. Most research on risk factors is constrained by the outcome of celiac disease diagnosis (vs. no diagnosis), which may be influenced by increased interactions with healthcare providers. Such studies may produce misleading associations between suggested exposures (e.g., infections) and the long-standing presence of celiac disease, even if these factors do not play a causative role, due to the time lag between the loss of gluten tolerance and the diagnosis of CD.

It is likely that some risk factors, such as those associated with gluten exposure, act early in life, while others, such as smoking, contribute to risk later in life. Uncertainty still surrounds the process behind the loss of gluten tolerance in adults. Identifying microbiome characteristics linked to the onset of celiac disease is of particular interest, as it may represent a modifiable risk factor (Leonard, Camhi, Huedo-Medina, & Fasano, 2015).

Given that elective cesarean delivery (Mårild et al., 2012) and the use of antibiotics (Mårild et al., 2013) have been associated with an increased risk of developing celiac disease, it is possible that these procedures alter the microbiome, contributing to the rising prevalence of the condition. Research examining the microbiomes of stool samples from infants who were exclusively breastfed supports the idea that the microbiome links environmental and genetic risk factors to celiac disease. Infants with the HLA DQ2 haplotype exhibited a distinct microbiome, characterized by higher proportions of *Proteobacteria* and *Firmicutes*, and lower levels of *Actinobacteria*, compared to those who tested negative for DQ2 or DQ8. These findings suggest that the microbiome may play a role in how the HLA haplotype influences the risk of celiac disease (Olivares et al., 2015).

While the exact mechanism by which the microbiome influences the risk of celiac disease remains unclear, potential mediators have been proposed, including the proteolytic activity of *Pseudomonas* species in the intestine (Caminero et al., 2019) and microbially produced gluten mimics (Petersen et al., 2020). Despite the lack of definitive evidence, there remains considerable interest in intervening along this pathway, particularly since early probiotic supplementation in the first year of life did not correlate with a lower risk of

CD in the TEDDY (The Environmental Determinants of Diabetes in the Young) cohort (Uusitalo et al., 2019).

Chapter 3

Pathophysiology and Immunology of Celiac Disease

Abstract

Celiac disease involves an immune-mediated response to gluten, resulting in inflammation and damage to the small intestine. This chapter delves into the underlying immunological mechanisms, focusing on the role of the adaptive immune system, particularly the involvement of T-cells and the HLA-DQ2/DQ8 molecules. It explains how gluten peptides, when deamidated by tissue transglutaminase, trigger an immune cascade that leads to villous atrophy. The chapter also addresses the molecular interactions that contribute to disease pathogenesis and the systemic effects of CD.

Immunoreactive Cereal Proteins

Global food security predominantly relies on cereal production, which occupies around 60% of agricultural land. In 2016, almost 2800×10^6 tons of cereals were harvested globally, with maize (1060×10^6 masses), wheat (749×10^6 tons), and paddy rice (741×10^6 tons) being the principal crops (Nakai, 2018). Wheat serves as a significant source of dietary nutrients, fulfilling approximately 30% of the daily requirements for carbs and proteins, 25% for dietary fiber, and 10-30% for vitamins (e.g., thiamin and niacin) and minerals (e.g., potassium, magnesium, iron, and zinc) (P. Shewry & Hey, 2016; P. R. Shewry, 2018).

Wheat consumption has been controversially linked to various health conditions, including type 2 diabetes mellitus, obesity, depression, autism, allergies, and other potential health risks, according to some studies and claims circulated on pseudoscientific platforms and social media (P. R. Shewry, Pellny, & Lovegrove, 2016). The resulting media response has generated significant confusion and ambiguity among consumers, with the removal of wheat (gluten) often touted as a miraculous remedy. Many consumers independently begin a gluten-free diet (GFD), which excludes common wheat, spelt, durum wheat, khorasan wheat, emmer, einkorn, triticale, rye, barley, and often oats, without any definitive medical justification. They do so under the belief that a GFD promotes health, enhances overall well-being, and aids in weight loss (Aziz, 2018). In doing so, they risk overlooking a potential genuine wheat allergy, which could lead to long-term health problems that might be mitigated with appropriate treatment. Moreover, there is a lack of credible scientific evidence supporting the benefits of a gluten-free diet. In fact, the opposite is often true, as many gluten-free products are deficient in essential nutrients, including vitamins, minerals, phytochemicals, protein, and dietary fiber, all of which are necessary for a balanced and nutritious diet (Babio et al., 2017).

Cereal Proteins

T. B. Osborne classified cereal proteins into sequentially extractable portions based on their solubility characteristics: albumins in water, globulins in dilute salt solutions, prolamins in 40–70% (v/v) aqueous ethanol, and glutelins in dilute acetic acid or alkali (Osborne, 1907). Albumins and globulins, which comprise 20–30% of Triticeae proteins, include metabolic and defensive proteins that play roles in grain development and resistance to diseases and pests. Prolamins and glutelins, making up 70–80% of Triticeae proteins, are storage proteins (gluten proteins) that function as reservoirs of amino acids and nitrogen during germination. Prolamins are primarily monomeric proteins, while glutelins are mainly polymeric proteins connected by intermolecular disulfide bonds (Schalk, Lexhaller, Koehler, & Scherf, 2017).

With the increasing availability of knowledge regarding grain proteins, the traditional Osborne fractions have been reinterpreted. Triticeae storage proteins are now classified based on sequence homologies and comparable relative molecular weights (Mr) into three categories: high-molecular-weight (HMW, Mr = $67–90 \times 10^3$), medium-molecular-weight (MMW, Mr = $34–51 \times 10^3$), and low-molecular-weight (LMW, Mr = $21–42 \times 10^3$). One example is γ-75k-secalins, which can reach a molecular weight of approximately 52×10^3 (Figure 1) (Lexhaller, Tompos, & Scherf, 2017).

Recent developments, such as the International Wheat Genome Sequencing Consortium (IWGSC) RefSeq v1.0, have provided the first annotated reference sequence for the hexaploid common wheat genome (Consortium et al., 2018). A diverse array of wheat proteins, along with closely related proteins from rye and barley, including both gluten and non-gluten proteins, have been identified as allergens or triggers for celiac disease (CD) and non-celiac gluten/wheat sensitivity (NCGS). A selection of the most significant causative proteins is presented in Table 1.

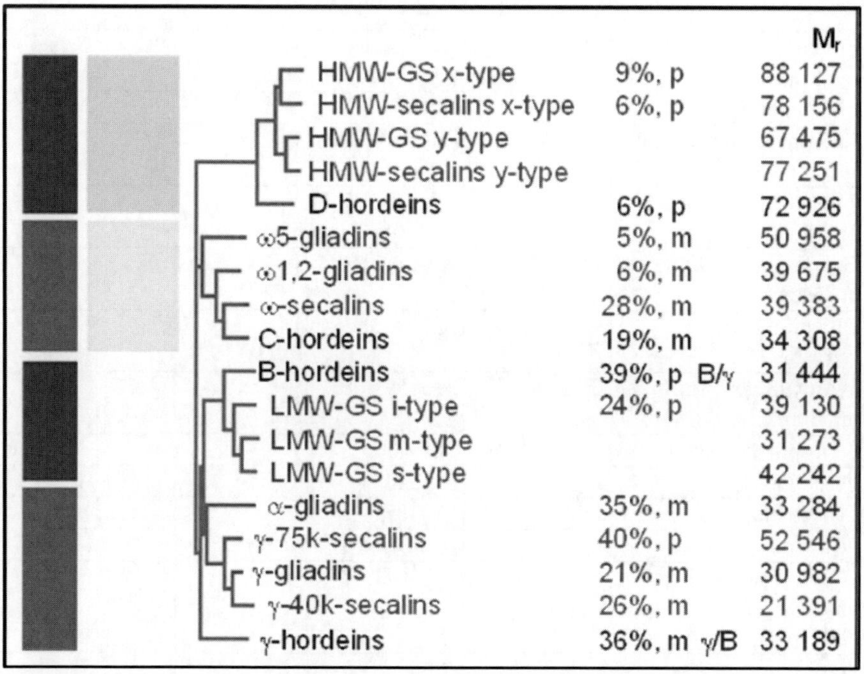

Figure 1. Gluten protein types assembled by homology using Clustal Omega and classification into groups with high-molecular-weight (HMW), medium- molecular-weight (MMW) and low-molecular-weight (LMW), as well as the alternative traditional classification into prolamins and glutelins. Percentages are typical values for amounts of each protein type relative to the total amount of gluten. The values for B-hordeins and g-hordeins also contain the respective other protein type (B/g and g/B), because they could not be separated by stepwise extraction/RP-HPLC. Relative molecular masses (M_r) are given as average masses of the protein without signal peptide. The following UniProtKB accessions of representative amino acid sequences were used: HMW-GS x-type, P10388, HMW-secalins x-type, Q94IK9, HMW-GS y-type, P10387, HMW- secalins y-type, Q94IL4, D-hordeins, Q40054, v5-gliadins, Q402I5, v1,2-gliadins, D2KKB1, v-secalins, C4NFN9, C-hordeins, Q41210, B-hordeins, P06470, LMW-GS i-type, P10385, LMW-GS m-type P16315, LMW-GS s-type Q9XGF0, a-gliadins, P18573, g-75k-secalins, E5KZP9, g-gliadins, P06659, g-40k-secalins, H8Y0K4, g-hordeins, P80198. m, mainly monomeric proteins, p, mainly polymeric proteins.

Table 1. Selected allergens in wheat (*Triticum aestivum*) flour, their allergen code according to the World Health Organization/International Union of Immunological Societies (WHO/IUIS) allergen nomenclature (allergen.org online database) and the accession (UniProtKB database) of one exemplary protein

Protein	Allergen code	Accession (UniProtKB)[a]	Wheat allergies	NCG	Celiac disease
Elongation factor	Tri a 45	W5AGF9	+		
Endosperm transfer cell specific PR60	Tri a 44	B2C4K0	+		
Grasses, group 43, uncharacterized	Tri a 43	A0A0G3F5F7	+		
Grasses, group 42, uncharacterized	Tri a 42	A0A0G3F2F5	+		
Ubiquitin ligase activator	Tri a 41	A0A0G3F2P1	+		
α-Amylase/trypsin - inhibitor CM16/CM17	Tri a 40	P16159	+	+	
Serin-protease-inhibitor	Tri a 39	P82977	+		
Purothionin	Tri a 37	P01543	+		
LMW glutenin subunit	Tri a 36	P10385	+		+
Dehydrin	Tri a 35	D2TE72	+		
Glyceraldehyde-3-phosphate dehydrogenase	Tri a 34	C7C4X1	+		
Serpin	Tri a 33	P93693	+		
1-Cys peroxiredoxin PER1	Tri a 32	Q6W8Q2	+		
Triosephosphate-isomerase	Tri a 31	Q9FS79	+		
α-Amylase-inhibitor CM2	Tri a 30	P17314	+	+	
α-Amylase-inhibitor CM3	Tri a 29	P16850	+	+	
α-Amylase-inhibitor 0.19/0.53	Tri a 28	P01085	+	+	
Thiolreductase	Tri a 27	D2TE73	+		
HMW glutenin subunit	Tri a 26	P08488	+		+
Thioredoxin	Tri a 25	Q9LDX4	+		
α-/β-Gliadin	Tri a 21	D2T2K3	+		+
γ-Gliadin	Tri a 20	P08079	+		+
ω5-Gliadin	Tri a 19	Q9FUW7	+		+

Protein	Allergen code	Accession (UniProtKB)[a]	Wheat allergies	NCG	Celiac disease
Wheat germ agglutinin	Tri a 18	P02876	+		
β-Amylase	Tri a 17	P93594	+		
α-Amylase-inhibitor 0.28	Tri a 15	P01083	+	+	
Lipid-transfer-protein	Tri a 14	D2T2K0	+		
Profilin	Tri a 12	D0PRB5	+		

[a] UniProt accession is given for one exemplary protein, but many different isoforms exist, especially of gluten proteins, +, known causative factor, no symbol, not a causative factor according to the current state-of-knowledge, NCGS, non-celiac gluten sensitivity, for references for each allergen, please see the allergen.org online database as well as Tatham and Shewry (Tatham & Shewry, 2008) and Juhasz et al., (Juhász et al., 2018) and references cited therein.

Gluten - Unique Protein with Two Faces

The term 'gluten' (derived from the Latin word for 'glue') carries different meanings depending on the context in which it is used. The original definition dates back to 1745, when J. B. Beccari first identified gluten in wheat flour and described it as the "rubber-like proteinaceous mass that remains after washing wheat dough with water." When wheat flour is combined with water, gliadins contribute to the viscosity and extensibility of the dough, while glutenins provide cohesion and elasticity. In the optimal gliadin/glutenin ratio of about 2:1, the dough exhibits superior gas retention, resulting in yeast-leavened bread with an elastic, uniformly porous crumb after baking (K. A. Scherf, Koehler, & Wieser, 2016).

A secondary definition of gluten pertains to the starch industry. Gluten is a byproduct of wheat starch production and is used in its dried powdered form as 'vital gluten' in both animal feed and food products. It serves multiple purposes, such as enhancing flours with low protein content, acting as a binding agent, or functioning as a meat substitute (K. A. Scherf, Umseher, Kieffer, & Koehler, 2016).

Third, In the context of hypersensitivities, gluten is defined as "a protein fraction derived from wheat, rye, barley, oats, or their hybrid varieties and derivatives, to which certain individuals exhibit intolerance, and which is insoluble in water and 0.5 M NaCl." Prolamins are specifically described as "the fraction of gluten extractable by 40-70% ethanol," with the "prolamin content of gluten typically regarded as 50%" (Commission, 2008). Gluten proteins are hydrophobic and characterized by repeated sequences that are rich in glutamine (26-53%) and proline (10-29%). Common repeated motifs include QQPQQPFP in v1,2-gliadins and g-gliadins, QQQFP in v5-gliadins, QPQPFP and PQQPYP in a-gliadins, QQQPPFS in LMW-GS, and QQPGQG and YYPTS in HMW-GS.

The majority of the approximately 1,000 identified CD-active gluten peptides originate from these repetitive sequences (Goodman et al., 2016), as human gastrointestinal enzymes - such as pepsin, trypsin, and chymotrypsin - cannot cleave before or after proline and glutamine. This results in the preservation of large peptides containing more than nine amino acid residues (Colgrave, Byrne, & Howitt, 2017; K. A. Scherf, Wieser, & Koehler, 2018). Incompletely digested gluten peptides pass through the small intestine brush border, penetrate the epithelial barrier via transcellular or paracellular pathways, and trigger disease-specific immunogenic cascades in the lamina propria.

Hypersensitivities towards Cereal Proteins

Hypersensitivities to cereal proteins can be categorized based on their pathomechanism into autoimmunogenic or innate immune responses, as well as immunoglobulin E (IgE)-mediated, non-IgE-mediated, or mixed (both IgE-mediated and non-IgE-mediated) allergies (Figure 2) (Dale, Biesiekierski, & Lied, 2019; Quirce, Boyano-Martínez, & Díaz-Perales, 2016).

Celiac Disease

CD is characterized as a chronic immune-mediated enteropathy of the small intestine triggered by the consumption of gluten from wheat, rye, and barley in genetically susceptible individuals (Dale et al., 2019). The global mean estimated prevalence of CD is 1.4% based on serology and 0.7% based on biopsy, while significant regional variations exist (P. Singh et al., 2018). The etiology of CD involves a confluence of environmental variables, including the ingestion of gluten from wheat, rye, or barley, and genetic predispositions, notably the presence of human leukocyte antigens (HLA)-DQ2 and (HLA)-DQ8. Nonetheless, this genetic tendency is observed in approximately 30% of the healthy population, suggesting that its presence alone is unable to induce

CD (Trynka, Wijmenga, & van Heel, 2010). Additional factors linked to the loss of gluten tolerance include infections (such as rotavirus and adenovirus 12), alterations in intestinal microbiota, heightened small intestinal permeability, and the hygiene hypothesis, which suggests that a reduced incidence of infections during early childhood accounts for the increase in immune-mediated hypersensitivities (Bach, 2018). As a complex condition, CD manifests in symptomatic, asymptomatic, prospective, or refractory forms (Leonard, Sapone, Catassi, & Fasano, 2017). All symptoms exhibit a genetic predisposition and the presence of CD-specific IgA and IgG antibodies in the bloodstream. Symptomatic celiac disease manifests with intestinal and/or extraintestinal symptoms such as diarrhea, steatorrhea, vomiting, and stomach discomfort, along with anemia, thyroid dysfunction, and reduced bone mineral density. The defining characteristic of CD is damage to the upper small intestine, characterized by increased infiltration of intraepithelial lymphocytes (IELs), crypt hyperplasia, and partial to complete villous atrophy. Asymptomatic celiac disease is defined by the existence of CD-specific mucosal lesions in the absence of usual symptoms associated with the condition. Patients are frequently diagnosed by case-finding procedures that involve screening at-risk populations, including first-degree relatives of individuals with CD, patients with autoimmune diseases (e.g., type I diabetes), or those with genetic disorders (e.g., Down syndrome) linked to CD (Hyun-seok Kim, Unalp-Arida, Ruhl, & Murray, 2019). Potential celiac disease is marked by the absence of symptoms, while the small intestinal mucosa remains normal. Due to the existence of CD-specific antibodies in the bloodstream, these individuals face an elevated chance of getting CD later in life, similar to the at-risk populations previously mentioned.

The diagnosis of CD depends on a synthesis of symptoms and patient history, identification of CD-specific antibodies in the bloodstream, histological evaluation of small intestinal biopsies, potential HLA-DQ genotyping, and monitoring subsequent to the initiation of a GFD. The daily consumption of gluten should not surpass trace amounts (20 mg) to prevent symptom recurrence and promote mucosal healing (Catassi et al., 2007). A recent study predicted that people with CD on a GFD may unwittingly consume 100-400 mg of gluten daily, quantities sufficient to induce ongoing mucosal damage (Syage et al., 2018).

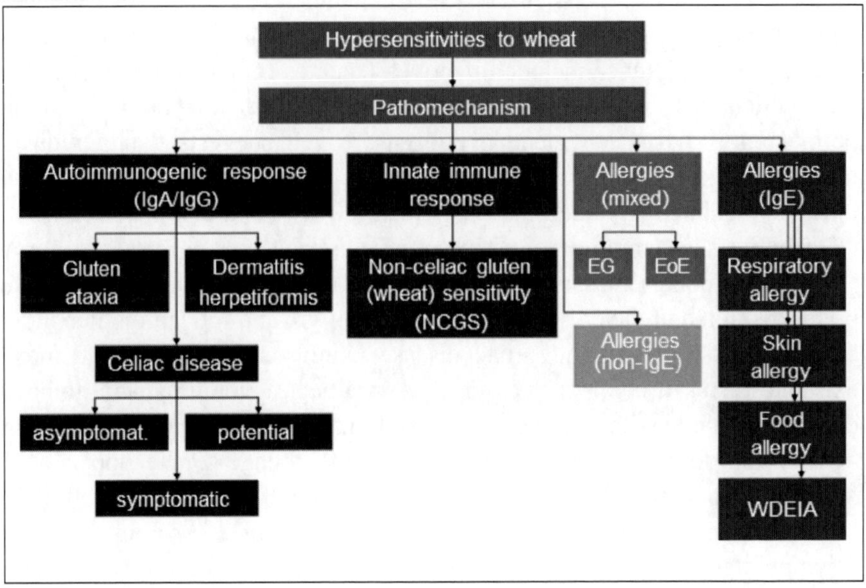

Figure 2. Classification of wheat hypersensitivities. EG, eosinophilic gastroenteritis, EoE eosinophilic esophagitis, Ig, immunoglobulin, WDEIA, wheat- dependent exercise-induced anaphylaxis.

Non-Celiac Gluten/Wheat Sensitivity

Among wheat hypersensitivities, non-celiac gluten sensitivity (NCGS) is the least well-defined, as its causal factors remain poorly understood and no precise biomarkers are available. The estimated prevalence ranges from 0.6% to 6% of the population; however, accurate figures are difficult to ascertain due to the previously mentioned complications and the significant overlap between NCGS and irritable bowel syndrome (IBS) (Catassi et al., 2017). Symptoms typically manifest several hours to a few days after the ingestion of wheat or gluten-containing foods, encompassing both intestinal and extraintestinal complaints (Uhde et al., 2016). Following the implementation of a gluten-free diet (GFD), symptoms resolve, and recent studies suggest that a reduction to 5-10% of the usual wheat intake may be sufficient to alleviate symptoms (Zevallos et al., 2019).

Unlike celiac disease (CD), NCGS patients exhibit normal small intestine mucosa (Leonard, Sapone, et al., 2017). The diagnostic approach for NCGS includes the elimination of CD, wheat allergy, and other food intolerances, alongside a detailed patient history, which typically shows symptom exacerbation after the consumption of gluten-containing products. NCGS should be confirmed with a double-blind, placebo-controlled crossover challenge; however, this methodology is difficult to implement in routine clinical practice, and many patients decline to reintroduce gluten into their diet.

The pathomechanism of non-celiac gluten sensitivity (NCGS) remains poorly understood. Wheat contains potentially harmful components such as gluten proteins, α-amylase/trypsin inhibitors (ATIs), wheat germ agglutinins, and fermentable oligosaccharides, disaccharides, monosaccharides, and polyols (FODMAPs). Wheat ATIs have been shown to stimulate the innate immune response (Zevallos et al., 2017) and act as adjuvants for pre-existing inflammatory adaptive immune responses (Bellinghausen et al., 2019; Zevallos et al., 2019).

Until the pathomechanism of NCGS is better understood, patients are advised to adhere to a gluten-free or gluten-reduced diet (Dieterich et al., 2019). The uncertainty surrounding NCGS is further complicated by individuals who eliminate gluten from their diet based on self-diagnosis rather than clinical validation. Individuals who identify as 'lifestylers,' 'free from,' or 'clean eaters' make up approximately 6-13% of the population in industrialized nations (Potter et al., 2018; P. R. Shewry et al., 2016).

Wheat Allergies

Wheat allergies are characterized by harmful immune reactions to wheat proteins, which consistently manifest in affected individuals within minutes to hours following exposure. Non-IgE-mediated food allergies are well recognized in children under three years old, although they are less commonly acknowledged in adults. However, there is a growing body of research suggesting that such allergies may be frequently overlooked, and that non-celiac gluten sensitivity (NCGS) could indeed represent a form of non-IgE-mediated food allergy (Catassi et al., 2017). Mixed food allergies involve both IgE-mediated and non-IgE-mediated immune responses. Wheat is a common allergen associated with eosinophilic esophagitis (EoE) and eosinophilic gastroenteritis.

IgE-mediated wheat allergies are triggered by inhaling flour and flour dust (respiratory allergy), skin contact (cutaneous allergy), or oral consumption of wheat products (wheat food allergy and wheat-dependent exercise-induced anaphylaxis, WDEIA) (K. Scherf, Brockow, Biedermann, Koehler, & Wieser, 2016). The prevalence estimates for wheat allergies vary depending on the evaluation method used, ranging from 0.1% (based on positive food challenges) to 3.6% (lifetime self-reported prevalence) (Nwaru et al., 2014). Standard diagnostic methods include documenting the patient history of reproducible symptoms following allergen exposure, skin prick testing, evaluation of specific IgE antibodies, and functional assays such as *in vitro* basophil activation tests and oral meal challenges.

The management of wheat allergy primarily involves avoiding allergenic exposure, whether through flours and flour dust or by excluding wheat products from the diet. Antihistamines or corticosteroids may be used to treat acute episodes.

Why Is the Prevalence of Wheat Hypersensitivities Increasing?

Despite a growing body of evidence indicating an increasing prevalence of wheat hypersensitivities (Almallouhi et al., 2017; Grode et al., 2018) - as well as allergies and autoimmune diseases in general (Verdu & Danska, 2018) - the underlying causal factors remain unidentified. The primary factors influencing the human immune system include reduced infection rates due to improved hygiene (Trynka et al., 2010), the use of antibiotics and vaccinations, altered intestinal permeability (Odenwald & Turner, 2017), diminished exposure to airborne bacteria, and changes in dietary practices. These dietary changes include increased consumption of omega-6 fatty acids, decreased intake of omega-3 fatty acids, and lower antioxidant levels, all of which subsequently affect gut microbiota (Blázquez & Berin, 2017; Olivares et al., 2018).

Alterations in the protein composition of cereals may have contributed to increased levels of immunoreactive components, due to varying protein expression patterns in diploid, tetraploid, and hexaploid wheat species (Geisslitz, Ludwig, Scherf, & Koehler, 2018; Prandi, Tedeschi, Folloni, Galaverna, & Sforza, 2017). Factors such as breeding (Boukid et al., 2017; Ribeiro et al., 2016), thermal and cryogenic stress (Juhász et al., 2018), and agricultural practices, including fertilization, may also play a role. The immunodominant 33-mer peptide has been exclusively identified in hexaploid common wheat and spelt, but is absent in tetraploid emmer, durum wheat, and diploid einkorn (Schalk, Lang, Wieser, Koehler, & Scherf, 2017).

The processing of ungerminated grains, refined white flour, and the use of fast yeast fermentation instead of prolonged sourdough fermentation (Muir, Varney, Ajamian, & Gibson, 2019) may have increased the overall gluten content in the diet, potentially exceeding a threshold that triggers hypersensitivities. However, as several studies have yielded divergent results, additional evidence is needed to establish clear cause-and-effect relationships.

Further fundamental research is needed to clarify the relationships between immunoreactive components in cereals and the human gastrointestinal and immune systems, including the role of gut bacteria. Only multidisciplinary research initiatives that involve specialists from plant science, food technology, cereal proteomics, bioinformatics, nutrition, dermatology, immunology, gastroenterology, and other relevant fields will be able to explain the reasons behind the rising prevalence of wheat hypersensitivities in the population. This research will help improve gluten-free products for individuals with celiac disease, develop more reliable methods for detecting gluten traces, and clarify structure–function–bioactivity relationships, ultimately leading to improved treatment and prevention strategies for wheat hypersensitivities.

The Etiology of CD with a Focus on the Role of Gluten in Autoimmunity

Gluten Structure

The three grains that are most often consumed worldwide are wheat, rice, and maize. Since its flour may be used to make a range of delectable and filling foods, wheat is the one of these that is most widely farmed. This is partially a result of wheat dough's special viscoelastic qualities, which let CO_2 be trapped during fermentation and so enable the creation of leavened bread as well as other bakery items. In addition to providing significant amounts of dietary fiber, vitamins, minerals, and phytochemicals, these items also significantly contribute to the intake of calories and protein (K. E. Lundin, 2014). However, consumption of wheat products can also lead to intolerances and allergies to the grain, including non-celiac gluten sensitivity and CD (Dale et al., 2019). These illnesses are linked to exposure to structural associated proteins called prolamins, which vary in name depending on the cereal: prolamins from wheat are known as gliadins and glutenins, while those from barley, rye, and oats are known as hordeins, secalins, and avenins, respectively. Prolamins are present in all cereals, but only those from wheat, rye, oat, and barley or any of their crossbred forms, which are detrimental to those who are gluten intolerant. Multiple proteins make up prolamins, which can be further classified into monomeric and polymeric groups. Monomeric prolamins can be dissolved in aqueous alcohols, whereas polymeric prolamins necessitate the reduction of interchain disulfide bonds through the use of a reducing agent, an acid, or an enzyme. Additionally, polymeric prolamins also include intermolecular disulfide bonds in addition to intramolecular links, whereas monomeric prolamins only have intramolecular bonds. These connections help to pack proteins more tightly into a given area by holding them together closer. Prolamins can also be categorized according to their sulfur concentration, size, or sequence homology. Prolamins were categorized by Shewry and Tatham (P. R. Shewry & Tatham, 1990) into S-poor, S-rich, and high-molecular-weight (HMW) prolamins based on their sulfur content, while Wieser (Wieser, 2000) separated prolamins into three groups based on their size: low-molecular-weight (LMW) (3052 kDa), medium-molecular-weight (MMW) (52-80 kDa), and HMW (-80 to 120 kDa) groups. The D-hordeins, HMW secalins, and HMW glutenin subunits of wheat make comprise the HMW group. The MMW group comprises barley C-hordeins, secalins, and gliadins of the ω-type. γ-secalins, γ-hordeins, and α/β- and γ-gliadins are all members of the LMW group (Leišová-Svobodová, Sovová, & Dvořáček, 2022). Interesting similarities exist between HMWs and LMW glutenin subunits from wheat (Pronin, Börner, & Scherf, 2021) (Figure 2). Avenins, on the other hand, are monomeric and may be categorized according to their molecular weights: α-avenins are around 12-18 kDa and γ-avenins are roughly 22-35 kDa.

Gluten Immunogenic Peptides Involved in CD

Due Prolamins are distinct from other proteins due to their high concentrations of proline (Pro, P) and glutamine (Gln, Q), which can reach 15% and 35%, respectively. Proline has a unique ability to form β-turns, resulting in a tighter helix than the α-helix, allowing proteins to be packed more densely and making it more difficult for enzymes to hydrolyze them. Consequently, gastric and pancreatic proteases in the digestive system are less effective at breaking down these proteins. In celiac disease (CD) patients with a genetic predisposition, certain partially hydrolyzed peptides may penetrate the intestinal epithelium and damage the lamina propria through an unidentified mechanism.

The two-signal model (Brandtzaeg, 2006), which explains CD immunopathogenesis, is the most widely accepted theory. According to this model, some peptides, including the 19-mer gliadin peptide, trigger an innate immune response (Maiuri et al., 2003). This response is primarily characterized by the generation of interleukin-15 by epithelial cells, which increases intestinal permeability and leads to enterocyte apoptosis, disrupting the epithelial barrier (Maiuri et al., 2000). As a result, immune-adaptive peptides like the 33-mer gliadin peptide, which contains multiple overlapping immunogenic T-cell epitopes, can reach the lamina propria. There, tissue transglutaminase 2 (TG2) deamidates these peptides. When gliadin peptides are deamidated, they acquire a negative charge, enhancing their ability to bind to HLA-DQ2/8, a protein produced on the surface of dendritic cells (DCs) and encoded by a susceptibility gene for CD (Tollefsen et al., 2006). DCs present the gluten antigen to T cells, promoting the development of a pro-inflammatory, antigen-specific adaptive immune response that contributes to the disease's symptomatology (Bernardo, 2013).

Genetics played a significant role in the emergence of CD. While the presence of certain HLA alleles is a required element, HLA alleles by themselves are inadequate for disease development in CD, a condition with a high genetic link, with HLA being the most significant genetic factor for disease development (Del Pozzo et al., 2021). When confronted with HLA-DQ2 /8 molecules linked to the illness, $CD4^+$ T cells from CD patients can detect gluten peptides, while $CD4^+$ T cells from healthy individuals cannot (Ø Molberg et al., 1997). The majority of patients have HLA-DQ2.5 haplotypes, whereas the remaining patients have HLA-DQ8 haplotypes. A tiny subset of CD patients who do not have either DQ2.5 or DQ8 molecules express HLA-DQ2.2 molecules. Recently, it was found that the intestinal mucosa of DQ2.2 individuals and a patient with an unusual cis-configuration of DQ8.5 also has gluten-reactive T cells (Bodd, Kim, Lundin, & Sollid, 2012). Therefore, via the action of TG2, deamidated gluten peptides bind with an enhanced affinity to DQ2.5 and DQ8, and it has been demonstrated that the rate at which they dissociate from DQ2.5 is significantly slower than that of their native equivalents (Camarca et al., 2009). The immunogenic properties of gluten have been confirmed by several investigations. It is not surprising that there are several unique T-cell epitopes produced from gliadin and glutenin given the variety of wheat gluten proteins (Table 2).

Table 2. Main investigated T-cell epitopes in regard to celiac disease

T-cell epitopes	Peptide sequence	Protein	Reference(s)
DQ2 .5	P F S Q Q Q Q P V	Low molecular weight glutenin	(W. Vader et al., 2002)
	F S Q Q Q Q S P F		(Stepniak et al., 2005; W. Vader et al., 2002)
DQ2 .2	P F S Q Q Q Q P V	High molecular weight glutenin	(Bodd et al., 2012)
DQ8	Q G Y Y P T S P Q		(van de Wal et al., 1999)
DQ8 .5	Q G Y Y P T S P Q		(Y. Kooy-Winkelaar et al., 2011)
DQ2 .5	P Y P Q Q Q Q P F	Avenin	(L. W. Vader et al., 2003)
	P Y P Q Q Q Q P F		(Arentz-Hansen et al., 2004)
	P Y P Q Q Q Q P I		(Hardy et al., 2015)
DQ2 .5	P Q Q S F P Q Q Q	γ-Gliadin	(Sjöström et al., 1998)
	I Q P Q Q P A Q L		(Qiao, Bergseng, et al., 2005)
	Q Q P Q Q P Y P Q		(Arentz–Hansen et al., 2002)
	S Q P Q Q Q F P Q		(Arentz–Hansen et al., 2002)
	P Q P Q Q Q F P Q		(Qiao, Bergseng, et al., 2005)
	Q Q P Q Q P F P Q		(Arentz–Hansen et al., 2002)
	P Q P Q Q P F C Q		(Qiao & Sollid, 2019)
	L Q P Q Q P F P Q		(Qiao & Sollid, 2019)
	Q Q P F P Q Q P Q		(Arentz–Hansen et al., 2002)
DQ2 .5	P F P Q P Q Q P F	Hordein	(J. A. Tye-Din et al., 2010)
	P Q P Q Q P F P Q		(L. W. Vader et al., 2003)
	P I P Q Q P Q P Y		(J. A. Tye-Din et al., 2010)
	P Y P Q Q P Q P Y		(Hardy et al., 2015)
DQ2 .2	Q G S V Q P Q Q L	α-Gliadin	(Dørum et al., 2014)
	Q Y S Q P Q Q P I		(Dørum et al., 2014)
DQ8 .5	Q G S F Q P S Q Q		(Y. Kooy-Winkelaar et al., 2011)
DQ8	Q G S F Q P S Q Q		(Van De Wal et al., 1998)
DQ2 .5	P F P Q P Q L P Y		(Arentz-Hansen et al., 2000)
	P Y P Q P Q L P Y		(Arentz–Hansen et al., 2002)
	P Q P Q L P Y P Q		(Arentz-Hansen et al., 2000)
	F R P Q Q P Y P Q		(W. Vader et al., 2002)
DQ2 .5	P F P Q P Q Q P F	Secalin	(J. A. Tye-Din et al., 2010)
	P Q P Q Q P F P Q		(L. W. Vader et al., 2003)
	P F P Q Q P Q Q I		(Hardy et al., 2015)

T-cell epitopes	Peptide sequence	Protein	Reference(s)
DQ2 .5	P F P Q P Q QPF	ω-Gliadin	(J. A. Tye-Din et al., 2010)
	PQP Q QPFPW		(J. A. Tye-Din et al., 2010)
DQ8 .5	P Q Q S F P Q Q Q		(Y. Kooy-Winkelaar et al., 2011)

The glutamate residues generated by transglutaminase 2-mediated deamidation, which are crucial for T cell recognition, are displayed in bold. T-cell epitopes have been reported from high-molecular-weight (HMW) and low-molecular-weight (LMW) glutenins, as well as from α-, γ-, and ω-gliadins. Additionally, T-cell epitopes from hordein, secalin, and avenin have been identified. Secalin and hordein epitopes closely resemble those found in wheat, while avenin epitopes are more distinct (J. A. Tye-Din et al., 2010).

T-cell epitopes are typically located within gluten peptide fragments that are 15–50 residues long and resistant to proteolytic degradation. These peptides are often effective substrates for TG2. In HLA-DQ2.5-restricted epitopes, the glutamate inserted by TG2 is commonly found at position 4 (P4), position 6 (P6), or position 7 (P7), and at position P1 and/or P9 in HLA-DQ8-restricted epitopes. The anchoring functions of these glutamate residues are crucial for peptide binding (Sollid et al., 2020a).

Most of the research on gluten epitopes has focused on individuals who are positive for HLA-DQ2.5, and thus further epitopes are expected to be discovered for HLA-DQ8 and HLA-DQ2.2. Due to the overlap in specificity between TG2, gluten characteristics, and the binding requirements of HLA-DQ2 and HLA-DQ8, highly immunogenic interactions between these molecules are formed.

Pathogenesis of CD

The consumption of gluten, including the insoluble prolamin polypeptides found in wheat (gliadins and glutenins), barley (hordein), rye (secalin), and other closely related cereals, plays a crucial role in the pathogenesis of celiac disease. Due to the high proline content of gluten, it is resistant to breakdown by digestive proteases in the stomach, pancreas, and intestine. The mechanisms by which these undigested gliadin polypeptides enter the intestinal submucosa are not fully understood, but they are thought to involve both transcellular and paracellular pathways (Ménard et al., 2012). In the lamina propria, transglutaminase 2 (TG2) deamidates the gluten peptides.

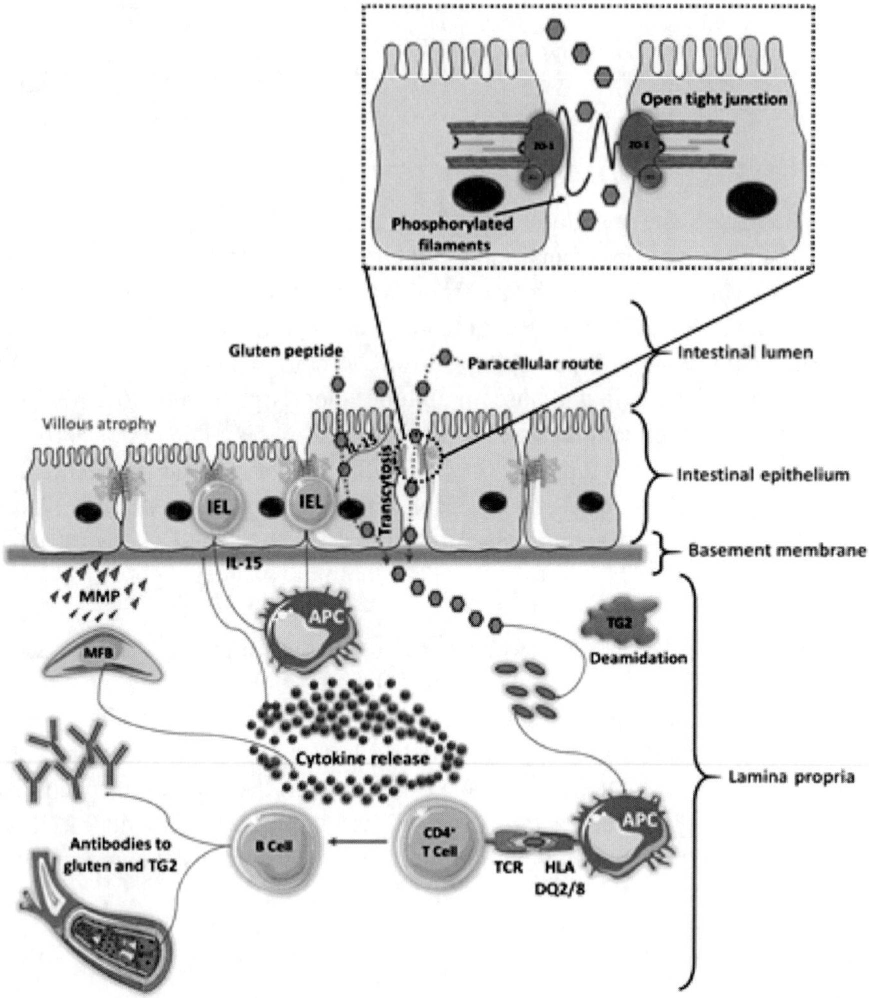

Figure 3. Simplified pathogenic pathways of celiac disease. Gluten peptides trigger an innate immune response, overexpressing interleukin-15 and activating intraepithelial lymphocytes (IELs). These cells destroy stressed enterocytes, and gluten peptides infiltrate the lamina propria, activating the adaptive immune system. Tissue transglutaminase (TG2) deamidates gluten peptides, enabling them to interact with HLA-DQ2/8 on antigen-presenting cells, leading to cytokine release, B cell activation, antibody production, and villous atrophy.

In vitro studies have shown that individuals with untreated celiac disease have elevated blood levels of Th1 and Th2 cytokines, including interferon-gamma (IFN-γ), interleukin-4 (IL-4), and IL-10. These levels significantly decrease following a gluten-free diet (GFD) (Manavalan et al., 2010). Similarly, tumor necrosis factor-alpha (TNF-α) is expressed in the mucosa by activated intraepithelial lymphocytes in CD. Studies have indicated that individuals with refractory celiac disease (RCD) have significantly higher levels of TNF-α RNA transcripts compared to those with active, uncomplicated CD. Therefore, anti-TNF-α drugs, such as infliximab, are not therapeutically effective in non-complex CD (Caruso et al., 2014).

Cytokines like interleukin-15 (IL-15) and IL-21 appear to play a central role in CD development. In pediatric CD lesions, particularly early or mild Marsh 1-2 lesions, a high number of lamina propria T cells producing IL-21 have been observed (Van Leeuwen et al., 2013). Moreover, CD generates increased levels of IL-21 in the presence of IL-15 (Sarra et al., 2013). In untreated CD and RCD, elevated IL-15 expression in the mucosa, lamina propria mononuclear cells, and enterocytes leads to the overexpression of the IL-15 receptor on intraepithelial lymphocytes (IELs), which enhances cell proliferation and the production of inflammatory cytokines. This process results in IEL cytotoxicity and reduced apoptosis (Mention et al., 2003).

Antiapoptotic signals induced by IL-15, involving Bcl-2, Bcl-xL, IL-15R, Jak3, and STAT5, have been identified as contributing to the survival of IELs. Animal studies have shown that administering antibodies targeting IL-15 to animals overexpressing human IL-15 in their gastrointestinal epithelium induces IEL death and eliminates the excessive IEL buildup (Malamut, El Machhour, et al., 2010).

Additionally, T lymphocytes' CD28 and CTLA-4 molecules interact with their respective ligands, B7-1 (CD80) and B7-2 (CD86), when T cells are activated by antigens through their T cell receptor (TCR). In this interaction, CTLA-4 acts as a repressive regulator of T cell activation, while CD28 serves as a costimulatory signal for T cell activation. Consequently, these molecules may play a role in the pathogenesis of CD and could potentially be targeted in CD treatments (A. King et al., 2002) (Figure 3).

Structural Bases of T Cell Antigen Receptor Recognition in Celiac Disease

T cells identify pathogens and hence safeguard against microbial infections. This function hinges on T cells' capacity to differentiate between self and non-self-peptide antigens. The heterodimeric αβ T cell receptor (TCR) on T cells identifies peptide (p) antigens shown by the human leukocyte antigen (HLA) molecule on antigen-presenting cells (Broughton et al., 2012; Goel et al., 2017). Each TCR chain has three complementarity determining regions (CDRs) that interact with the pHLA complex to variable extents, allowing the TCR to detect the peptide and the HLA (Petersen et al., 2016; Zareie et al., 2021). A consensus docking polarity underlies this TCR-HLA interaction, which is associated with T cell signaling limitations (Zareie et al., 2021).

The identification of non-self-peptide antigens activates T lymphocytes to initiate an inflammatory response to eliminate infection (Bodd et al., 2012; J. A. Tye-Din et al., 2010). A disruption in tolerance can result in an abnormal immune response against self-peptides, leading to autoimmune disorders such as multiple sclerosis, rheumatoid arthritis, and diabetes (Lim et al., 2021; Quarsten et al., 2001; M. T. Tran et al., 2021). Many autoimmune illnesses exhibit a significant genetic correlation with the HLA locus (Lim et al., 2021; M. T. Tran et al., 2021). Nonetheless, elucidating the mechanistic foundations of T cell-mediated autoimmunity has been difficult due to the highly polymorphic characteristics of HLA, the vast diversity of the T cell repertoire, the necessity to identify the auto-antigens that provoke the immune response, and other complicating factors such as environmental influences (Ashorn et al., 2008; Dahal-Koirala et al., 2021; Lim et al., 2021; Petersen et al., 2020; Ting et al., 2020; M. T. Tran et al., 2021). Significant advancements have been achieved in comprehending the foundations of CD.

CD is a T cell-mediated autoimmune-like disorder that results in tissue destruction in the small intestine (Dubé et al., 2005). CD is initiated by the ingestion of dietary gluten, the primary storage protein found in wheat, barley, and rye, along with other proteins (Abadie, Sollid, Barreiro, & Jabri, 2011; Jabri & Sollid, 2009; Koning, 2005). CD represents a substantial health issue, especially in westernized nations where approximately 1% of the population is affected (Abadie et al., 2011; Riddle, Murray, & Porter, 2012). Unrecognized CD, which is increasing (Anderson, 2011) in prevalence, is linked to a three-fold spike in all-cause death, primarily due to upper digestive tract malignancies, lymphoma, and sepsis. The sole available treatment is the elimination of gluten-containing foods, specifically those derived from wheat, barley, or rye (Dicke, Weijers, & KAMER, 1953; KAMER, Weijers, & Dicke, 1953). In longitudinal investigations, less than fifty percent of adults attain complete histological remission on a GFD (Bardella et al., 2007), which is associated with a heightened risk of cancer and osteoporosis relative to individuals with normal small intestinal histology (Kaukinen et al., 2007). CD predominantly affects genetically predisposed individuals, specifically those with HLA-DQ2 .5 (~95% of patients) or HLA-DQ8 (~5% of patients), as CD patients lacking both HLA-DQ2+ and HLA-DQ8+ are exceedingly rare (<5%) (Karell et al., 2003; Sollid, 2002). CD4+ T cell responses specific to gluten peptides given by HLA-DQ2.5 or HLA-DQ8 molecules are critically implicated in CD, as these T cells are regularly identified in the small intestine of CD patients (Abadie et al., 2011).

Presentation of Gluten Epitopes by HLA-DQ2.5 and HLA-DQ8

The proline-rich composition of gluten inhibits its complete digestion by gastric proteases in the gastrointestinal system (Arentz–Hansen et al., 2002; Henderson et al., 2007). Patients with CD possess gluten-reactive T lymphocytes that identify highly immunogenic epitopes inside proteolytically stable areas of gluten (Dørum et al., 2014; J. A. Tye-Din et al., 2010). In HLA-DQ2 .5-mediated celiac disease, peptides originating from the diverse array of proteins constituting wheat gluten (a, b, g, and u gliadins and glutenins), as well as analogous sequences in rye secalins and barley hordeins, can stimulate T lymphocytes (Anderson, Degano, Godkin, Jewell, & Hill, 2000; Arentz-Hansen et al., 2000; J. A. Tye-Din et al., 2010; W. Vader et al., 2002; van de Wal et al., 1999). The peptides are ineffective binders for HLA-DQ2.5; rather, glutamine residues are deamidated to glutamate by tissue transglutaminase 2 (TG2) (Figure 4a), resulting in chemically advantageous residues that enhance binding affinity to HLA-DQ2.5 (Høydahl et al., 2019). Gluten epitopes are generally deamidated at specific glutamine residues located at positions P4 or P6 of the HLA peptide binding pocket register (Figure 4b) (Qiao, Piper, et al., 2005). Structural studies have demonstrated that a hydrogen bond network is crucial, as the presence of glutamate enhances binding affinity to HLA-DQ2.5 (Figure 4c) (C.-Y. Kim, Quarsten, Bergseng, Khosla, & Sollid, 2004; Petersen et al., 2014). In HLA-DQ2.5-associated celiac disease, the majority of T cell activity targets five gluten epitopes identified in three peptides (J. A. Tye-Din et al., 2010). Concerning wheat, the four principal gluten peptides include two overlapping T cell epitopes within a-gliadin (LQPFPQPELPYPQPQ and epitopes within: DQ2).5-glia-a1a, PFPQPELPY, and DQ2.5-glia-a2, PQPELPYPQ) and u-gliadin (QPFPQPEQPFPWQP and epitopes within: DQ2.5-glia-u1, PFPQPEQPF, and DQ2.5-glia-u2, PQPEQPFPW) (Anderson et al., 2000; Arentz–Hansen et al., 2002; Dahal-Koirala et al., 2021; Goel et al., 2017; Sollid et al., 2020b; J. A. Tye-Din et al., 2010).

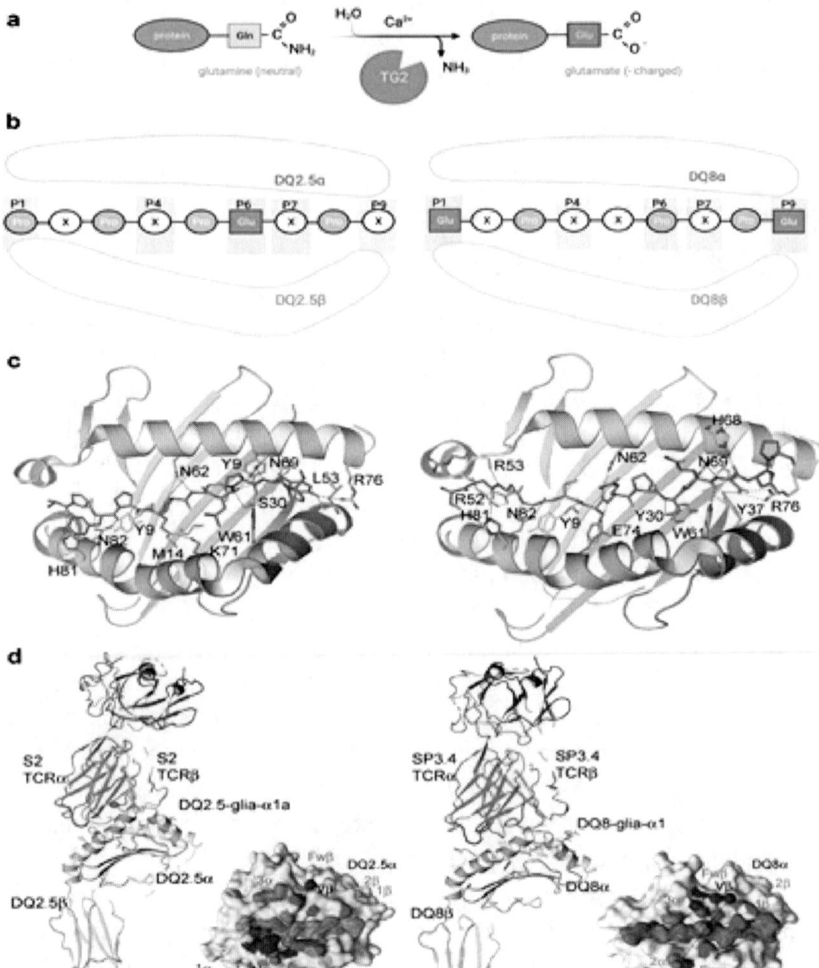

Figure 4. Deamidation of gluten peptides enhances binding to HLA molecules. (a) Tissue transglutaminase (TG2) mediates the Ca^{2+}-dependent deamidation of specific glutamines to glutamates in the "Gln-X-Pro" motif. (b) Left panel: HLA-DQ2.5 prefers negatively charged glutamate residues at pockets P4 and P6. Right panel: HLA-DQ8 prefers glutamate at P1 and P9. (c) Structural overview of HLA-DQ2.5-glia-a1a and HLA-DQ8-glia-a1 structures. (d) TCR docking on peptide-HLA structures for S2-HLA-DQ2.5-glia-a1a and SP3.4-HLA-DQ8-glia-a1. The peptide and HLA residues interacting with deamidated peptides are labeled.

The third peptide obtained from barley hordein (PEQPIPEQPQPYPQQ) contains the fifth epitope, DQ2 .5-hor-3a (PIPEQPQPY) (Goel et al., 2017; Sollid et al., 2020b; J. A. Tye-Din et al., 2010). Several of these immunodominant epitopes are located inside other gluten peptides (Sollid et al., 2020b).

The DQ8 -glia-a1 (EGSFQPSQE) epitope is the principal immunogenic peptide linked to T cell reactivity in HLA-DQ8þ CD patients (Tollefsen et al., 2006; Van De Wal et al., 1998). HLA-DQ8 exhibits a pronounced affinity for acidic residues located in the P1 and P9 pockets of the antigen-binding cleft (Figure 4b) (M. T. Tran et al., 2021). Consequently, the glutamic acid residues at the P1 and P9 positions facilitate the formation of the DQ8-glia-a1 epitope (EGSFQPSQE), endowing this peptide with a strong affinity for HLA-DQ8, as evidenced by the presence of salt bridges between the peptide and HLA-DQ8 in the positively charged P1 and P9 anchor pockets (Henderson et al., 2007).

The discovery of peptide antigens associated with CD development has facilitated the isolation of gluten -reactive T lymphocytes with HLA-DQ2 .5+ or HLA-DQ8 + gliadin epitope tetramer reagents (Bodd et al., 2013; Broughton et al., 2012; Asbjørn Christophersen et al., 2014; Dahal-Koirala et al., 2016; Leonard et al., 2021; Petersen et al., 2016; Petersen et al., 2014; Petersen et al., 2015; Quarsten et al., 2001; Sarna, Lundin, et al., 2018; Sarna, Skodje, et al., 2018). pHLA tetramers, produced by combining biotinylated recombinant pHLA molecules with fluorescently tagged streptavidin, exhibit enhanced avidity for the pHLA-TCR interaction. Consequently, these reagents have demonstrated significant use in identifying gliadin-reactive T cells, which would be unattainable with the use of pHLA monomers (Bodd et al., 2013; Quarsten et al., 2001). Tetramers containing one of five epitopes (DQ2.5-glia-α1a, DQ2.5-glia-α2, DQ2.5-glia-ω1, DQ2.5-glia-u2, or DQ2.5-hor3a) (J. A. Tye-Din et al., 2010) have been mostly utilized, as they represent the primary T cell antigen response to wheat gliadin and barley hordein in CD (Bodd et al., 2013; Broughton et al., 2012; Asbjørn Christophersen et al., 2014; Dahal-Koirala et al., 2016; Dahal-Koirala et al., 2021; Leonard et al., 2021; Petersen et al., 2015; Qiao et al., 2011; Quarsten et al., 2001; Sarna, Lundin, et al., 2018; Sarna, Skodje, et al., 2018). This has enabled the quantification and characterization of T cells in gluten-sensitive individuals, specifically in CD patients, derived from peripheral blood and affected tissue. This includes the analysis of TCR repertoires, such as T cell TRAV/TRBV gene usage and CDR3α/β sequences, facilitating structural studies of TCR interactions crucial to CD (Bodd et al., 2013; Asbjørn Christophersen et al., 2014). These structural investigations provide insight into the molecular characteristics of pathogenic T cells within the responsive CD repertoire (Broughton et al., 2012; Petersen et al., 2020; Petersen et al., 2016; Petersen et al., 2014; Petersen et al., 2015). Research indicates that tetramers can delineate immunological markers of the gluten-specific CD4+ T cell response for the diagnosis of CD and assess the effectiveness of epitope-specific immunotherapies targeting these T cells in CD (Asbjørn Christophersen et al., 2014; Dahal-Koirala et al., 2021; Goel et al., 2017; Leonard et al., 2021; Sarna, Lundin, et al., 2018; Sarna, Skodje, et al., 2018).

Structural Basis of HLA-DQ8 -Mediated CD

The T cell response to HLA-DQ8-glia-α1 is characterized by biased TCR utilization, with the predominant population of HLA-DQ8-glia-α1-restricted T cells primarily using the TRBV9*01 gene, which is commonly associated with TRAV26-2 (Broughton et al., 2012). The majority of TRBV9-TCRs used TRBV6-1, with no significant preference for TRAV genes. The crystal structure of a TRBV9-TCR complexed with HLA-DQ8-glia-α1 (Figure 5) (Broughton et al., 2012) provided a structural basis for understanding the rationale behind the TRBV9 bias and the specific recognition of the DQ8-glia-α1 peptide by these TCRs (Broughton et al., 2012).

The TCR repertoire exhibited a non-germline-encoded arginine residue in the TRAV26-1 CDR3α loop, which was critical for interaction with both the DQ8-glia-α1 epitope and HLA-DQ8 (Petersen et al., 2015). The non-germline-encoded CDR3β arginine identified in the TRBV9-TCRs had a similar function in ternary complex formation. The structure of a TRAV20/TRBV9+ TCR, which lacked a non-germline-encoded CDR3α or CDRβ arginine, was shown to compensate for this deficiency by using a germline-encoded CDR1α arginine in a structurally comparable manner, in association with HLA-DQ8-glia-α1 (Petersen et al., 2016).

In the studied HLA-DQ8-glia-α1-restricted TCRs, mutation of the non-germline-encoded CDR3 arginine or the germline-encoded CDR1α arginine resulted in a complete loss of antigen recognition (Broughton et al., 2012; Petersen et al., 2016; Petersen et al., 2015). The collective data indicated a notable conserved selection of this residue, encompassing both non-germline and germline elements, in the recognition of HLA-DQ8-glia-α1.

Structural Basis of HLA-DQ2.5-Mediated CD

Biased T cell receptor use towards specific gluten epitopes is a characteristic of HLA-DQ2β CD. The DQ2 .5-glia-α2 specific T cell repertoire exhibits a preferential pairing and utilization of TRAV26-1/TRBV7-2 genes, conservation of a CDR3β motif featuring a non-germline encoded Arg residue, and a TRAV4 bias across several unrelated individuals with CD (Dahal-Koirala et al., 2016; Dahal-Koirala et al., 2021; Gunnarsen et al., 2017; Petersen et al., 2014; Qiao, Christophersen, Lundin, & Sollid, 2014). Although there is significant sequence homology between the DQ2.5-glia-α2 and DQ2.5-glia-ω2 epitopes, the repertoire specific to DQ2.5-glia-ω2 is distinct and non-overlapping, yet both exhibit a similar TRAV4 bias (Dahal-Koirala et al., 2016).

Biased utilization of TRAV4 and TRBV20-1 or TRBV29-1 genes was noted for both DQ2 .5-glia-α1a and DQ2.5-glia-ω1 epitopes (Dahal-Koirala et al., 2019; Gunnarsen et al., 2017). Furthermore, almost 5% of the responding T cells exhibited cross-reactivity, enabling them to detect both DQ2.5-glia-α1a and DQ2.5-glia-ω1 epitopes (Gunnarsen et al., 2017). The structures of TRBV7-2+ TCR-HLA-DQ2.5-glia-α2 and TRAV4*01+ TCR-DQ2.5-glia-α1a complexes have been elucidated, offering a structural foundation for these TCR biases (A. Han et al., 2013; Petersen et al., 2014; Qiao et al., 2014; Qiao et al., 2011), and revealed distinct docking geometries among these ternary complexes (Figure 5).

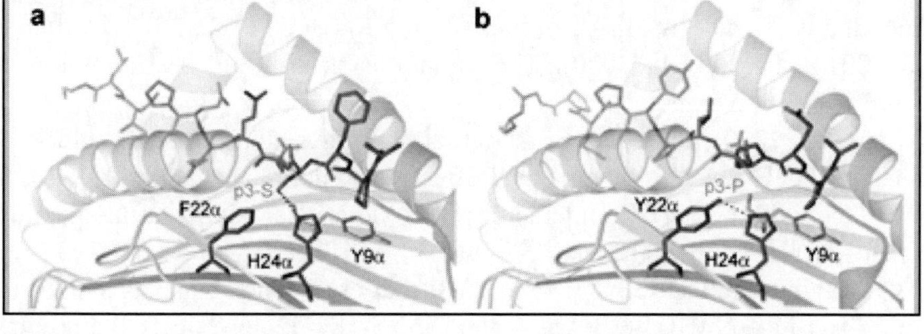

Figure 5. The single HLA-DQa22 polymorphism affects epitope specificity of HLA-DQ2 molecules. (a) Interactions between HLA-DQ2.2 and DQ2.2-glut-L1 peptide in the 594-HLA-DQ2.2-glut-L1 complex (PDB: 6PY2). (b) Interactions between HLA-DQ2.5 and DQ2.5-glia-a2 in the JR5.1-HLA-DQ2.5-glia-a2 complex (PDB: 4OZF). Peptide residues are shown as grey sticks.

The conserved presence of the non-germline-encoded Arg in the HLA-DQ2.5-glia-α2 limited response paralleled that seen in the HLA-DQ8 -glia-α1. The non-germline CDR3β Arg established essential connections with both the gliadin epitope and HLA-DQ2.5, functioning as a pivotal element. Mutation of the CDR3β Arg in TRAV26-2/TRBV7-2+ TCRs eliminated recognition of HLA-DQ2.5-glia-α2 (Petersen et al., 2014; Qiao et al., 2011). The extent to which conservation in TCR use patterns influences the response to specific gluten factors is uncertain.

Structural Basis of HLA-DQ2.2-Mediated CD

HLA-DQ2.5 exhibits a robust association with CD, but HLA-DQ2.2, differing from HLA-DQ2.5 by a solitary polymorphism residue (HLA-DQ2.2-Phe22α, HLA-DQ2.5-Tyr22α), demonstrates a weak association as a risk factor for CD (Bodd et al., 2012). The binary structures of HLA-DQ2.2-glut-L1 and HLA-DQ2.5-glia-α2 demonstrated that the disparity in epitope binding affinity between HLA-DQ2.5 and HLA-DQ2.2 molecules is attributable to a singular polymorphism residue at position 22 of the HLA-DQ2 α-chain (Figure 5) (Ting et al., 2020). The DQα22 polymorphism disrupts an essential hydrogen bonding network with the gluten epitope main chain necessary for stability (Bodd et al., 2012; Dørum et al., 2014). HLA-DQ2.2-Phe22α is incapable of participating in the hydrogen bond network, in contrast to HLA-DQ2.5-Tyr22α. Consequently, HLA-DQ2.2 imposes an extra selectivity constraint on epitopes containing p3-Ser, which is necessary for compensatory hydrogen bonding with adjacent HLA residues (Figure 5) (Bodd et al., 2012; Dørum et al., 2014; Ting et al., 2020). The variations in epitope specificity led to significantly divergent T cell responses to HLA-DQ2.2 (Bodd et al., 2012; Ting et al., 2020). Nonetheless, the ternary configurations of DQ2.2-glut-L1-specific TCRs revealed that the CDR3b loops predominated at the TCR-HLA interface, with both TCRs interacting with the critical p5-Gln of the peptide (Ting et al., 2020). The DQ2.2-glut-L1-specific TRAV9-2+-TRBV11-2+ TCR exhibited a CDR3β Trp (Trp111β) that established contacts similar to those facilitated by CDR3β Arg of the DQ2.5-glia-α2-specific TCRs, despite the distinct characteristics of the peptides (Petersen et al., 2014; Ting et al., 2020). A solitary variation in the antigen-binding cleft of HLA-DQ2.2 influences disease penetrance by modifying the binding frequency of peptides, which in turn affects the characteristics of the T cell response.

Evidence for TCR Cross-Reactivity to Gliadin and Microbial Peptides in CD

The presence of HLA-DQ2.5, HLA-DQ8, or HLA-DQ2.2 alleles alone is insufficient to cause disease; thus, environmental risk factors likely contribute to the disease burden, although the mechanisms behind these correlations remain poorly understood. Several studies suggest a link between gastrointestinal infections, altered gut microbiota (dysbiosis), and celiac disease (CD) (Ashorn et al., 2008; Caminero et al., 2016; D'argenio et al., 2016; Riddle, Murray, Cash, Pimentel, & Porter, 2013a; Riddle et al., 2012; Sánchez, Donat, Ribes-Koninckx, Fernández-Murga, & Sanz, 2013; Viitasalo et al., 2020; Viitasalo et al., 2018; Viitasalo et al., 2014; Wacklin et al., 2014). Recent findings suggest that the proteolytic activity of *Pseudomonas aeruginosa*, an opportunistic pathogen isolated from CD patients, processes gluten into T cell-reactive epitopes. In contrast, bacterial species from healthy controls inactivate these reactive epitopes through additional proteolytic degradation (Caminero et al., 2016).

These observations prompted a structurally-driven inquiry into TCR cross-reactivity between gluten and bacterial epitopes. Prior structural and functional investigations of TCR-HLA-DQ2 .5 complexes (Petersen et al., 2014) identified the portions of the DQ2.5-glia-α1a and DQ2.5-glia-α2 peptides critical for HLA-DQ2.5 or TCR binding. Utilizing these limitations, bacterial protein databases were analyzed to identify matches with DQ2.5-glia-α1a and DQ2.5-glia-α2 peptides (Petersen et al., 2020). A collection of candidate "hits" from various bacteria, including Pseudomonas sp. and Bordetella sp., clinically relevant pathogens, was acquired.

Notably, two *Pseudomonas* peptides originated from the identical parent protein, succinylglutamate desuccinylase (SGDS), exhibiting a sequence overlap that resembled those of DQ2 .5-glia-α1a and DQ2.5-glia-α2 in gliadin. CD TCC exhibited cross-reactivity with several peptides in the panel, including the two *Pseudomonas* SGDS peptides and the original protein, suggesting accurate antigen processing and presentation of the peptides (Petersen et al., 2020). The crystal structures of T cell receptors (TCRs) complexed with two distinct bacterial peptides provided by HLA-DQ2.5 exhibited very analogous interactions to those observed for the same TCRs coupled to HLA-DQ2.5 showing the original gluten epitopes (Figure 6) (Høydahl et al., 2019). The data indicated that molecular mimicry underpinned the cross-reactivity of gliadin-restricted T lymphocytes with bacterial peptides. This study suggests that previous exposure to microbial antigens may contribute to the development and/or persistence of CD.

All ternary structures of CD-related TCR-HLA-DQ2 -gluten and TCR-HLA-DQ8 -gluten complexes identified to date exhibit a conventional TCR docking mode over pHLA, despite variations in TRAV/TRBV use and CDR3 loop sequences (Broughton et al., 2012; Petersen et al., 2020; Petersen et al., 2016; Petersen et al., 2014; Petersen et al., 2015; Ting et al., 2020). These structures demonstrate that the varied TCR gene use for TCRs specific to DQ2.5-glia-α1a, DQ2.5-glia-α2, DQ2.2-glut-L1, DQ8-glia-α1, or DQ8.5-glia-γ1 establishes distinct contacts; nonetheless, a convergence into a consensus binding solution is noted among numerous

TCRs, especially those utilizing Arg residues in pHLA recognition (Petersen et al., 2014). These findings have established a foundation for the biased employment of TRAV/TRBV, the selection of CDR3 motifs, and insights into the epitope specificity of responding T cells in HLA-DQ2 /8-mediated CD. The degree of TCR cross-reactivity among gluten epitopes has yet to be determined, although it is noteworthy that TCR cross-reactivity was observed with bacterial mimics of gluten epitopes.

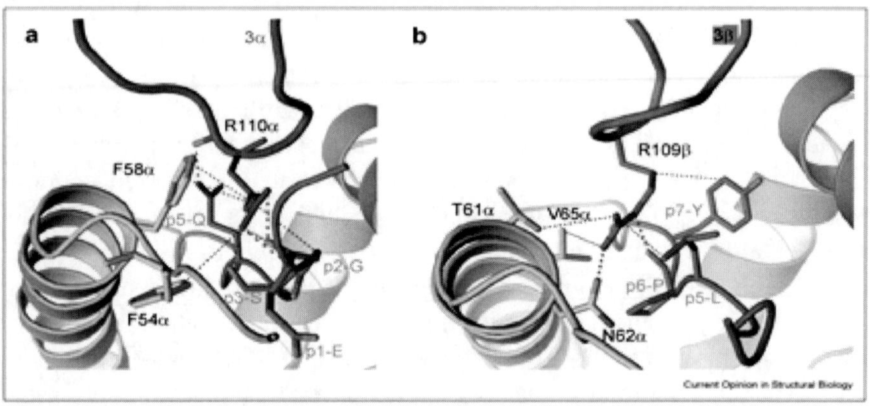

Figure 6. Convergent non-germline CDR3–arginine interactions at TCR–pHLA interface. (a) SP3.4 TCR-HLA-DQ8 -glia-a1 complex (PDB: 4GG6) and (b) S16 TCR-HLA-DQ2 .5-glia-a2 complex (PDB: 4OZH). Amino acid residues are denoted by single-letter codes.

An essential factor is how this structural information may facilitate future diagnostics and therapies for monitoring or treating CD. The similarities at the TCR-HLA interface indicate that small molecule inhibitors could be a viable option. Creating biologics that target the HLA-DQ2 .5-gluten combination is a viable option. Recent findings indicate that an antibody selectively targeting HLA-DQ2.5-glia-α2 on gut plasma cells exhibits very high affinity, binds in a TCR-like manner, and inhibits T cell activation at minimal concentrations (Frick et al., 2021). The crystal structure of the Fab segment of a TCR-like antibody coupled to HLA-DQ2.5-glia-α2 exhibited interactions analogous to those of archetypal DQ2.5-glia-α2-specific TCRs. Additional structural research is necessary to achieve a more thorough and widespread comprehension of the core TCR-HLA interactions that drive CD. This may have ramifications for comprehending the pathophysiology of other autoimmune illnesses with significant HLA genetic connections.

Single-Cell Approaches in CD

Single-cell analysis has transformed numerous research domains, particularly in the examination of adaptive immune responses and autoimmunity. Understanding the antigens targeted in an immune response facilitates the isolation of antigen-specific T cells and B cells through the use of T- and B-cell receptor (TCR and BCR) binding ligands as baits. B cells can be identified using monovalent or multivalent BCR ligands (Franz, May Jr, Dranoff, & Wucherpfennig, 2011). Nevertheless, owing to diminished TCR-ligand affinities, the identification of T cells only became practicable through multimer technologies that enhance receptor avidity (Crawford, Kozono, White, Marrack, & Kappler, 1998; Jd, 1996).

The rapidly advancing field of sequencing technology has revolutionized the profiling of TCR and BCR repertoires through deep sequencing of amplified RNA or DNA from the variable (V) region of immune receptor loci (AIRR-seq). Single-cell AIRR-seq (scAIRR-seq) incorporates chain-pairing data and allows for the quantification of cells possessing identical receptors. The expression cloning of human monoclonal antibodies (hmAbs) from individual disease-relevant plasma cells (PCs) (Di Niro et al., 2010) enables the investigation of binding affinity, specificity, target epitopes, and binding mechanisms. Furthermore, complete, paired TCR or BCR sequences facilitate the study of epitope-paratope interactions, such as through mutational and structural analyses.

Lineage Tracing

TCRs and BCRs, being highly diverse molecules formed through somatic rearrangements, can be used to trace the lineage of an individual T cell or B cell, referred to as clones. The identification of similar TCRs across multiple time points and tissues indicates a systemic and sustained immune response to the target antigen. During somatic hypermutation (SHM), clonally related B-lineage cells share similar, though not necessarily identical, B cell receptors (BCRs). The mutations acquired during affinity maturation can be computationally reconstructed into phylogenetic trees and analyzed at the clone or repertoire level (Hoehn et al., 2019; Stern et al., 2014). Paired chain data from individual cells provides the most accurate representation of lineage trees.

Flow Cytometry

Flow cytometry is an essential tool for examining cell-surface markers and intracellular targets in large populations of individual cells. Currently, traditional flow cytometry can assess over 20 markers simultaneously (McKinnon, 2018). It enables the rapid analysis of millions of cells, with the evaluated cells being categorized and utilized for subsequent analyses. Prior knowledge of marker expression is crucial, and the simultaneous detection of multiple markers requires careful adjustment for fluorescence spillover between channels, a complex task. As a result, traditional flow cytometric analyses have often been limited to a small number of markers, allowing researchers to differentiate specific cell lineages. Recent advancements, particularly in spectral flow cytometry, have expanded this capability, enabling the detection of up to 40 markers, potentially altering current practices (Bonilla, Reinin, & Chua, 2021).

Mass Cytometry

Mass cytometry, also known as cytometry by time-of-flight (CyTOF), has emerged as a powerful tool that enables the concurrent study of approximately 40 markers in millions of individual cells. This technology combines flow cytometry with mass spectrometry, utilizing metal isotopes instead of fluorescently tagged antibodies, thus eliminating the need for signal spillover adjustment. However, mass cytometry can result in significant cell loss and ideally requires prior knowledge of marker expression. Notably, the technique also enables high-dimensional imaging.

Single-Cell RNA-Sequencing

Single-cell RNA sequencing (scRNA-seq) enables the identification and characterization of cellular subpopulations within diverse samples by analyzing their whole transcriptional profiles (Stubbington, Rozenblatt-Rosen, Regev, & Teichmann, 2017). scRNA sequencing (scRNA-seq) is particularly effective for identifying unusual cell types, which cannot be discerned from the average gene expression levels derived by bulk RNA sequencing. Moreover, scRNA-seq enables the exclusion of contaminated cells from subsequent analysis of specific subpopulations. A multitude of library preparation procedures (Svensson et al., 2017) and sequencing platforms provides significant flexibility in throughput and sequencing depth. Although prior knowledge of markers is unnecessary, genes with low expression may go undetected, and mRNA levels do not always precisely reflect protein expression in a cell. scRNA-seq can be integrated with several methods for multi-omics single-cell investigations, including index-sorting (Wilson et al., 2015), barcoded antibody labeling of proteins (Stoeckius et al., 2017), or simultaneous sequencing of transcriptomes and genomes (Macaulay et al., 2015) and/or epigenomes. Single-cell RNA sequencing can be linked with spatial transcriptomics to ascertain the geographical distribution of cell populations inside a tissue, thereby elucidating local networks of cellular communication (Macaulay et al., 2015).

TCR and BCR sequences can be computationally rebuilt directly from scRNA-seq data, (Afik, Raulet, & Yosef, 2019; Afik et al., 2017; Canzar, Neu, Tang, Wilson, & Khan, 2017; Eltahla et al., 2016; Lindeman et al., 2018; Rizzetto et al., 2018; Stubbington et al., 2016; Upadhyay et al., 2018) enabling integrated investigation of antigen specificity and phenotype. This information is also accessible through commercial platforms, such as the Chromium Single Cell Immune Profiling service offered by 10x Genomics.

Detection of Antigen-Specific Cells in CD

Gluten-Specific CD4+ T Cells

Historically, the stimulation of gut biopsies with gluten antigens facilitated the isolation of gluten-specific CD4+ T lymphocytes, which notably utilized the disease-associated HLA-DQ variations as restriction molecules (K. Lundin et al., 1993). Gluten-specific CD4+ T lymphocytes are epitope-specific, and several gluten epitopes are present (Sollid et al., 2020b). A select number of epitopes, referred to as immunodominant, elicit the most robust memory reactions and are recognized by the majority of patients (Nilsen et al., 1998).

Recombinant soluble HLA-DQ molecules complexed with gluten peptides serve as ligands for gluten-specific CD4+ T lymphocytes, and their multimerization facilitates the separation of these cells at both bulk and single-cell levels (Multimers, 2001; Petersen et al., 2015). HLA-DQ: gluten tetramers have been utilized to identify T lymphocytes that are specific for the immunodominant gluten epitopes. DQ2 .5-glia-α1a, 54, 55 DQ2.5-glia-α2, 55–57, DQ2.5-glia-ω1,54 DQ2.5-glia-ω2,57 DQ2.5-hor358, or DQ8 -glia-α153,59, derived from small intestine biopsies (Broughton et al., 2012; Dahal-Koirala et al., 2019; Dahal-Koirala, Neumann, Jahnsen, Lundin, & Sollid, 2020; Petersen et al., 2015; Qiao et al., 2014) and/or peripheral blood (Broughton et al., 2012; Dahal-Koirala et al., 2019; Dahal-Koirala et al., 2016; Dahal-Koirala et al., 2020; Qiao et al., 2014; Ráki et al., 2007) of untreated patients, treated patients, or treated patients following gluten challenge. The bead enrichment of tetramer-binding cells facilitates the identification of gluten-specific CD4+ T cells in the blood of treated patients, indicating that tetramer analysis may serve as a diagnostic instrument for those adhering to a GFD (Brottveit et al., 2011; Asbjorn Christophersen, 2014; Sarna, Lundin, et al., 2018).

Numerous investigations of gluten -specific T cells have concentrated on individual T-cell epitopes, while others have employed a combination of immunodominant HLA-DQ: gluten tetramers to obtain a broader understanding of the T-cell response to gluten (Risnes et al., 2018; Sarna, Lundin, et al., 2018; Sarna, Skodje, et al., 2018; Zühlke et al., 2019). The findings collectively demonstrate that gluten-specific CD4+ cells are selectively prevalent in CD patients, can be readily detected in the blood and gut following a short-term oral gluten challenge, and exhibit a drop-in prevalence in treated individuals.

TG2-Specific B-Lineage Cells

The identification of TG2-specific serum autoantibodies in patients with CD suggests the presence of TG2-specific antibody-secreting cells in these people. TG2 was utilized as bait to identify TG2-specific PCs using immunohistochemistry of duodenal biopsy cryosections and flow cytometry of lamina propria lymphocytes. TG2-specific PCs constitute, on average, 10% of all duodenal PCs in untreated CD (Di Niro et al., 2012). Although TG2-specific antibodies were commonly detected in the intestine, serum antibody titers did not correspond with the prevalence of intestinal TG2-specific PCs, suggesting that some serum autoantibodies in CD may be generated outside the small intestine (Di Niro et al., 2016; Hietikko et al., 2018). This concept was further validated by comparative proteomic analysis of TG2-specific and DGP-specific antibodies in serum and those generated in mucosal explants, demonstrating that the antigen-specific serum IgA antibodies predominantly existed as monomers, unlike the customary dimeric form derived from mucosal sources (Iversen et al., 2017).

TG2-specific PCs are exclusively present in CD patients (Di Niro et al., 2012). Notably, they have been identified before the onset of villous atrophy, and their frequency increases as overt disease manifests (Hietikko et al., 2018). This finding is consistent with the frequent presence of autoantibodies before the onset of symptoms in CD (Green, 2005). Despite a reduction in the frequency of TG2-specific PCs on a GFD (Di Niro et al., 2012; Di Niro et al., 2016; Hietikko et al., 2018; Lindeman et al., 2020; Snir et al., 2015), some cells can still be detected in well-managed individuals who have adhered to a gluten-free regimen for years (Di Niro et al., 2016; Lindeman et al., 2020; Snir et al., 2015). Knowledge about TG2-specific B-cell populations in the bloodstream is limited, likely due to their sparse presence. Rare TG2-specific memory B cells have been indirectly identified in CD patients (Snir et al., 2015), and we are currently studying these cells at a single-cell level.

Gluten-Specific B-Lineage Cells

Gluten-specific intestinal PCs have been discovered with a high staining specificity of 75–80% through the use of tetramerized synthetic gluten peptides as antigens (Steinsbø et al., 2014). About 1% of intestinal IgA+ PCs in untreated CD patients bound a peptide with the sequence PLQPEQPFP, whereas, on average, 0.5% recognized a 33-mer peptide (LQLQPFPQPELPYPQPELPYPQPELPYPQPQPF) (Steinsbø et al., 2014). The prevalence of gluten-specific PCs is contingent upon gluten intake

(Lindeman et al., 2020). Similar to TG2-specific PCs, certain gluten-specific PCs persist even after prolonged adherence to a GFD (Lindeman et al., 2020).

Gluten-Specific CD4+ T Cells

Biased TCR repertoires targeting specific pHLA class II complexes have been documented in numerous disorders and may encompass preferential V-gene utilization, chain pairing, conserved CDR3 motifs, and/or identical TCR sequences among people (Miles, Douek, & Price, 2011; Turner, Doherty, McCluskey, & Rossjohn, 2006). scAIRR-seq has demonstrated preferential V-gene utilization and chain pairing in gluten -specific CD4+ T lymphocytes that recognize each immunodominant epitope. Furthermore, TCRs exhibiting analogous V-gene use and sequences have been identified among different individuals, designating these TCRs as public receptors (Dahal-Koirala et al., 2021).

The TCR repertoires of gluten -specific CD4+ T cells exhibit significant utilization of public TCRs. T cells identifying the analogous DQ2 .5-glia-α1a and DQ2.5-glia-ω1 epitopes exhibit a common V-gene bias, favoring the use of TRAV35, TRAV4, TRAV12-2, and either TRBV29-1, TRBV20-1, or TRBV5-1 (Dahal-Koirala et al., 2019). DQ2.5-glia-α2-specific T cells predominantly utilize TRAV26, TRAV4, and TRBV7 (Dahal-Koirala et al., 2016; A. Han et al., 2013; Qiao et al., 2014; Qiao et al., 2011). whereas T cells specific for the analogous DQ2.5-glia-ω2 epitope primarily employ TRAV4 and TRBV4 (Dahal-Koirala et al., 2016). The DQ2.5-glia-α2-specific TCRs utilizing the canonical TRAV26-1/TRBV7-2 pair generally possess a conserved CDR3β arginine motif (Dahal-Koirala et al., 2016; Dahal-Koirala et al., 2021; Qiao et al., 2014; Qiao et al., 2011). T lymphocytes targeting the immunodominant barley-derived gluten epitope DQ2.5-hor-3 commonly utilize TRAV26-1 and either TRBV20-1 or TRBV29-1 (Dahal-Koirala et al., 2020). Comparable V-gene biases have been documented for DQ8 -restricted gluten epitopes, wherein DQ8-glia-α1-specific T lymphocytes predominantly utilize TRBV9/TRAV26-2, characterized by a conserved CDR3 arginine motif (Broughton et al., 2012; Petersen et al., 2015).

CD8+ αβ and γδ IELs

Unlike the well-defined gluten -specific CD4+ T cells, the antigen specificities of CD8+ αβ and γδ IELs, which proliferate in prevalence in CD, remain unclear (Mayassi & Jabri, 2018). A scAIRR-seq investigation conducted by Han and associates, utilizing TCRβ or TCRγ sequencing of activated (CD38+) and gut-homing (CD103+) CD8+ αβ T cells and γδ T cells in the blood of CD patients six days post-gluten challenge, demonstrated significant clonal expansion and preferential utilization of TRBV7-8, TRBV7-9, and TRBV28 in CD8+ αβ T cells, as well as TRDV1 (i.e., Vδ1) in γδ T cells (A. Han et al., 2013). scAIRR-seq analyses of γδ IELs and peripheral blood gut-homing γδ T cells revealed a preference for TRGV4 (i.e., Vγ4) and TRDV1 use in healthy subjects, while indicating that CD patients exhibited a more diversified γδ TCR repertoire, lacking the TRGV4 bias (Eggesbø et al., 2020). The alteration in the γδ TCR repertoire was almost identical for both untreated and treated persons. In contrast to γδ T cells, no permanent alteration of the TCR repertoire associated with CD has been observed in CD8+ αβ T cells (Eggesbø et al., 2021). A recent study (Eggesbø et al., 2021), in contrast to a prior publication (A. Han et al., 2013), demonstrated that the CD8+ αβ T cell repertoire is markedly polyclonal and diversified in untreated compared to treated CD and controls.

TG2-Specific B-Lineage Cells

A single-cell analysis of the BCRs from 60 intestinal tissue transglutaminase 2 (TG2)-specific PCs revealed a skewed usage of V-genes and a restricted quantity of somatic mutations (Di Niro et al., 2012). The characteristic features were further examined through high-throughput AIRR-seq of the immunoglobulin heavy-chain variable (IGHV) region in both gut and blood (Snir et al., 2015), large-scale scAIRR-seq of intestinal IgA PCs (Roy et al., 2017), and computational BCR sequence reconstruction from scRNA-seq information about intestinal PCs (Lindeman et al., 2020). This provided substantial evidence of preferential V-gene usage and chain pairing, restricted somatic mutations and affinity maturation, clonal expansion, low diversity, and biased isotype usage.

TG2-specific PCs exhibit a notable preference for the IGHV5-51: IGKV1-5 pair, along with biases for several additional heavy- and light-chain V-gene combinations, including IGHV3-48: IGLV5-45 and IGHV4-34: IGKV1-39 (Roy et al., 2017). Furthermore, TG2-specific PCs are predominantly of the IgA isotype (Steinsbø et al., 2014), particularly IgA1 (Iversen et al., 2017; Lindeman et al., 2020), in contrast to the overall PC population in CD and controls (Chiba, Ohta, Yagisawa, & Masamune, 1987). The frequencies of somatic mutations are correlated for both heavy and light chains in TG2-specific PCs and the overall plasma cell population, suggesting that the limited acquisition of mutations is associated with the cell's developmental history (Lindeman et al., 2020; Roy et al., 2017). Generally, several mutations preserve the physicochemical characteristics of the amino acid, suggesting restricted affinity maturation and conservation of germline-encoded residues (Roy et al., 2017).

Gluten-Specific B-Lineage Cells

Gluten-specific B-lineage cells have received less attention than their TG2-specific equivalents due to their relative scarcity. A study of 38 gluten -specific PCs72 and IGHV bulk sequencing of IgA+ PCs revealed repertoire characteristics that closely resemble those of TG2-specific PCs, exhibiting restricted V-gene utilization and few alterations (Snir et al., 2017). Recently, paired BCR sequences of 232 gluten-specific intestinal PCs were rebuilt from scRNA sequencing data (Lindeman et al., 2020). These investigations indicate a markedly stereotypical antibody response to gluten, predominantly consisting of the chain pairings IGHV3-23/IGLV4-69, IGHV3-15/IGKV4-1, or IGHV3-74/IGKV4-1. Mutational study revealed that, although there is a correlation between the mutational burden in the heavy and light chains, their tendency to undergo somatic hypermutation relative to the general PC population differs based on V-gene usage (Lindeman et al., 2020). This work further validated flow cytometry results (Steinsbø et al., 2014) indicating that gluten-specific PCs are predominantly of the IgM isotype in comparison to TG2-specific PCs.

TCR: pHLA-DQ Binding

TCR: pHLA-DQ binding from individual CD4+ T cells of CD cases has led to the resolution of various disease-relevant TCR structures in ternary complexes of TCR: pMHC, specifically for TCRs restricted by HLA-DQ2 .5 (Petersen et al., 2014), HLA-DQ2.2 (Ting et al., 2020), and HLA-DQ8 (Broughton et al., 2012; Petersen et al., 2016; Petersen et al., 2015). This research elucidates the structural foundation for V-gene biases and the rationale for the conserved CDR3β arginine motif in T-CRs utilizing TRAV26-1/TRBV7-2. The general deamidation dependency of gluten - specific CD4+ T cells in CD remains unclear at this juncture.

TG2-Specific BCRs/Antibodies

The restricted mutation of TG2-specific antibodies suggests strong affinity in the germline structure. Reverting several TG2-specific hmAbs to their germline sequences has shown that, although diminished, the affinity for TG2 remains comparatively high (Di Niro et al., 2012). Consequently, affinity maturation appears to be non-essential for the formation of CD.

CD patient-derived TG2-specific hmAbs preferentially target the enzyme in its catalytically active conformation, recognizing primarily four N-terminal conformational epitopes that are exclusively accessible on soluble TG2 and correspond with the IGHV gene use of the antibodies (Di Niro et al., 2012; Iversen, 2013; Iversen et al., 2019). The antibodies exhibited no cross-reactivity with other transglutaminases (Iversen, 2013). The structural foundation for TG2 binding has been examined with an epitope 1-specific hmAb utilizing IGHV5-51/IGKV1-5, uncovering numerous residues in both the heavy and light chains that participate in epitope recognition (X. Chen et al., 2015; Roy et al., 2017).

TG2-specific antibodies can be crosslinked by TG2 when presented as IgD or IgM, but not as IgA1 or IgG1, thereby facilitating the recruitment of PCs from naive or IgM memory cells (Di Niro et al., 2012). The functional implications of antibody binding to TG2 differ according on the epitope, which may account for preferences toward specific epitopes (Hnida et al., 2016). Antibodies that recognize C-terminal epitopes have been shown to inhibit TG2-mediated crosslinking (Iversen et al., 2019). Moreover, *in vitro* modified B cells targeting N-terminal epitopes, but not C-terminal epitopes, were capable of internalizing TG2-gluten complexes and functioning as APCs for gluten-specific T cells. Consequently, the bias towards the N-terminal epitope may arise from the collaboration of B- and T-cells (Iversen et al., 2019).

Gluten-Specific BCRs/Antibodies

The epitopes identified by gluten -specific serum antibodies have been delineated through the assessment of their reactivity to gluten peptide libraries (Ballew et al., 2013; Osman et al., 2000). Notably, the B-cell epitopes are situated next to or overlapping with T-cell epitopes within the gluten protein sequences. DGPs demonstrate greater antibody reactivity than their native counterparts (Aleanzi, Demonte, Esper, Garcilazo, & Waggener, 2001; Osman et al., 2000), highlighting the significance of deamidation in epitope recognition in CD. The expression cloning of 38 gluten-specific human monoclonal antibodies from individual intestinal PCs verified that the antibodies generally interacted with gluten peptides associated with T-cell epitopes, with many exhibiting a preference for deamidated gluten peptides (DGP) (Steinsbø et al., 2014). Although the hmAbs were not polyreactive, certain ones shown cross-reactivity with several DGPs. The binding of the hmAbs to synthetic gluten peptides was inhibited by patient-derived serum, indicating the recognition of shared gluten epitopes (Steinsbø et al., 2014). A study utilizing the same hmAb panel revealed that the antibodies typically attach to elongated deamidated peptide fragments containing multivalent B-cell epitopes, TG2 recognition sequences, and diverse T-cell epitopes (Dørum et al., 2016). There appears to be a link between V-gene use and gluten epitope specificity for TG2-specific antibodies (Steinsbø et al., 2014).

The stereotypical antibody response to gluten has facilitated the investigation of the structural foundation for antibody detection of DGP in CD. Crystal structures of two antibodies utilizing IGHV3-23/IGLV4-69 or IGHV3-15/IGKV4-1 demonstrate that germline-encoded residues in both heavy and light chains participate in binding to the DGP with the sequence PLQPEQPFP (Snir et al., 2017). Certain sequences may be significant among a group of gluten-specific antibodies. DGP-specific antibodies utilizing IGHV3-15/IGKV4-1 or IGHV3-74/IGKV4-1 possess a conserved arginine residue in the heavy chain (R55), critical for the binding of PLQPEQPFP (Lindeman et al., 2020; Snir et al., 2017). R55 is nonpolymorphic in five IGHV genes, while seven more genes possess one or more R55-containing alleles (Lefranc, 2011). The significance of conserved germline residues may suggest a role for polymorphisms in the antibody response in CD. As a proof of concept, it was proven that a patient-derived gluten-specific antibody utilizing the R55-containing IGHV4-4*07 allele in conjunction with IGKV4-1 was unable to bind to DGP upon changing R55 to the allelic variation E55 (Lindeman et al., 2020).

Lineage Tracing

For an extended while, it remained uncertain if the circulating gluten -specific T cells accurately represented the broader population of CD4+ T cells located in the lamina propria. Bulk and scAIRR-seq of tetramer-sorted CD4+ T cells in CD demonstrated that the two compartments comprised almost similar T-cell clonotypes in both untreated and treated CD, suggesting a shared origin and migration of clones between blood and gut (Risnes et al., 2018).

Disease-associated T-cell clonotypes in CD are shared not only between the gut and blood but also across several time points. This has been demonstrated for gluten -specific CD4+ T cells (Risnes et al., 2018) as well as for CD103+ γδ and CD8+ T cells (Risnes, Eggesbø, Zühlke, et al., 2021). Moreover, an analysis of individual T cells from intestinal biopsies collected years apart revealed that gluten-specific CD4+ T-cell clonotypes can endure for decades in patients with CD adhering to a GFD (Risnes et al., 2018). Furthermore, the recall response during the gluten challenge was primarily characterized by preexisting clonotypes. Consequently, the disease-specific

TCR repertoire remains consistent over the years in treated individuals. Although long-lived intestinal memory T cells are present (Bartolomé-Casado et al., 2019; Bartolomé-Casado et al., 2021), tiny quantities of gluten may occasionally contribute to these persistent T-cell responses. As of now, only two studies have examined the evolution of intestinal CD-specific PC lineages at a single-cell level, demonstrating restricted affinity maturation and recurrent proliferation of cells possessing identical BCRs within each clone (Lindeman et al., 2020; Roy et al., 2017). Notably, PCs exhibiting various isotypes and longevity-related characteristics were identified within single clones, suggesting persistent immunological responses to TG2 and DGP characterized by isotype class switching and possible reactivation of memory B cells (Lindeman et al., 2020). Combined lineage tracking of PCs and memory B cells may serve as a crucial method to determine if the reactivation of memory B cells adds to the reservoir of TG2- or DGP-specific PCs. The sole published investigation to date employing this methodology was conducted at the bulk level, revealing a restricted overlap between TG2-specific plasma cells and circulating memory B cells (Snir et al., 2015). Clonal overlaps have been demonstrated by a combination of bulk IGHV sequencing of intestinal PCs and proteomic analysis of the heavy-chain CDR3 region of serum antibodies (Iversen et al., 2017). Comprehensive investigations at single-cell resolution, ideally across many time points and tissues, regarding both GFD and gluten challenges, are necessary.

Single-Cell Phenotyping of Adaptive Immune Cells in CD

Numerous studies have sought to characterize adaptive immune responses in CD at a single-cell level to enhance understanding of their function and discover possible treatment targets. In the past few years, robust single-cell "omics" investigations have surfaced, illuminating T-cell and B-cell responses at the protein and mRNA levels.

Assessing Phenotypes by Immunohistochemistry and Flow Cytometry

T-Cell Populations

Modified compositions of T-cell subtypes have been seen in the intestinal and blood of CD patients in comparison to controls (Cianci et al., 2012; SABATINO et al., 1998; Steenholt et al., 2017). A study utilizing immunohistochemistry revealed that intestine CD4+ T cells do not display the proliferation marker Ki-67, yet express the activation marker CD25 when exposed to gluten (Halstensen & Brandtzaeg, 1993).

Gluten-Specific CD4+ T Lymphocytes

The imaging of tetramers for gluten-specific CD4+ T cells has enabled a more detailed analysis of disease-relevant T cells in celiac disease (CD). Circulating DQ2.5-glia-α1a-specific T cells in CD patients undergoing a gluten challenge exhibited integrin β7 expression, indicating their gut-homing capability (Ráki et al., 2007). Additionally, phenotyping of gluten-specific CD4+ T subsets in blood using tetramer labeling of naive, TEM, and central memory (TCM) cells revealed elevated frequencies of gluten-specific TEM cells, particularly gut-homing cells, in both untreated and treated CD patients compared to controls (Asbjorn Christophersen, 2014). A significant fraction of circulating gluten-specific CD4+ T cells are Tregs, characterized by the expression of FOXP3 and CD39. The counterintuitive increase in these cells among CD patients is attributed to their compromised suppressive abilities (Cook et al., 2017). Elevated frequencies of gluten-specific TH17 cells have also been observed in CD (Fernández et al., 2011). While minimal gluten-reactive TCM or TEM cells are detectable in controls, gluten-specific naive T cells are present in both controls and CD patients (Asbjorn Christophersen, 2014). Functional analyses of HLA-DQ:gluten tetramer-positive cells demonstrated that healthy HLA-DQ2.5+ controls lack gluten-specific regulatory and memory T cells (Asbjørn Christophersen et al., 2016).

IELs

A subset of IELs expresses Ki-67 following gluten exposure, suggesting proliferation, however their antigen specificity remains unidentified (Halstensen & Brandtzaeg, 1993). Activated (CD38+), gut-homing (CD103+) γδ and CD8+ αβ T cells have been identified in the bloodstream subsequent to gluten challenge (A. Han et al., 2013). CD8+ αβ T cells consistently express activating natural killer receptors (Bauer et al., 1999; Billadeau, Upshaw, Schoon, Dick, & Leibson, 2003), with the highest expression of the activating receptor NKG2D observed in the intestines of untreated compared to treated CD patients (Bertrand Meresse et al., 2004). Although the majority of small intestine γδ IELs express the activating natural cytotoxicity receptors NKp46 and/or NKp44, their expression is markedly diminished in patients with CD, even after prolonged adherence to a GFD (Mayassi et al., 2019). Moreover, individuals adhering to a GFD exhibit elevated frequencies of CD8+ γδ IELs that express the inhibitory receptor NKG2A and intracellular TGF-β1 in comparison to untreated individuals (Bhagat et al., 2008). Although the frequencies of CD8+ αβ IELs normalize on a GFD, this phenomenon does not occur for γδ IELs (Calleja et al., 2011).

The dynamic control of various T-cell populations during gluten challenge remains a topic of ongoing debate. Han et al., and others have reported elevated frequencies of gluten-specific CD4+ T cells, γδ T cells, and CD8+ αβ T cells in the bloodstream following gluten challenge (A. Han et al., 2013; López-Palacios et al., 2018). However, recent findings suggest that not all patients show an increase in all three T-cell subsets. Nevertheless, all patients who exhibited an increase in γδ and/or CD8+ αβ T cells also showed heightened frequencies of gluten-specific CD4+ T cells (Risnes, Eggesbø, Zühlke, et al., 2021). The variations across studies may be due to differences in gluten challenge protocols and laboratory techniques, underscoring the need for standardized challenge protocols (Núñez & Fernández-Bañares, 2021; Risnes, Eggesbø, Christophersen, & Sollid, 2021).

Intestinal PCs

The substantial population of intestinal antibody-secreting cells in patients with CD and controls predominantly consists of end-differentiated PCs, as evidenced by their expression of CD138 and absence of CD20 or intracellular Ki-67 staining (Di Niro et al., 2010; Di Niro et al., 2012). PCs of the IgA and IgM isotypes have a functioning BCR (Di Niro et al., 2010; Pinto et al., 2013), and a subset of intestinal PCs maintains surface expression of HLA class II (Di Niro et al., 2010; Di Niro et al., 2012; Høydahl et al., 2019) and costimulatory molecules (Høydahl et al., 2019). Intestinal PCs can, contrary to prior assumptions, endure for years. Retrospective carbon-14 dating of bulk-sorted populations, categorized by the cell surface proteins CD19 and CD45, has identified three groups of PCs: short-lived, intermediate-lived, and long-lived, with median ages of 0, 11, and 22 years, respectively (Landsverk et al., 2017). Consistent with this theme, new findings indicate that the majority of PCs in untreated CD, particularly those specific to TG2 or DGP, exhibit a short- or intermediate-lived phenotype, likely due to the significant proliferation of PCs within the celiac lesion (Lindeman et al., 2020). This was equally applicable to patients who had adhered to a GFD for several years, but individuals treated for over a decade predominantly exhibited long- and intermediate-lived TG2- or DGP-specific PCs. The elevated prevalence of transient TG2- or DGP-specific PCs in patients undergoing prolonged treatment was unexpected and may suggest that these individuals have inadvertently encountered trace amounts of gluten (Freeman, 2017).

Memory B Lymphocytes

No research has delineated the phenotype of memory B cells in celiac disease.

Regulatory B Cells

Regulatory B cells (Bregs) have been associated with multiple autoimmune disorders (Fillatreau, 2019). While TG2- or gluten -specific Bregs have not been discovered in CD, the overall population of peripheral blood CD24hi CD38hi Bregs is much greater in CD patients than in controls or individuals with Hashimoto's thyroiditis (Santaguida et al., 2018). The same authors have suggested that these Bregs may exhibit functional deficiencies in CD due to their restricted capacity to manufacture interleukin (IL)-10 following *in vitro* stimulation with CpG.

Phenotyping by Mass Cytometry

Van Unen et al., (Van Unen et al., 2016) conducted a study employing mass cytometry to examine the comprehensive composition of innate and adaptive immune cells in intestinal biopsies and corresponding PBMCs from healthy subjects and patients with inflammatory intestinal disorders, including CD. The results corroborated earlier findings of an elevated γδ IEL population in CD and additionally discerned variations in innate lymphocyte populations.

T Cells

A restricted quantity of mass cytometry investigations has concentrated on the T-cell response in CD. This technology was employed in a study examining activated and gut-homing γδ and CD8+ αβ T cells following gluten exposure (A. Han et al., 2013). A further study integrated HLA tetramer labeling with mass cytometry to characterize gluten-specific CD4+ T cells (Asbjørn Christophersen et al., 2019). This study demonstrated that gluten-specific CD4+ T lymphocytes exhibit a unique phenotype characterized by the elevation of activation markers CD38, CD161, CD28, HLA-DR, and OX40, along with CXCR3, CD39, and PD-1 in both the gut and blood. Notably, the identical CD4+ T-cell phenotype was observed in patients with systemic sclerosis or systemic lupus erythematosus, indicating that pathogenic CD4+ T cells in autoimmune disorders with unidentified target antigens may be discerned by their phenotype.

B-Lineage Cells

No research utilizing mass cytometry to analyze B-cell responses in CD have been published to date. The work by van Unen et al., included certain B-lineage cells but lacked markers to analyze the B-lineage response. Although investigations of antigen-specific B-lineage cells in CD are necessary, the characterization of B-cell subsets and their marker expression in healthy intestinal and blood samples may provide a valuable reference (Nair et al., 2016). Mass cytometry has been employed alongside the labeling of antigen-specific cells to characterize rotavirus-specific intestinal and circulating B-lineage cells (Nair et al., 2016).

Single-Cell RNA-Sequencing

Single-cell RNA sequencing (scRNA-seq) can enhance prior bulk RNA sequencing studies of CD (Asbjørn Christophersen et al., 2019; Leonard et al., 2019; Snir, Kanduri, Lundin, Sandve, & Sollid, 2019) by analyzing the cellular composition of celiac lesions, identifying rare cell types that may contribute to disease pathology, and eliminating contaminating cells from in-depth examinations of specific cell populations. To characterize the composition of immune cells in celiac lesions, Atlasy and colleagues sequenced immune cells from duodenal biopsies of celiac patients and controls (Atlasy et al., 2019). The authors confirmed earlier findings, indicating a higher quantity of total lamina propria immune cells and CD3+ IELs in untreated CD patients relative to controls.

T Cells

Current scRNA-seq investigations of T cells with established antigen specificity in CD are deficient; the sole RNA-seq data accessible for gluten - specific T cells derives from bulk populations, which essentially corroborates mass cytometry findings (Asbjørn Christophersen et al., 2019). The preprint by Atlasy et al., discovered that the majority of CD4+ T cells exhibit transcriptional differences between CD patients and controls, while no information on antigen specificity is provided. Moreover, the majority of CD8+ T lymphocytes in the epithelium and lamina propria exhibited an activated phenotype in CD relative to controls, demonstrating expression of genes linked with cytotoxic activity, including KLRC2 and KLRD1.

B-Lineage Cells

A recent scRNA-seq investigation of intestinal PCs in CD and controls substantially validated bulk RNA-seq findings (Snir et al., 2019) and demonstrated that TG2- and DGP-specific PCs exhibit some differences compared to PCs of unspecified specificity (Lindeman et al., 2020; Snir et al., 2019). A subset of the PCs, irrespective of antigen specificity, exhibited low levels of mRNA transcripts for HLA class II and costimulatory molecules. The intestinal PC population in CD patients may have transcriptional differences compared to controls (Lindeman et al., 2020; Snir et al., 2019). The disparities among PCs in untreated and treated CD patients and controls may suggest potentially harmful functions of PCs, including non-disease-specific roles, in CD. PCs are generally characterized as CD27high, along with elevated expression of CD38 or CD138. Similarly, CD27 has been extensively utilized as a marker for memory B cells. The definitions are evolving, as CD27−/dim B-cell subsets are receiving increased attention (Guikema et al., 2003; Kerkman et al., 2021), particularly with autoimmune disorders. Our RNA-seq experiments demonstrated that CD27 expression is diminished in TG2- or DGP-specific PCs relative to other PCs, and in PCs of CD patients compared to controls. The protein level has also revealed an enrichment of CD27−/dim TG2-specific PCs and circulating memory B cells.

T-Cell Functions in CD

Helper Cell Functions

The accumulation of evidence from comprehensive celiac disease (CD) research indicates that gluten-specific CD4+ T lymphocytes play a central role in CD pathogenesis by aiding B cells in antibody production and by promoting cytotoxic intraepithelial lymphocytes (IELs) that target enterocytes (Jabri & Sollid, 2017). Bulk RNA-seq data from HLA-DQ:gluten tetramer-staining cells in gut lesions demonstrated the expression of IL-21 and CXCL13, cytokines typically associated with follicular helper cells that assist B cells (Crotty, 2011); however, the absence of CXCR5 expression challenges the idea of a germinal center function for these cells (Asbjørn Christophersen et al., 2019). The interaction between T cells and B cells not only influences B-cell antibody production but also leads to T-cell activation and clonal proliferation. Research involving transfectants, in which TCRs and BCRs from CD patients were introduced, showed that gluten-specific T cells can be activated by TG2-specific B cells in the presence of TG2-gluten complexes (Di Niro et al., 2012).

Regulatory T Cell Function

Tregs are a subpopulation of CD4+ T lymphocytes crucial for sustaining peripheral tolerance. It is so hypothesized that in a healthy condition, Treg activity regulates the reaction to gluten (Jabri & Sollid, 2009; B Meresse, Ripoche, Heyman, & Cerf-Bensussan, 2009; Pabst & Mowat, 2012). Although the presence of the transcription factor FOXP3 is a defining characteristic of regulatory T cells in mice, there is a deficiency of reliable markers for human Tregs. In humans, Tregs are typically identified as FOXP3+ CD25+ CD127low, however activated human CD4+ T cells can also express FOXP3 without possessing regulatory activities (Kmieciak et al., 2009). The observation of elevated levels of gluten-specific CD4+ memory T cells in CD patients, exhibiting characteristic Treg markers after gluten stimulation of blood samples, is perplexing. The cells exhibited compromised suppressive function during *in vitro* growth, indicating that Treg malfunction may contribute to CD (Cook et al., 2017). The study's findings contrast comprehensive phenotyping of gluten-specific T cells via mass cytometry, indicating that whereas certain gluten-specific T cells express FOXP3, they do not express CD25 (Asbjørn Christophersen et al., 2019). The variance among studies may be elucidated by the observation that *in vitro* activation of gluten-specific FOXP3+ CD25- T cells induces CD25 expression in these cells (Asbjørn Christophersen et al., 2019). Individuals expressing healthy HLA-DQ2 .5 possess seldom CD4+ T cells in their blood that react with HLA-DQ: gluten tetramers. These cells lack expression of FOXP3 and CD25, indicating they are not Tregs (Asbjørn Christophersen et al., 2016).

Cytotoxic Functions and Other Functions by IELs

CD8+ αβ IELs. IELs often enhance gut immune defense by obstructing pathogen ingress into the epithelium through the preservation of barrier integrity. In CD, the augmented population of CD8+ αβ IELs is believed to be accountable for the destruction of epithelial cells, facilitating the development of the disease lesion. The cytokine interleukin IL-15 is deemed crucial for the proliferation of CD8+ αβ IELs (Jabri & Abadie, 2015; Bertrand Meresse, Korneychuk, Malamut, & Cerf-Bensussan, 2015). IL-2 and IL-21, among other cytokines, are probably also involved (Y. M. Kooy-Winkelaar et al., 2017; Korneychuk et al., 2014). It has been proposed that CD8+ IELs in CD are activated in a TCR-independent manner through the binding of ligands to activating natural killer receptors (Jabri & Sollid, 2017). This hypothesis is substantiated by the observed polyclonal TCR repertoire and absence of V-gene bias in CD8+ IELs in CD (Eggesbø et al., 2021), the shift in expression towards activating natural killer receptors in untreated CD (Bhagat et al., 2008), and the capacity to respond to stress signals through activating natural killer receptors independent of TCR specificity (Jabri & Abadie, 2015; Jabri & Sollid, 2009). Consequently, it is likely that CD8+ IELs detect intestinal stress and inflammation, receive authorization to eliminate enterocytes with the assistance of pro-inflammatory CD4+ T cells, and enhance their cytolytic activity.

γδ IELs

γδ IELs are crucial for immunological monitoring of the intestinal epithelium (van Konijnenburg et al., 2017). Their involvement in CD pathogenesis is inadequately comprehended. In CD, intraepithelial lymphocytes are likely recruited to the intestinal epithelium in response to stress or damaged epithelial cells. A subpopulation of γδ IELs, distinguished by the expression of CD8 and NKG2A, is posited to have a regulatory function in CD due to their capacity to restrain the cytotoxic potential of IL-15-induced CD8+ αβ IELs (Bhagat et al., 2008). Moreover, it was shown that gluten -induced inflammation results in the depletion of naturally occurring Vγ4+/Vδ1+ IELs possessing innate cytolytic capabilities and selectivity for enterocyte-expressed butyrophilin-like (BTNL) molecules BTNL3 and BTNL8 (Mayassi et al., 2019). The diminished expression of BTNL8 in enterocytes and the depletion of Vγ4+/Vδ1+ IELs were associated with the proliferation of gluten-sensitive, interferon-γ-producing Vδ1+ IELs that do not recognize BTNL3/BTNL8 and may have a pathogenic effect.

B-Cell and Plasma-Cell Functions in CD

Antibody Secretion

Although autoantibodies exhibit a definitive pathogenic function in many autoimmune illnesses, the pathogenicity of antibodies specific to TG2 or gluten as circulating immunoglobulins remains ambiguous (Iversen, Mysling, Hnida, Jørgensen, & Sollid, 2014; Lindfors, Kaukinen, & Mäki, 2009) The observation that gluten-specific PCs are more abundant in IgM-expressing cells than TG2-specific PCs may have implications for the potential pathogenicity of these antibodies in CD, given that IgM antibodies can activate complement via the classical pathway (Macaulay et al., 2015).

Antigen Presentation

Although circulating immunoglobulin may not be harmful in CD, immunoglobulin as a BCR on antigen-presenting B cells undoubtedly plays a significant pathogenic function. The interaction between antigen-presenting B cells and T cells in CD likely occurs within organized lymphoid structures, such as Peyer's patches, isolated lymphoid follicles, or mesenteric lymph nodes. The swift reduction of serum antibody levels upon initiation of a GFD (Sugai et al., 2006; Sulkanen et al., 1998) and the restricted extent of SHM in TG2-specific (Di Niro et al., 2012; Lindeman et al., 2020; Roy et al., 2017; Snir et al., 2015) and DGP-specific (Lindeman et al., 2020; Snir et al., 2017; Steinsbø et al., 2014) PCs concurrently suggests transient germinal center or extrafollicular responses (Jenks, Cashman, Woodruff, Lee, & Sanz, 2019). The potential connection between B-lineage cells and T cells in the lamina propria remains an unresolved inquiry. At this location, PCs predominate, with a minimal presence of B cells (Mesin, Sollid, & Niro, 2012). PCs are believed to downregulate surface BCR and HLA class II expression, and hence, these cells have not been regarded as APCs. Significantly, IgA- and IgM-expressing plasma cells, unlike IgG-expressing plasma cells, maintain functioning cell-surface B cell receptors (Di Niro et al., 2010; Pinto et al., 2013). A low to medium expression of HLA class II molecules was seen at both the protein and mRNA levels in a subset of intestinal PCs (Høydahl et al., 2019; Lindeman et al., 2020; Snir et al., 2019), together with the expression of costimulatory molecules (Høydahl et al., 2019), suggesting that the increased lamina propria plasma cell population may function as antigen-presenting cells in CD. Utilizing pHLA-specific hmAbs, it was established that PCs are the predominant cell type expressing gluten peptides on their surface (Høydahl et al., 2019). Consequently, intestinal PCs possess the necessary apparatus to display pertinent T-cell epitopes on HLA-DQ molecules on their surface. Crucially, the actual detection and activation of T-cells by gluten peptides presented on PCs has not yet been demonstrated.

Cytokine and Chemokine Secretion

The role of B-lineage cells in secreting chemicals that contribute to the formation of celiac lesions remains uncertain, as the predominant B-lineage cells in CD are plasma cells (PCs), whose roles beyond antibody production are not well explored. Recent research has highlighted the release of cytokines and chemokines by PCs, especially regulatory PCs (Fillatreau, 2019). Although scRNA-seq shows no evidence of intestinal regulatory PCs in CD, a subset of intestinal PCs, regardless of specificity, synthesizes mRNA for IL-

15 and IL-16 (Lindeman et al., 2020; Snir et al., 2019), while small populations of PCs exhibit elevated levels of CCL3 and CCL4 (Lindeman et al., 2020). This is noteworthy given the presumed critical role of IL-15 in the pathogenesis of CD (Jabri & Abadie, 2015; Bertrand Meresse et al., 2015) and the ability of IL-16 to recruit and activate CD4+ T cells (Cruikshank et al., 1994). It remains unclear whether the mRNA expression of these cytokines corresponds to their secretion; for instance, the translation of IL-15 is tightly regulated (Bamford, DeFilippis, Azimi, Kurys, & Waldmann, 1998; A. Mishra, Sullivan, & Caligiuri, 2014; Nishimura et al., 2000), and several isoforms with distinct functions and subcellular localizations are present (Nishimura et al., 2000; Tagaya et al., 1997).

Chapter 4

The Clinical Manifestations of Celiac Disease

Abstract

Celiac disease presents with a wide range of clinical manifestations, from classic gastrointestinal symptoms like diarrhea and malabsorption to extra-intestinal symptoms including neurological and psychiatric disorders. This chapter explores the diverse clinical presentation of CD, including its effects on children and adults. It also highlights the diagnostic challenges posed by atypical forms of CD, which may be asymptomatic or present with non-specific symptoms. The chapter discusses how these manifestations complicate diagnosis and impact the patient's quality of life.

Physiological Symptoms of CD

Anemia brought on by a lack of iron, digestive issues such as diarrhea and constipation, and fatigue and laziness are the three main signs of CD. In adult CD patients, weakness, vomiting, weight loss, diarrhea, loose stools, and an enlarged belly are common physiological signs. Children with CD exhibit failure, dental enamel abnormalities, and small height (J. Kumar, Kumar, Pandey, & Chauhan, 2017). Arthralgias, steatorrhea, osteoporosis, skin rash (dermatitis herpetiformis), hypothyrosis, and postprandial stomach discomfort have also been recorded in CD as additional general symptoms of type 1 diabetes (N. E. Castillo, Theethira, & Leffler, 2015; K. E. Lundin, Qiao, Snir, & Sollid, 2015). In order to better understand the family history of the disease (if any), it is also essential to screen the immediate family, including siblings, the mother, and the father. In the absence of an etiology factor, elevated serum aminotransferase levels are frequently used to diagnose CD (K. E. Lundin & Sollid, 2014). Using celiac disease-specific antibodies, serological testing is used as the initial screening method for CD.

Neuropsychiatric Manifestations in CD

Children with CD are at risk of developing neurological issues, but the risk is smaller than in maturity. The differential can be attributable to short disease duration, early elimination of gluten from the diet, stricter adherence to diet, or differing sensitivity to immune-mediated disorders (Lionetti et al., 2010). Several neurological symptoms are substantially related with CD in the pediatric population. The most common is headache, that is present in up to one-fifth of the patients. Rarer disorders in the pediatric population are ataxia, neuropathy, and brain white matter abnormalities (Lionetti et al., 2010; Nardecchia, Auricchio, Discepolo, & Troncone, 2019). The relationship between epilepsy and CD remains largely unknown. The most prevalent seizure patterns are the complex partial, followed by tonic–clonic seizures.

Epilepsy

The relationship between epilepsy and celiac disease (CD) remains unclear and contentious; however, a correlation between the two is documented, with an elevated risk of epilepsy observed in both children and adults (Chapman, Laidlow, Colin-Jones, Eade, & Smith, 1978; Cronin et al., 1998; Fois, Vascotto, Di Bartolo, & Di Marco, 1994; G. Holmes, 1996). The majority of patients experience complex partial seizures originating from the occipital or temporal lobes, although secondarily generalized seizures, along with other seizure types and episodic headaches, have also been reported (Arroyo, De Rosa, Ruggieri, de Dávila, & Fejerman, 2002; Crosato & Senter, 1992). The incidence in children varies significantly, from 0% (Cakir et al., 2007) to 7.2% (Zelnik, Pacht, Obeid, & Lerner, 2004), with a definitive estimate depending on the selected criteria, as febrile convulsions are often included. A frequency of 3.41% was found in a cohort of children with atypical CD (Sel, Aksoy, Aksoy, Yüksel, & Özbay, 2017). A pediatric meta-analysis identified a 2.1-fold increased risk of seizures in children with CD (Lionetti et al., 2010). In 2012, Ludvigsson et al., determined hazard ratios (HRs) for epilepsy in individuals with CD and reported that CD was associated with a 1.43-fold increased risk of epilepsy, irrespective of temporal factors. The incidence of epilepsy was higher both before and after the diagnosis of CD, suggesting a potential shared underlying etiology or predisposition, rather than CD itself, as the cause of epilepsy (Ludvigsson, Zingone, Tomson, Ekbom, & Ciacci, 2012).

The impact of a gluten-free diet (GFD) on epilepsy management in CD has been inconsistent. In most patients, beneficial effects have been documented, including improved seizure control and a reduction in antiepileptic medication, though complete cessation of seizures is rare (Cernibori & Gobbi, 1995; R. L. Chin et al., 2004; Giuseppe Gobbi, 2005; Pratesi, Modelli, Martins, Almeida, & Gandolfi, 2003). The triad "Celiac disease, epilepsy, and cerebral calcification" (CEC) was likely first presented by Sammaritano et al., in 1985 (Sammaritano, 1985). The first explicit study describing the distinctive CEC syndrome was conducted by Gobbi et al., in an Italian multicenter investigation in 1992, where they identified 29 individuals (age range: 4.6–30.7) exhibiting these distinct characteristics (Giuseppe Gobbi, 2005). The authors concluded that CD must be considered in the differential diagnosis for all cases of epilepsy and cerebral calcifications of unknown cause. Subsequent cases of CEC were reported in Italy (age range: 6–23), including one instance of partial epilepsy (Calvani Jr, Parisi, Guaitolini, Parisi, & Paolone, 2001; Cernibori & Gobbi, 1995; Magaudda et al., 1993), as well as in other countries among both pediatric (Arroyo et al., 2002; Bye et al., 1993) and young adult populations (Hernandez, Colina, & Ortigosa, 1998). This syndrome occurs in 0.7% of children examined in a pediatric meta-analysis (Lionetti et al., 2010). Some studies indicate that cerebral calcification may manifest later in life, and early intervention for CD can reduce the risk of calcification development (Lionetti et al., 2010). The frequency of CD is significantly higher in patients with epilepsy, being 2.3 times greater than in control subjects (Riccardo Pratesi et al., 2003). Consequently, individuals with epilepsy should be evaluated for CD (Ghadami, 2016).

Gluten Ataxia

Gluten ataxia is a prevalent neurological symptom of gluten -related diseases, first documented in 1966 (L. Di Cagno & Ravetto, 1966). A recent consensus publication indicated that GA constituted 15% of all ataxias and 41% of idiopathic sporadic ataxias (Mitoma et al., 2016). Dysarthria, dysphonia, pyramidal signs, and problems of eye and gaze movement are distinctive manifestations; nonetheless, these symptoms are indistinguishable from other forms of cerebellar ataxia. Ataxia associated with CD is infrequently linked to conventional gastrointestinal symptoms or indicators of malabsorption (Fasano et al., 2003). Ataxia in CD frequently does not exhibit specific clinical characteristics of identifiable forms of ataxia (cerebellar and sensory ataxias) (Pellecchia et al., 1999). In numerous people with ataxia, cerebellar involvement may manifest alongside low levels of vitamin E (Mauro, Orsi, Mortara, Costa, & Schiffer, 1991). The majority of patients will either stabilize or improve with rigorous compliance to a GFD, contingent upon the duration of ataxia previous to treatment. As many as 60% of individuals with GA exhibit signs of cerebellar atrophy on MR imaging (Marios Hadjivassiliou, Sanders, & Aeschlimann, 2015); postmortem examinations have revealed gliosis, loss of Purkinje cells, atrophy, and degeneration of the posterior column of the spinal cord (Cooke & Smith, 1966). If rigorous GFD does not alleviate ataxia symptoms, intravenous immunoglobulins appear to offer advantageous results. The prevalence of this condition significantly differs between adults and children, potentially reaching 40% in adults, whereas it is minimal or negligible in children (Lionetti et al., 2010). Ataxia may manifest as a pancerebellar syndrome due to the occurrence of enteropathy-associated T-cell lymphoma and lymphomatous metastases to the cerebellum. This diagnosis must be considered for individuals with CD-related enteropathies prior to attributing cerebellar symptoms to various vitamin or nutritional deficits or an associated autoimmune cause (Shams, Waldman, Dogan, MacKenzie, & Plant, 2002).

Peripheral Neuropathy

Peripheral neuropathy is the second most prevalent neurological manifestation in adults with CD, occurring in up to 49% of affected individuals (Cicarelli et al., 2003). Neuropathy is characterized as chronic, distal, symmetric, and primarily sensory, manifesting as distal sensory loss, paresthesias, and unbalance; however, isolated motor neuropathy, mononeuritis multiplex, Guillain-Barré-like disease, and autonomic neuropathy have also been reported (R. Chin et al., 2003; M Hadjivassiliou et al., 1997; Kaplan et al., 1988; USAI et al., 1997). Motor weakness is infrequent and limited to the ankles (Cooke & Smith, 1966). The primary presentation of peripheral neuropathy during the physical examination of individuals with CD is sensory neuropathy, exhibiting varied involvement of both big and small fibers (R. Chin et al., 2003; Cross & Golumbek, 2003). Electrophysiologic studies reveal a wide range of manifestations among people with CD; indeed, some patients exhibit no electrical signs of neuropathy, while others present with a mixed sensorimotor axonal peripheral neuropathy (R. Chin et al., 2003; M

Hadjivassiliou et al., 1997; Kaplan et al., 1988; USAI et al., 1997). In 2005, Tursi et al., reported the presence of antineuronal antibodies (anti-GM1 antibodies) in adults; however, symptoms persisted despite the absence of antibodies during subsequent follow-up (Tursi et al., 2006). The efficacy of the gluten-free diet (GFD) remains unclear; some studies have characterized the diet as beneficial (R. Chin et al., 2003; Cross & Golumbek, 2003; M Hadjivassiliou et al., 1997; Kaplan et al., 1988; Polizzi, Finocchiaro, Parano, Pavone, & Musumeci, 2000; Usai et al., 1997), while others have observed the continuation and progression of neuropathy despite adherence to an appropriate GFD (Luostarinen, Himanen, Luostarinen, Collin, & Pirttilä, 2003; Simonati, Battistella, Guariso, Clementi, & Rizzuto, 1998; Tietge, Schmidt, & Manns, 1997). Only two studies have examined the prevalence of peripheral neuropathy in children, yielding conflicting results: Cakir et al., (Cakir et al., 2007) reported a prevalence of 4.7%, while Ruggieri et al., (Ruggieri et al., 2008) identified only one female among 835 infants assessed.

Headache

Several research delineate the correlation between CD and headache in both adults and children (Cicarelli et al., 2003; Gabrielli et al., 2003; Parisi et al., 2015; Zelnik et al., 2004). The incidence of headache in people with CD appears to be greater than in controls (46% compared to 29%) (Cicarelli et al., 2003). Serratrice et al., (1998) identified headache as a symptom of CD in its classic, atypical, and silent forms, which responds to a GFD (Serratrice, Disdier, De Roux, Christides, & Weiller, 1998). In 2009, Lionetti et al., reported a high prevalence of headaches (24.8%) in a juvenile population and indicated that headaches considerably improved in 77.3% of children with CD adopting a GFD; analogous findings were previously documented. A pediatric meta-analysis (Lionetti et al., 2010) indicated that the relative risk (RR) of patients with CD developing headaches is 3.2 (95% confidence interval [CI]: 2.2–4.7), the odds ratio (OR) is 4.0 (95% CI: 2.6–6.1; p b 0.001; I2 b 27.6%), and the risk difference (RD) is 0.08 (95% CI: 0.06–0.11; p b 0.001; I2 = 99.7%), suggesting that children with CD may have an elevated risk of headaches compared to controls. The prevalence of CD is twice as high in people with chronic headache, akin to epilepsy. Screening for CD may be recommended as a component of the diagnostic evaluation in these pediatric patients, especially those who do not respond to pharmacological therapy (Nenna et al., 2016).

Rare Neurological Manifestations of CD

In literature, case reports document several neurological manifestations in CD. A 2015 case report detailed a 14-year-old girl presenting with constipation and pseudotumor cerebri, characterized by headache and papilledema without structural abnormalities. She was diagnosed with CD due to significant constipation. The patients commenced a GFD, resulting in the alleviation of both gastrointestinal symptoms and symptoms of pseudotumor cerebri (Rani, Imdad, & Beg, 2015). In 2015, Plant et al., documented a case of a patient with CD and cerebral occipital calcification who had a gradual and apparently selective inability to detect visual cues (Plant, James-Galton, & Wilkinson, 2015). In 2016, a case report described a 17-month-old girl with CD and transverse myelitis diagnosed with magnetic resonance imaging. Following the initiation of both GFD and methylprednisolone, she achieved full recovery (Krom, Sprangers, van den Berg, Benninga, & Kindermann, 2017). Instances of transverse myelitis have been previously documented in adults (Iyer et al., 2014). In 2006, Belgian investigators documented a case involving a 2-year-old male exhibiting opsoclonus-myoclonus syndrome characterized by action myoclonus, palpebral flutter, opsoclonus, and ataxia. Magnetic resonance imaging of the brain was unremarkable on two instances, while oligoclonal bands were detected in the cerebrospinal fluid. Serum screening for CD was positive, and duodenal biopsies corroborated the physician's determination of CD (Deconinck, Scaillon, Segers, Groswasser, & Dan, 2006). Additionally, a case report from 2004 detailed a child exhibiting recurrent transitory hemiplegia, with CD serology showing high positivity and a duodenal biopsy confirming the diagnosis (Goodwin, Beattie, Millar, & Kirkham, 2004).

Neurological Investigation

EEG Findings

The range of electroencephalography (EEG) characteristics linked to CD is extensive; focused activity, including unilateral or bilateral spikes or slow waves mostly situated in the occipital regions, has been documented in the majority of awake EEG investigations (Aksoy, Tıraş-Teber, Kansu, Deda, & Kartal, 2016; Dai, Akcali, Varan, & Demiryürek, 2014; Labate et al., 2001; Magaudda et al., 1993; Riccardo Pratesi et al., 2003). Epilepsy is one of the most prevalent neurological complications in childhood (Lionetti et al., 2010).

Only a single study (Parisi et al., 2015) has examined the incidence of neuronal hyperexcitability and subclinical EEG abnormalities in asymptomatic children with newly diagnosed CD. This study's EEG exams identified aberrant findings, including focal or generalized sharps and/or spikes and spike-waves in 47.4% of cases, without distinct medical symptoms. Pennisi et al., asserted the existence of a "hyperexcitable brain" in CD based on these grounds (Pennisi et al., 2017).

Electrophysiological Tests

In adults, people with CD exhibit a heightened prevalence of chronic axonal neuropathy, even while following a long-term stringent GFD. Timely identification of CD may avert the onset of overt neuropathy. Subclinical peripheral neuropathy in patients with CD, despite the absence of electrophysiological alterations, is evidenced by diminished pain thresholds and impaired heat and tactile sensations; 23.1% of those with CD exhibited characteristics of chronic axonal neuropathy on quantitative needle EMG; furthermore, two CD people displayed indications suggestive of myopathy; an elevated prevalence of axonal neuropathy was noted in well-managed CD, further suggesting that neurological manifestations can arise even in patients without overt malabsorption (Luostarinen et al., 2003). The involvement of the peripheral nervous system in children with CD is infrequent (refer to the specific paragraph). Electrophysiological investigations are unnecessary in asymptomatic patients of CD. A new study examined 167 asymptomatic patients and 100 control cases for predisposing variables of polyneuropathy, utilizing electrophysiological testing for peripheral nervous system disorders. Motor nerve conduction investigations, including F-waves, were conducted for the median, ulnar, peroneal, and tibial nerves; also, sensory nerve conduction studies were executed for the median, ulnar, and sural nerves, along with unilateral H reflex assessment of the soleus muscle. Electrophysiological tests did not reveal indications of subclinical neuropathy (Işikay & Kocamaz, 2015).

Imaging

Individuals with CD referred for neurological evaluation exhibit notable abnormalities on MR imaging of the brain and cerebellum. People with CD exhibit markedly reduced gray matter volume across many brain regions, including the cerebellum, and a greater prevalence of cerebral white matter abnormalities, particularly among those experiencing headaches (Currie et al., 2012). Unilateral and bilateral focal T2 hyperintense white matter lesions were previously identified (Kieslich et al., 2001). Neuroimaging is crucial for diagnosing CEC syndrome (CD, epilepsy, and bilateral occipital calcification) (G Gobbi, 1993; Giuseppe Gobbi et al., 1992). CEC syndrome is a localized or complicated partial epilepsy typically starting in the occipital lobe. TC and MR data indicate bilateral cortical and subcortical occipital calcification, with no evidence of lobar or hemispheric atrophy, and no contrast enhancement linked to atrophy or vascular abnormalities (Magaudda et al., 1993). Radiograph spectroscopy revealed the presence of calcium and silica in these calcifications (Toti et al., 1996).

Psychiatric and Psychological Manifestations of CD

Psychiatric illnesses have been documented as a consequence of CD in numerous people, and various investigations have indicated symptom amelioration following the initiation of a GFD. Patients with CD typically exhibit psychiatric symptoms such as depressed manifestations, apathy, heightened anxiety, irritability, eating disorders, and attention-deficit/hyperactivity disorders (ADHD) (Karwautz et al., 2008). A study indicated that individuals with CD exhibited a considerably higher prevalence of state anxiety compared to controls (G Addolorato et al., 2000). A meta-analysis regarding anxiety and depression in CD revealed that depression is more prevalent and more severe in individuals with CD compared to healthy controls (D. Smith & Gerdes, 2012). Social phobia appears to be elevated in individuals with CD (Giovanni Addolorato et al., 2008), and a greater lifetime frequency of panic disorders has been identified (Carta et al., 2002). Campagna et al., indicated that patients with CD exhibited markedly elevated scores in anxiety, harm avoidance, separation panic, and somatic symptoms, even following the implementation of a GFD (Campagna et al., 2017). The implementation of GFD generates significant anxiety, which may exhibit varying characteristics based on gender, leading to depression in females and aggressive conduct and irritability in males. The correlation between schizophrenia and CD has been recognized since the 1950s; symptoms of schizophrenia appear to ameliorate with rigorous adherence to a GFD. There is no conclusive data indicating whether CD precedes the start of schizophrenia or the reverse (Eaton et al., 2004; Samaroo et al., 2010). A recent multicentric research in Sweden indicates an increased risk of psychiatric illnesses in children. Children with CD exhibited a 1.4-fold increased risk of developing future psychiatric illnesses compared to the general population. Childhood CD has been recognized as a risk factor for mood disorders, anxiety disorders, eating disorders, behavioral disorders, ADHD, ASD, and intellectual disability (Butwicka et al., 2017). The TEDDY Study Group indicated that celiac disease autoimmunity correlates with heightened instances of childhood sadness and anxiety, aggressive behavior, and sleep disturbances when mothers are uninformed of their children's CD autoimmune status (L. B. Smith et al., 2017). A recent comprehensive review determined an association between CD and psychiatric disorders with varying levels of evidence: substantial evidence supports a link between CD and depression, and to a lesser degree, eating disorders; a potential association exists between CD and panic disorder, autism, and ADHD, although the evidence is limited; data concerning the association of CD with schizophrenia or other anxiety disorders is conflicting (Slim, Rico-Villademoros, & Calandre, 2018).

Present data indicates that patients with CD have an elevated risk of developing neurological and mental diseases. The current incidence of these disorders in adults and children remains unclear, necessitating further research to elucidate their pathophysiology. A GFD appears to have advantageous effects on neurological disorders, epileptic activity, and neuropsychiatric symptoms, as it may ameliorate these conditions. Neurological involvement in CD is prevalent, necessitating more precise testing in these patients to achieve an appropriate diagnosis. Gastroenterologists and other healthcare professionals involved in the diagnosis and ongoing therapy of individuals with CD should conduct routine surveillance for potential neurological and psychiatric symptoms. A meticulous evaluation is essential to appropriately refer the child or adult to the neurology or psychiatry departments, facilitating an accurate early diagnosis and corresponding therapy. The neurologist should similarly consider CD in patients exhibiting the previously stated neurological symptoms. Given the established elevated risk ratio of epilepsy and headache in patients with CD (and conversely), these individuals should be screened for CD at the time of diagnosis and during subsequent follow-up.

Chapter 5

Diagnosis of Celiac Disease

Abstract

Accurate diagnosis of celiac disease (CD) is critical for effective management. This chapter covers the diagnostic criteria, including serological testing for anti-TTG antibodies, HLA genotyping, and duodenal biopsies. It explores the challenges in diagnosing CD due to its diverse clinical manifestations and the overlap with other gastrointestinal disorders. Emerging diagnostic techniques such as genetic screening and novel biomarkers are discussed, along with the role of differential diagnosis. This chapter emphasizes the importance of early detection for preventing long-term complications of CD.

Serological Testing

Serological testing for celiac disease exhibits sensitivities, specificities, and diagnostic accuracies over 90%, with enhanced accuracy when people are assessed while consuming a gluten -containing diet (Di Sabatino et al., 2017; Rubio-Tapia, Hill, Kelly, Calderwood, & Murray, 2013). Autoantibody titers often decrease substantially within a year following the commencement of a gluten-free diet in individuals with celiac disease. This is beneficial for monitoring dietary compliance, indicative of gastrointestinal healing, and correlated with enhanced clinical symptoms (Midhagen et al., 2004). Serological assays may exhibit diminished accuracy regarding mucosal inflammation and healing in RCD (Adriaanse & Leffler, 2015; Leonard, Weir, et al., 2017; Silvester et al., 2017). These issues have led to the creation of supplementary diagnostics such as microbead-based technologies, chemiluminescence, autoantibody profiling, and regression tree analysis, which seek to enhance sensitivity and forecast biopsy needs (Belei, Iacob, Iacob, Amaricai, & Marginean, 2020; Ermarth et al., 2017; Sowa et al., 2017).

Duodenal Biopsies

The "lifecycle" of a duodenal biopsy has three primary phases: (Dicke et al., 1953) preanalytic, (Abadie et al., 2011) analytical, and (Paulley, 1954) postanalytic. Processes must be improved and, preferably, standardized at every level to guarantee optimal outcomes.

Preanalytic Phase

The paramount preanalytic variable is biopsy sampling. This is due to two factors. Similar to Crohn's disease, mucosal changes in CD may be irregularly distributed (Hopper, Cross, & Sanders, 2008). Secondly, tiny intestinal biopsies are often not oriented prior to processing in the majority of institutions across the United States. It is advised that four to six biopsy specimens be collected from both the second segment of the duodenum and the duodenal bulb to guarantee appropriate sampling, particularly when considering a diagnosis of celiac disease (Hopper et al., 2008). The American College of Gastroenterology advises obtaining four biopsies from the postbulbar duodenum and two from the duodenal bulb; nevertheless, it is widely recognized that some endoscopists fail to collect the recommended quantity of biopsies, which may result in false-negative diagnosis (Lebwohl, Kapel, Neugut, Green, & Genta, 2011; Rubio-Tapia et al., 2013). A critical consideration is that the patient must be ingesting gluten during the biopsy, as the negative predictive value of a normal biopsy is significantly diminished when a gluten-free diet is followed (Rubio-Tapia et al., 2013).

A biopsy of the duodenal bulb, formerly deemed unfavorable due to the potential for artifacts (mostly from large Brunner glands), assists in identifying a small subset of individuals with celiac disease (13%) who would be overlooked by postbulbar biopsies alone (Gonzalez et al., 2010). The quality of the biopsies may be enhanced by acquiring one sample at a time rather than numerous samples each pass. This method demonstrated an improvement in the yield of properly orientated samples (66% vs 42%) in a prospective trial (Latorre et al., 2015). Acquiring six levels from each small intestine biopsy block, rather than the standard three levels for other gastrointestinal biopsies, is suggested for thorough assessment. Hematoxylin and eosin staining of biopsies is adequate for standard morphological evaluation. Based on our experience, immunohistochemistry (IHC) for T-cell antigens, particularly cluster of differentiation 3 (CD3), to emphasize elevated intraepithelial lymphocytes is not beneficial in routine treatment (Mino & Lauwers, 2003). Certain researchers have proposed that CD3 immunohistochemistry is "essential" in instances when intraepithelial lymphocytes are detected (Volta & Villanacci, 2011). Certain laboratories do CD3 IHC on all small intestine samples as a first step, a practice that contradicts existing data (Hudacko, Kathy Zhou, & Yantiss, 2013). Occasionally, CD3 IHC can emphasize a little elevation in IEL density and may reveal their distribution mostly at the villus tips. This examination is reserved for the infrequent instances that remain really borderline despite meticulous hematoxylin and eosin evaluation. Additionally, immunohistochemistry for CD3 and CD8 is beneficial in assessing refractory Crohn's disease. In this context, the presence of CD8 positivity in the majority (> 50%) of CD31 IELs serves as evidence against refractory celiac disease type 2, a clonal lymphoproliferative illness, or enteropathy-associated T-cell lymphoma, which are uncommon consequences of celiac disease (Chander, Leeman-Neill, & Bhagat, 2018).

Analytical Phase

The biopsy examination must commence with a meticulous and systematic inspection of the slide at low-power magnification (×4 objective), assessing all mucosal compartments. This facilitates the assessment of the architecture and manifest inflammatory alterations. For proper evaluation, a minimum of one biopsy specimen must be "well-oriented," meaning that four consecutive parallel crypt-villus units are observable (Perera, Weinstein, & Rubin, 1975). The interpreting pathologist must be familiar with the spectrum of normal morphological changes in small intestine mucosal architecture. In the duodenum, the villi should be three to five times higher than the depth of the crypts (Dickson, Streutker, & Chetty, 2006; Serra & Jani, 2006). Failure to maintain this ratio results in villus atrophy and/or crypt hyperplasia. No criteria exist to delineate an aberrant density of lamina propria lymphocytes and plasma cells. These are typical components of the intestinal lamina propria, and their quantities elevate in ACD and other inflammatory states. An expert pathologist possesses an intuition for distinguishing between the normal and the excessive. Neutrophilic granulocytes are not regarded as a standard element of the small intestine lamina propria (Villanacci, Ceppa, Tavani, Vindigni, & Volta, 2011). The low-power assessment should involve examining the interstitial area between the villi, if present, for parasites.

Giardia organisms are frequently seen at low magnification, although may be overlooked if the biopsy is not examined systematically.

Upon concluding the low-power assessment, all biopsies must undergo high magnification analysis. This aims to investigate characteristics that may not be easily discernible at low magnification, including IEL density, the existence of goblet and Paneth cells, gastric metaplasia and heterotopia, subepithelial fibrosis, and the presence and qualitative evaluation of granulocytes and plasma cells, as well as the identification of pathogens. Despite considerable contention in the literature over the typical quantity of intraepithelial lymphocytes in the duodenum, the majority of specialists concur on a maximum of 25 per 100 enterocytes (Hayat, Cairns, Dixon, & O'Mahony, 2002). A rise beyond this threshold defines IEL. The distribution of the IELs is crucial as well. The normal duodenal mucosa has a "decrescendo" pattern of intraepithelial lymphocytes, with increased density observed near the basal region of the villi (Goldstein & Underhill, 2001). Consequently, elevated intraepithelial lymphocytes at the tips of villi, quantified as an average of 12 IELs per 20 enterocytes in five villus tips, are associated with celiac disease, but elevations in IELs along the lateral borders of villi exhibit lower specificity (Goldstein & Underhill, 2001). This modified pattern may also aid in identifying people with probable celiac disease (seropositivity without symptoms or villous atrophy) (Biagi et al., 2004). The assessment of normal and pathological IEL distribution patterns, as well as an increase in IELs, is insufficient in unoriented biopsies or when the villi are detached or entirely atrophic.

Upon completion of the low- and high-power inspection, the observations must be systematically arranged. Definitive assertions should be articulated wherever feasible (e.g., "Duodenal mucosa, within normal limits," or "Duodenal mucosa with giardiasis"). It is not unusual to observe inflammatory alterations that indicate a disease, yet are not diagnostically definitive on their own. A differential diagnosis should be incorporated in the report in such contexts. If the pathologist has access to the medical records and/or the gastroenterologist, the differential diagnosis should be customized to the patient's specific situation.

Differential Diagnosis

Considering the differential diagnosis of CD in conjunction with the Marsh-Oberhuber pattern is advantageous. In other terms, when a pathologist evaluates a Marsh-Oberhuber type 1 pattern (normal architecture with enhanced intraepithelial lymphocytes), the differential diagnosis differs from that associated with a Marsh-Oberhuber type 3C pattern (flat mucosa).

Preserved Architecture with Intraepithelial Lymphocytosis

The differential diagnosis of the Marsh-Oberhuber type 1 (or Corazza A) pattern is extensive and has been observed with increasing frequency in recent years. As the incidence of elevated IELs has risen, the positive predictive value of this pattern for celiac disease (CD) has diminished (Shmidt, Smyrk, Boswell, Enders, & Oxentenko, 2014). While many cases are idiopathic, alternative etiologies include inadequately managed celiac disease, tropical sprue, Helicobacter pylori infection (of the stomach), pharmacological effects (e.g., proton pump inhibitors, selective serotonin reuptake inhibitors, nonsteroidal anti-inflammatory drugs), small intestinal bacterial overgrowth, viral gastroenteritis, morbid obesity, autoimmune disorders, inflammatory bowel disease, and others (Aziz, Evans, Hopper, Smillie, & Sanders, 2010; I. S. Brown, Bettington, Bettington, & Rosty, 2014; Harpaz, Levi, Yurovitsky, & Kini, 2007; Lauwers, Fasano, & Brown, 2015; Masia, Peyton, Lauwers, & Brown, 2014; Memeo et al., 2005; Patterson, Shmidt, Oxentenko, Enders, & Smyrk, 2015; Shmidt et al., 2014).

Identifying the underlying or causative agents is challenging due to the prevalence of common etiological factors, such as drug usage, and the possibility that the patient may have multiple concurrent conditions. Comprehensive clinical data and laboratory analyses, including genetic testing, may be required to rule out CD in certain cases. In patients with a documented history of celiac disease, the finding may be attributed to limited gluten exposure. This trend is unusual in newly diagnosed Crohn's disease (I. S. Brown, Smith, & Rosty, 2012). Research indicates that 5% to 10% of individuals without a documented history of celiac disease, whose biopsies display the Marsh-Oberhuber type 1 pattern, may eventually be diagnosed with celiac disease (I. S. Brown et al., 2012; Kakar, Nehra, Murray, Dayharsh, & Burgart, 2003).

In one study, over 16% of children with stomach pain, but no celiac disease, H. pylori gastritis, or other identifiable gastrointestinal disorders, had more than 25 intraepithelial lymphocytes per 100 enterocytes (Guz-Mark, Zevit, Morgenstern, & Shamir, 2014). Therefore, when a physician receives a pathology report indicating a Marsh-Oberhuber type 1 pattern, further investigations should be conducted to rule out celiac disease. However, it is essential to recognize that this result is common, nonspecific, and frequently idiopathic.

Villus Atrophy

The occurrence of villus atrophy is a troubling discovery that should not be deemed "idiopathic" without thorough evaluation and maybe referral to a specialist facility. The differential diagnosis of villus atrophy and elevated intraepithelial lymphocytes (IELs) encompasses celiac disease; drug-induced enteropathy, notably Olmesartan-associated enteropathy (OAE), which may also relate to other angiotensin receptor blockers (ARBs); mycophenolate-based therapies; colchicine; collagenous sprue; common variable immunodeficiency; autoimmune enteropathy; lymphoma; inflammatory bowel disease; and specific infections (DeGaetani et al., 2013).

Among these entities, OAE has recently attracted the greatest interest. Rubio-Tapia and associates reported a cohort of 22 individuals exhibiting severe diarrhea and significant weight loss after to olmesartan exposure. Biopsies of the small intestine revealed pronounced villus atrophy and inflammation. Fifteen had complete villus atrophy, whereas fourteen demonstrated elevated intraepithelial lymphocytes. Serologic testing for celiac disease was consistently negative, and a gluten -free diet did not alleviate symptoms or mucosal abnormalities. Seven individuals were diagnosed with collagenous sprue. Among 14 individuals who had stomach biopsies, five (36%) demonstrated lymphocytic gastritis, whereas two (14%) revealed characteristics of collagenous gastritis. Colon biopsies from 5 of the 13 patients (38%) revealed microscopic colitis, comprising two cases of lymphocytic colitis and three cases of collagenous colitis. Clinical symptoms rapidly vanished with discontinuation of the drugs in all instances, and the histological alterations subsided in the majority (Rubio-Tapia et al., 2012). Numerous supplementary case reports, series, and reviews have corroborated these findings and linked various angiotensin receptor blockers (ARBs) (Abdelghany, Gonzalez III, Slater, & Begley, 2014; Burbure et al., 2016; deFonseka, Tuskey, & Moskaluk, 2012; DeGaetani et al., 2013; Dreifuss, Tomizawa, Farber, Davison, & Sohnen, 2013; Fiorucci et al., 2014; Freeman, 2016; Herman, Rubio-Tapia, Wu, & Murray, 2015; Ianiro et al., 2014; A. S. Khan, Peter, & Wilcox, 2014; Malfertheiner, Ripellino, & Cataldo, 2018; Marthey et al., 2014; Nielsen, Steephen, & Lewin, 2013; Scialom et al., 2015;

Stanich, Yearsley, & Meyer, 2013; Talbot, 2012; Théophile, David, Miremont-Salamé, & Haramburu, 2014; T. H. Tran & Li, 2014). In 2013, the US Food and Drug Administration authorized a modification of the label for olmesartan to recognize the risk of enteropathy.

Based on the above description of the histology of OAE, it is challenging (and occasionally impossible) to differentiate OAE from ACD only on morphological characteristics. In certain OAE instances, histological indicators exist that enable the observant pathologist to propose the diagnosis. The initial factor is the density of IELs. Research indicates that many cases of ARB-enteropathy do not show significantly elevated IELs, a characteristic almost ubiquitous in celiac disease (CD) (Ianiro et al., 2014; Rubio-Tapia et al., 2012). Secondly, OAE patients often present with elevated subepithelial collagen, resembling characteristics of collagenous sprue, which is an uncommon finding in CD (DeGaetani et al., 2013; Rubio-Tapia et al., 2012; Vakiani et al., 2010). Ultimately, seronegativity and medication exposure are the most significant factors in differentiating between CD and ARB enteropathy, with the clinical and histopathologic response to a change in drug class reinforcing medication exposure as the primary causative factor. Consequently, OAE exemplifies a scenario where understanding the clinical history enables the pathologist to provide a more significant assessment of the etiology and the correct diagnosis.

Common variable immunodeficiency is an immunodeficiency condition marked by the inability of B cells to mature into plasma cells, resulting in reduced blood immunoglobulin levels. Patients may exhibit diarrhea and malabsorption and are susceptible to diseases such as giardiasis and bacterial overgrowth (Ament, Ochs, & Davis, 1973; Washington, Stenzel, Buckley, & Gottfried, 1996). Duodenal biopsies may reveal various alterations, such as elevated intraepithelial lymphocytes and differing extents of villus atrophy (Malamut, Verkarre, et al., 2010). Common variable immunodeficiency often exhibits a lack of significant reduction in the quantity of lamina propria plasma cells. This contrasts with CD, in which plasma cells are elevated. The proliferation of lamina propria lymphocytes can occasionally be substantial, complicating the identification of absent plasma cells.

The phrase "autoimmune enteropathy "denotes a collection of uncommon autoimmune disorders that predominantly affect newborns, while they may occasionally manifest in adults. A severe X-linked illness in young boys is connected to immunological dysregulation and polyendocrinopathy due to a germline mutation in the FOXP3 gene on the X chromosome (Le Bras & Geha, 2006). Patients with this condition may exhibit failure to thrive, secretory diarrhea, weight loss, and malabsorption, necessitating whole parenteral feeding. AE typically impacts the proximal small intestine; however, instances of involvement of the stomach, distal small intestine, and colon have been reported. Duodenal biopsies reveal varied villus atrophy and crypt hyperplasia, frequently accompanied by a reduced quantity of Paneth and goblet cells. A prominent lymphoplasmacytic infiltration in the lamina propria is prevalent, and neutrophils with crypt abscesses are seen in severe instances (Gino R Corazza et al., 1997; Montalto et al., 2009; Russo, Brochu, Seidman, & Roy, 1999). The rise in IELs is particularly pronounced in the crypts. This trait may assist in differentiating AE from CD, which often exhibits a significant rise in surface IELs. Crypt apoptosis is frequently observed in autoimmune enteropathy (AE), however this observation is not exclusive, since it is also present in other conditions like Crohn's disease (CD) (Shalimar et al., 2013). Laboratory testing may reveal the existence of antienterocyte antibodies, and certain individuals may also exhibit anti-goblet cell, anti-parietal cell, and anti-smooth muscle antibodies. Antigliadin and antireticulin antibodies have been identified in autoimmune encephalitis (AE) (Gino R Corazza et al., 1997). We have observed a case of OAE in which the ileal biopsy revealed a near-total depletion of goblet and Paneth cells, prompting concerns regarding AE. Nevertheless, these cells were easily recognized in a second biopsy following the cessation of Olmesartan (Burbure et al., 2016). Significant morphological overlap exists across these entities, underscoring the necessity for meticulous attention and clinical correlation.

Postanalytical Phase

Postanalytic factors regarding duodenal biopsies mostly pertain to reporting wording. Numerous facilities employ "quick texts" to articulate gastrointestinal biopsy results; unfortunately, significant information is frequently overlooked as a result (Arguelles-Grande, Tennyson, Lewis, Green, & Bhagat, 2012). To guarantee the inclusion of all pertinent data in pathology reports, we utilize a worksheet for biopsies, accompanied by a request to screen for CD or to investigate the source of persistent symptoms or response to medication. The concept involves employing a framework akin to tumor staging checklists, comparable to the staging forms. The worksheet was created by collaboration between physicians and pathologists.

Supplemental Testing

Celiac disease exhibits a significant hereditary component, with a familial recurrence rate of 10-15% and a concordance rate of 75-80% among monozygotic twins (Green & Jabri, 2003; K. E. Lundin & Wijmenga, 2015). The HLA-DQA1*05:01-DQB1*02:01 haplotype, which encodes the DQ2 molecule, is found in 90–95% of individuals with celiac disease. In the remaining about 5% of individuals with CD, the HLA-DQA1*03:01-DQB1*03:02 haplotype is present, which encodes the DQ8 protein. Five percent of patients have at least one of the DQ2/DQ8 alleles (E. Liu et al., 2014). This organization offers an effective screening instrument for celiac disease using genotyping. The HLA DQ2/DQ8 genes are necessary but insufficient to induce celiac disease, hence restricting their use as an independent diagnostic test (Charlesworth, 2020; Green & Jabri, 2003).

In the realm of CD diagnosis, flow cytometry is primarily employed to identify and quantify IELs for the diagnosis of RCD when serological tests are inadequate (Kakar et al., 2003; Rostami et al., 2017; Sanchez-Muñoz et al., 2008). The characterization of RCDII IEL is often signified by the presence of clonal T-cells as seen using flow cytometry (Cellier et al., 2000; Ludvigsson et al., 2014). Clonal T-cells generally do not display surface CD3, CD4, or CD8, nevertheless they exhibit both cytoplasmic CD3 and CD103. The absence of surface CD3 and CD8, together the retention of cytoplasmic CD3 and monoclonal rearrangement of the T-cell receptor chain, are the principal criteria used in diagnosis (Ludvigsson et al., 2014; Rubio-Tapia & Murray, 2010; Sanchez-Muñoz et al., 2008). While the identification of IELs is largely employed for diagnosing RCD, they can also aid in the diagnosis of challenging instances of CD with ambiguous serology and histology (Arregui et al., 2016; Valle et al., 2017).

Diagnostic Algorithms for CD

Global criteria for Crohn's disease diagnosis have mostly been shaped by European, British, and North American recommendations (Caio et al., 2019; Husby, Murray, & Katzka, 2019; Ludvigsson et al., 2014; Rubio-Tapia et al., 2013). This diagnostic method employs five antibodies for serological assessment: IgA-tTG, total IgA, IgA-endomysial antibodies (EMA), IgA-DGP, and either IgG-tTG or IgG-DGP. Serology is then complemented by a duodenal biopsy for definitive confirmation and HLA genotyping as an exclusionary test when serological and biopsy results are inconclusive. Canada, New Zealand, and Australia adhere to analogous criteria (J. Tye-Din, 2018). The recent recommendations from the European Society for Paediatric Gastroenterology Hepatology and Nutrition (ESPGHAN) advise against biopsy when tTG levels exceed tenfold the normal threshold and a subsequent sample tests EMA positive. Nonetheless, there is a paucity of documented recommendations in underdeveloped nations. The South African methodology primarily comprises IgA-tTG and IgA-DGP serology, followed by a biopsy for confirmation. Diagnostic problems in resource-limited settings, such as South Africa, encompass patient follow-up attrition and diminished access to diagnostic tests.

Novel Directions

Numerous novel biomarkers are under research and may enhance the diagnostic, prognostic, and monitoring efficacy of CD testing. Nevertheless, the majority of these investigations were performed outside of Africa. Essential biomarkers encompass inflammatory indicators (cytokines, reactive oxygen species (ROS), and genetic fingerprints of lymphocyte activation), biochemical markers of intestinal damage (such as IFABP), and the identification of intraepithelial lymphocyte populations. Recently, there has been heightened interest in the gastrointestinal microbiome due to its probable pathogenic involvement in Crohn's disease. Surveillance and forecasting are essential in RCD due to the potential for malignant change (Ludvigsson et al., 2014; Rubio-Tapia et al., 2016). Promising research avenues encompass phospholipid profiling and miRNA identification (Auricchio et al., 2019; Bascuñán et al., 2020). Auricchio et al., (2019) established a blood phospholipid profile that differentiates those predisposed to developing CD prior to the manifestation of symptoms or antibodies (Auricchio et al., 2019). mRNA-146a, miRNA-155, miRNA-21, and miRNA-125b exhibit elevated specificity and sensitivity for both active and inactive Crohn's disease, regardless of therapy. Research on these biomarkers in South African populations is essential, given the recent studies on CD diagnoses have predominantly taken place in Europe and the USA.

In conclusion, the growing understanding of CD pathology has enabled the development of a sophisticated diagnostic algorithm that can precisely identify individuals with CD, a feat not achieved for many other autoimmune illnesses. Nonetheless, several limitations must be resolved by more study into the multiple pathways that might enhance the diagnosis, prognosis, and monitoring of individuals with CD. The existing diagnostic method in Iran necessitates revision to optimize resource use and effectively identify high-risk people.

Challenges of CD Diagnosis

Despite being first thought of as a childhood illness, current research indicates that 25% of CD cases occur in people over 60. Additionally, the median diagnosis age is rising, which has sparked interest in learning more about CD pathogenesis. Recent evidence of the prevalence of specific types of malignancies among CD patients is what has caused the pressure to properly identify and design appropriate therapies. This comprises esophageal and oropharyngeal squamous carcinoma, enteropathy-related T-cell lymphoma, small intestinal adenocarcinoma, and non-Hodgkin lymphoma. However, the fact of the matter is that following a GFD has been demonstrated to reduce the risk of malignancies (K. E. Lundin, Brottveit, & Skodje, 2022). A greater range of villous architecture - from near-normal to entire villous atrophy, with multiple intermediate stages - complicates the diagnosis of CD. Additionally, there are instances where CD clinical symptoms and serology and biopsy results are inconsistent. Reexamining the diagnosis and considering HLA typing may be an option in such complicated circumstances. The HLA-DQ2 and/or HLA-DQ8 alleles are carried by virtually all celiac patients (and between 25% and 40% of the general population), hence the lack of either marker has a very strong negative predictive significance. A relevant metric to use in addition to CD confirmation is progress in reaction to GFD (Marsh, 1992; Molina-Infante & Carroccio, 2017). It is important to note that there are instances where CD patients do not improve as a result of adhering to the GFD. In such cases, it may be advisable to do a biopsy on the CD patients again and to make sure that the GFD is not contaminated with grains containing gluten (Thompson, 2004). As a result, it is crucial to establish and abide by gold standards at every phase of the disease given the diversity in regards to diagnosis, therapy, pathophysiology, and prognosis.

Chapter 6

Nutritional Considerations in Celiac Disease

Abstract

The management of celiac disease largely relies on strict adherence to a gluten-free diet (GFD), which is crucial for symptom relief and intestinal healing. This chapter addresses the nutritional challenges faced by CD patients, including the risk of deficiencies in vitamins and minerals such as iron, calcium, and vitamin D. The impact of CD on bone health, including metabolic bone disease, is also discussed. Furthermore, the chapter explores strategies for optimizing nutrition and managing the dietary restrictions associated with a gluten-free lifestyle.

Nutritional Considerations in Regard to CD

In the treatment of individuals with CD, a professional dietician or nutritionist plays a crucial role. They may be the most crucial part of the patient's follow-up treatment and the main figure in any celiac center. Their responsibilities include general education about celiac disease, label reading instruction, advice on dining out, and cross-contamination prevention. A professional dietician or nutritionist is also a valuable resource for patients who have a poor or nonexistent reaction to a GFD. Patients who are often diagnosed with non-responsive celiac disease may have unintentionally consumed gluten -free commodities with the help of a thorough addition of history from a dietician or nutritionist.

Patients with CD are at risk for malabsorption and other related nutritional deficits. Numerous nutritional deficits might occur in young celiac disease patients. Deora et al., investigated the frequency of nutritional inadequacies in individuals with CD at diagnosis, at 6 months following the commencement of a GFD, and at 18 months after that. Additionally, they looked for any connections between mucosal injury at diagnosis, serum tissue transglutaminase immunoglobulin A antibody titers, and nutritional deficiencies. A number of 140 CD individuals under the age of 17 were enrolled, 87 of them were females (621%). At the time of diagnosis and 6 and 18 months after beginning a GFD, the blood levels of vitamins, minerals, and anti-tTG IgA antibodies were assessed. Using a modified Marsh classification, the histopathological alterations of duodenal samples upon diagnosis were recorded. At diagnosis, the average age was 7.8 ± 4.01 years. Seventy percent of children had vitamin D deficiency at the time of their diagnosis. Only 12 (10.9%) children developed iron deficiency anemia, but 34.5% of children's serum ferritin levels and 18.6% of children's zinc levels were subnormal. There was no association between the degree of villous atrophy, serum tTG IgA antibody titers, or nutritional deficits at diagnosis. Furthermore, most of the tested serum levels of micronutrients had returned to normal after six months of commencing the GFD, with the exception of vitamin D, which enhanced but remained subnormal (Deora, Aylward, Sokoro, & El-Matary, 2017). It has been assumed that the impaired uptake of fat-soluble vitamins in celiac disease is what causes the risk of vitamin A insufficiency. There are no substantial studies evaluating the scope of the alleged relationship, and the data that is available is restricted to letters to the editor (ALWITRY, 2000). In individuals with iron deficiency (ID), the CD is thought to occur somewhere between 0-6% of the time. In the USA, nothing is known about the frequency of celiac disease in those who are iron deficient. To further investigate this, Abdalla et al., utilized the NHANES database, a nationwide survey health study carried out between 2009 and 2010. They surveyed 2105 females who were at least 6 years old. Serum ferritin levels below 20 ng/mL were considered iron deficient, and CD was diagnosed in patients who tested positive for both IgA endomysial antibody, and IgA tissue transglutaminase antibody. Both the ID and non-ID groups of subjects were separated. Out of the 2105 participants, 559 patients had an ID, while 1536 did not. CD was diagnosed in five members of the ID group and two members of the non-ID group. After controlling for a few variables, female participants with ID had a greater frequency of CD, with an OR of 12.5 (95% CI 1.74-90). According to their research, just a small percentage of US females have CD generally; however, the frequency is greater in people with ID. Since only females were involved in the study, the findings might not be generalizable (Abdalla et al., 2017).

In a recent prospective observational research, CD among individuals with severe acute malnutrition (SAM) was examined for prevalence and clinical characteristics in an Indian patient cohort by Beniwal et al., All SAM-affected kids who had been hospitalized in a row were recruited. IgA-tTG antibodies were used to test subjects for CD. For confirmation, those who tested positive had an upper gastrointestinal endoscopy along with a small bowel biopsy. Individuals with and without CD were assessed in terms of their clinical characteristics. Children with SAM were reported to have a seroprevalence (IgA-tTG positive) of CD of 15.38% and a prevalence of biopsy-confirmed CD of 14.42%. In contrast to individuals without CD, patients with CD were more likely to experience mouth ulcers, edema, clubbing, diarrhea, anorexia, constipation, abdominal pain, and vitamin deficiencies. Only stomach distension and pain, however, were statistically significantly different from the control group (Beniwal, Ameta, & Chahar, 2017).

CD-Mediated Metabolic Bone Disease

Metabolic Bone Disease in CD

The principal cause of decreased bone mineral density (BMD) in celiac disease is secondary hyperparathyroidism resulting from loss of calcium and vitamin D. In people with gastrointestinal malabsorption, poor calcium absorption results in heightened fecal calcium losses, decreased urine calcium excretion, and a negative calcium balance (Harrison, Hitchman, Finlay, & McNeill, 1969). In cases of steatorrhea, the absorption of oral vitamin D is inversely correlated with the severity of steatorrhea (Gertner, Lilburn, & Domenech, 1977). Elevations in blood parathyroid hormone (PTH) subsequently augment the activity of renal 1-alpha-hydroxylase, facilitating the conversion of 25-hydroxyvitamin D into its active form, 1,25-hydroxyvitamin D, to promote calcium absorption from the small intestine. The inflow of luminal calcium is hindered by decreased levels of intracellular calcium-binding proteins in the context of CD, resulting in less facilitated diffusion of intracellular calcium. Moreover, in the context of steatorrhea, calcium is chelated to intraluminal fat, resulting in increased fecal losses, whereas secondary lactose intolerance causes a decrease in calcium intake (Plotkin & Isselbacher, 1964). Hypocalcemia subsequently results in compensatory elevations of serum parathyroid hormone levels, which have been shown to be increased in newly diagnosed patients with celiac disease (CD), but can normalize on a gluten -free diet (GFD) (Taranta et al., 2004).

As a result of the typical association between bone production and resorption, an increase in bone turnover leads to the acceleration of both processes, resulting in elevated markers for each phase of bone turnover. Markers of bone resorption, such as serum bone-specific alkaline phosphatase and urinary pyridinoline cross-links, as well as markers of bone formation like osteocalcin, have been shown to be elevated in individuals with celiac disease, newly diagnosed patients, and those with refractory celiac disease compared to patients on a gluten -free diet or healthy controls. Discrepancies in bone resorption and creation, especially in persons with Crohn's disease and ongoing disease activity, ultimately result in bone loss and compromised mineralization. The implementation of a gluten-free diet in newly diagnosed celiac disease patients correlates with increased bone mass, which is linked to elevated indicators of osteosynthetic activity before the GFD commences, indicating a period during which bone mineral metabolism in CD may be reversible (GINO ROBERTO Corazza et al., 1997). In addition to poor calcium absorption resulting in elevated PTH levels, increased proinflammatory cytokines such as IL-1 beta, IL-2, IL-6, and tumor necrosis factor alpha have been observed in newly diagnosed Crohn's disease, associated with decreased bone mineral density and improving with therapy. These cytokine abnormalities further affect the equilibrium between osteoclastogenesis and osteoblast growth (Taranta et al., 2004).

In terms of microarchitectural study of bone composition, high-resolution peripheral quantitative computed tomography revealed a reduction in trabecular bone volume, density, and thickness in newly diagnosed premenopausal patients with CD when compared to age and sex-matched controls (María Belén Zanchetta et al., 2015). In persons under 65 years of age, the predominant surface accessible for bone remodeling is the trabecular bone (Osterhoff et al., 2016). Osteoporotic bone loss is contingent upon the surface area available for bone remodeling on osseous surfaces. As aging advances, trabeculae become perforated and may entirely vanish, resulting in more active remodeling on the endocortical surface compared to other trabecular surfaces (Seeman & Delmas, 2006). Consequently, while constituting only 20% of skeletal bone mass, trabecular bone, due to its surface area, is accountable for the majority of bone turnover and is the most metabolically active bone compartment in the early stages of osteoporosis (Osterhoff et al., 2016). Zanchetta et al conducted a 1-year and 3-year follow-up research to illustrate the metabolic activity of trabecular bone in 26 and 24 newly diagnosed patients with celiac disease, respectively, after the initiation of a gluten -free diet and vitamin D supplementation. At both follow-up intervals, enhancements were observed in the trabecular bone compartment regarding volume, density, and thickness; nevertheless, these metrics remained substantially inferior compared to healthy controls at the one-year follow-up (María B Zanchetta et al., 2018; María Belén Zanchetta et al., 2017).

Fracture Risk in CD

Research on fracture risk in persons with CD initially yielded inconsistent findings (Jafri et al., 2008; Thomason, West, Logan, Coupland, & Holmes, 2003; West, Logan, Card, Smith, & Hubbard, 2003). In a comparison of people exhibiting classic symptoms of celiac disease to age and sex-matched controls, as well as those with subclinical or silent CD, patients with classical symptoms had a heightened risk of fractures in the peripheral skeleton. In questionnaire-based case-control research with a mean age of 60.2 ± 10.1 years among patients with celiac disease, Thomason et al., revealed a numerically but not statistically significant risk of fracture and low-trauma fracture in this population. A comprehensive registry study from Sweden involving over 13,000 individuals with celiac disease and 65,000 controls revealed an elevated risk of hip fracture (hazard ratio 2.1, 95% CI 1.8-2.4) and any fracture (hazard ratio 1.4, 95% CI 1.3-1.5). Additionally, a meta-analysis of nine cross-sectional and case-control studies indicated an overall pooled odds ratio of 1.92 (95% CI 1.29-2.84) for any fracture risk and a pooled odds ratio of 1.75 (95% CI 0.78-3.89) for hip fractures from four studies. Incorporating only prospective studies, the risk of hip fracture reached statistical significance (pooled odds ratio 1.69, 95% CI 1.1-2.59) (Heikkilä, Pearce, Mäki, & Kaukinen, 2015). A study from Argentina showed that the risk of peripheral skeletal fractures was elevated in individuals with celiac disease compared to control subjects (odds ratio 3.5, 95% CI 1.8-7.2); however, the majority of fractures (80%) occurred before the diagnosis of CD or in those non-compliant with a gluten-free diet. Similarly, although there is no definitive evidence supporting routine endoscopy to biopsy the small intestinal mucosa during CD follow-up, the presence of persistent villous atrophy in duodenal biopsies taken 6 months to 5 years after CD diagnosis was associated with an increased risk of hip fracture in a large study involving over 7,000 individuals with paired biopsy samples (Lebwohl, Michaëlsson, Green, & Ludvigsson, 2014).

Skeletal Disease in CD

Patients with celiac disease, when compared to age and sex-matched controls, have reduced bone mineral density, which correlates with elevated Fracture Risk Assessment Tool (FRAX) scores in male patients, indicating a higher risk of osteoporotic fractures (Kamycheva, Goto, & Camargo, 2017). Among newly diagnosed patients with Crohn's disease, 43%-63% exhibit osteopenia, whereas 12%-21% present with osteoporosis (Chakravarthi et al., 2012; T Kemppainen, Kröger, Janatuinen, Arnala, Kosma, et al., 1999; Walker et al., 2020). Among adult patients, 26% to 50% will subsequently develop osteoporosis (McFarlane, Bhalla, Reeves, Morgan, & Robertson, 1995; Meyer, Stavropolous, Diamond, Shane, & Green, 2001). In comparison to people exhibiting a typical illness presentation, patients with subclinical celiac disease exhibit a greater bone mineral density, but still lower than that of healthy controls (Corazza et al., 1996). Decreased bone mineral density is associated with an earlier illness start, Marsh grading of duodenal histology, and elevated anti-tTG levels, along with traditional osteoporosis risk factors such as menopausal status, low body mass index, insufficient blood vitamin D, and inadequate dietary calcium consumption (T Kemppainen, Kröger, Janatuinen, Arnala, Kosma, et al., 1999; McFarlane et al., 1995). Osteoporosis is more prevalent in males than in females, with variations in the sites of bone mineral density evaluation, since males have a higher incidence of distal forearm osteoporosis (17.6% vs 8.8%, $p < 0.001$) (Walker et al., 2020).

Screening for CD in Osteoporosis

Although screening for celiac disease (CD) is advised in some high-risk populations, including children with type I diabetes mellitus and those with first- or second-degree relatives diagnosed with CD, the practice of screening for CD in patients presenting with osteoporosis is still contentious. While celiac disease is acknowledged as a secondary cause of osteoporosis, the American Association of Clinical Endocrinologists recommends screening just in the presence of clinical or biochemical indicators of malabsorption. A study involving 978 unselected referral patients undergoing dual energy X-ray absorption, all of whom underwent serologic testing for celiac disease with confirmatory endoscopy if positive, revealed a prevalence of CD of 0.7% in individuals with normal bone mineral density, 1.4% in those with osteopenia, and 2.1% in those with osteoporosis ($p = 0.25$ compared to normal BMD), indicating no justification for universal screening for CD in osteoporosis. Moreover, all people with celiac disease had secondary illness symptoms, including anemia, bloating, or alternating bowel patterns (Sanders et al., 2005). A study involving 100 consecutive patients referred to an endocrinology practice for low bone mineral density underwent serologic testing using the highly specific anti-EMA, revealing a prevalence of 7.3% (7 of 96 patients); however, subsequent duodenal biopsies were nondiagnostic for celiac disease (Mather, Meddings, Beck, Scott, & Hanley, 2001), which is now classified as potential CD (Rubio-Tapia et al., 2013). patients exhibiting a positive anti-EMA did not demonstrate enhanced intestinal permeability or elevated urine N-telopeptide indicative of heightened bone resorption, so reinforcing the notion that screening for celiac disease in patients with low bone mineral density offers no advantage (Mather et al., 2001). Supplementary case-finding investigations of postmenopausal women with poor bone mineral density have revealed prevalence rates of celiac disease in osteoporosis as low as 0.5% (Kavuncu, Dundar, Ciftci, Evcik, & Yigit, 2009). A new meta-analysis indicates a 1.6% prevalence of biopsy -confirmed celiac disease in osteoporosis, consistent with the findings of its low incidence in this condition. A modeling study regarding population screening for celiac disease in adolescents found no cost savings or quality-adjusted life year benefits from universal screening compared to screening symptomatic individuals for the prevention of hip and vertebral fractures (K. Park et al., 2013). Consequently, based on the existing evidence, universal screening for celiac disease in patients with diagnosed osteoporosis is not advised unless additional clinical indicators of malabsorption are present, such as concurrent vitamin and mineral deficiencies or symptoms including abdominal discomfort, skin rash, or diarrhea.

Screening for Metabolic Bone Disease in CD

Given that celiac disease is a recognized contributor to secondary osteoporosis, it is advisable to test for metabolic bone disease in individuals with celiac disease. Although the American College of Gastroenterology's guidelines do not provide a clear evaluation regarding the timing and effects of screening for bone disease in celiac disease (Rubio-Tapia et al., 2013), both a technical review by the American Gastroenterological Association and recommendations from the British Society of Gastroenterology suggest conducting a bone density assessment after one year on a gluten-free diet (GFD) or one year following the commencement of a GFD in individuals over 55 years of age or those with additional osteoporosis risk factors (Bernstein, Leslie, & Leboff, 2003; Gastroenterology, Lewis, & Scott, 2008; Ludvigsson et al., 2014).

Previous guidelines from the British Society of Gastroenterology regarding osteoporosis in Crohn's disease recommended bone mineral density (BMD) screening at diagnosis; however, some argue that this approach may lack cost-effectiveness due to the generally low fracture risk and the inability to identify all at-risk cases through BMD assessment alone (J Compston, 2003; Scott, Gaywood, & Scott, 2000). According to the British Society of Gastroenterology guidelines, a follow-up bone density assessment may be conducted more than two years after starting a gluten-free diet, particularly for individuals with low BMD on initial screening, those exhibiting persistent villous atrophy, or individuals with inadequate dietary adherence (Ludvigsson et al., 2014).

Management of Bone Disease in CD

The aim of addressing decreased bone density in CD is to decrease the risk of fragility fractures and to fortify the skeleton (JE Compston, McClung, & Leslie). In newly diagnosed patients with celiac disease with evidence of diminished bone mineral density, the commencement of a gluten -free diet leads to substantial enhancements in bone mineral density in over 80% of cases within only one year of follow-up, alongside observable increases in blood parathyroid hormone, bone alkaline phosphatase, and vitamin D levels. Preliminary enhancements in bone mineral density have been shown to be more pronounced in the lumbar spine (trabecular bone), with more significant increases observed in women compared to males and in younger persons prior to treatment. Low baseline blood calcium levels, indicative of heightened malabsorption, predict improvements in bone mineral density on a gluten-free diet (Zylberberg, Lebwohl, RoyChoudhury, Walker, & Green, 2018).

During a median follow-up of 37 months, a mean Z-score enhancement of 1 ± 0.2 was seen in the lumbar spine, corresponding to an annual Z-score increment of 0.3 ± 0.1 (Bai et al., 1997). At the five-year follow-up, 46%-68% of assessed locations by dual energy X-ray absorptiometry remain unchanged or exhibit improvement (T Kemppainen, Kröger, Janatuinen, Arnala, Lamberg-Allardt, et al., 1999). Consequently, in an adult demographic, enhancements, but not normalization, of bone density are anticipated on a gluten -free diet. A study of children with a mean duration of gluten-free diet of 10.7 ± 4.3 years revealed no difference in bone mineral density between persons with celiac disease and healthy controls, indicating that the age at which GFD is initiated is crucial for attaining normal bone density. Addressing the underlying intestinal illness appears to be the logical approach to restore abnormal bone metabolism in people with Crohn's disease (von Tirpitz & Reinshagen, 2003).

In addition to a GFD, it is advisable to consume 800-1500 mg of calcium daily and aim for a blood 25-hydroxyvitamin D level of no less than 50 nmol/L (> 20 ng/mL) (91). Supplementation of calcium and vitamin D in persons who are already sufficient in these nutrients offers minimal or no advantage (JE Compston et al.). A limited trial with 11 individuals with newly diagnosed celiac disease found no improvement in bone mineral density with the supplementation of 1 g/d of calcium and 32,000 IU/wk of vitamin D alongside a gluten -free diet, compared to a control group adhering only to a gluten-free diet. Despite being advised for osteoporosis care, enhanced physical activity did not show additional advantages to a gluten-free diet for bone mineral density at the 2-year and 5-year follow-ups (Passananti et al., 2012).

Antiresorptive therapy, frequently employed in osteoporosis management, may be initiated after the commencement of a gluten -free diet and the normalization of calcium and vitamin D levels; however, the early administration of a bisphosphonate (zoledronic acid) has not been shown to confer additional advantages over a GFD in newly diagnosed celiac disease and may pose risks in individuals with significant malabsorption and hypocalcemia (M. Kumar et al., 2013).

Although bisphosphonates are a cornerstone of treatment for postmenopausal osteoporosis, their effectiveness in addressing osteoporosis associated with Crohn's disease remains uncertain, necessitating extrapolation from relevant studies involving pre-/postmenopausal women, men, and patients with inflammatory bowel disease (Gastroenterology et al., 2008). In studies involving males with osteoporosis, alendronate and zoledronic acid exhibited enhancements in measured bone mineral density and a reduction in vertebral fractures over two years (Boonen et al., 2012; Orwoll et al., 2000). In individuals with Crohn's disease, oral bisphosphonate therapy showed improvements in hip and vertebral BMD over one year (Haderslev, Tjellesen, Sorensen, & Staun, 2000). Likewise, teriparatide, a human recombinant parathyroid hormone, has been investigated in cases of glucocorticoid-induced osteoporosis and in premenopausal women with fragility fractures, showing enhancements in bone mineral density (A. Cohen et al., 2013; Saag et al., 2007).

Although there is no evidence to suggest that persons with celiac disease and osteoporosis would get lesser benefits from pharmacologic therapy compared to those with other etiologies of osteoporosis, formulating recommendations for premenopausal women and men under 55 years of age remains particularly challenging. Therapies may be considered for young people with a T-score < -2.5 or a history of fragility fractures, provided that sufficient emphasis has been placed on lifestyle adjustments, a gluten -free diet, and calcium/vitamin D supplementation. Consequently, we often do not endorse treatment beyond lifestyle adjustments and a gluten-free diet for a duration of two years to facilitate anticipated enhancements in bone mineral density. Future pharmacological therapies are evaluated depending on individual history and ongoing fracture risk.

In conclusion, metabolic bone disease frequently manifests in CD, with most patients exhibiting osteopenia or osteoporosis at the time of diagnosis. Deteriorated bone mineral density is associated with early illness start, increased intestinal damage, postmenopausal condition, reduced body mass index, diminished blood vitamin D levels, and insufficient dietary calcium consumption. Compliance with a gluten-free diet results in enhanced malabsorption and, therefore, an elevation in bone mineral density. Formal evaluation of bone density is advised for CD patients exhibiting supplementary risk factors for metabolic bone disease, with subsequent surveillance intervals according to the patient's age, risk factors, and overall dietary compliance.

Chapter 7

Therapeutic Management of Celiac Disease

Abstract

Currently, the gluten-free diet (GFD) remains the cornerstone of celiac disease treatment. However, many patients continue to experience symptoms or complications despite adherence to GFD. This chapter discusses the limitations of the GFD and explores alternative therapeutic strategies, including pharmacological interventions such as enzyme supplementation, immunomodulation, and potential gluten tolerance therapies. It provides an overview of the evolving treatment landscape, emphasizing the importance of a multi-faceted approach to managing celiac disease beyond diet alone.

Therapeutic Management of CD

Lifelong GFD is currently the only effective treatment for CD. The diet of a person with celiac disease must exclude all foods and dietary supplements that contain gluten and its derivatives because even a tiny amount of gluten (50 mg/d) can be immunogenic. The Food and Agricultural Organization, and the Codex Alimentarius Commission of the World Health Organization both oversee the GFD standards. According to this, GFD shouldn't have prolamines from *Triticum* species like wheat, rye, barley, or oats and shouldn't have more than 20 ppm of gluten (Rajpoot & Makharia, 2013). However, maintaining lifetime GFD is quite difficult. Other characteristics that affect GFD adherence include blandness, low nutritional value, increased cost of GFD meals, and ease of access. Therefore, patient-friendly alternative CD therapy requires focus.

Various studies have shown the intervention of probiotics, prebiotics, synbiotics, postbiotics, viromebiotics, gluten vaccination, gluten tolerance and immunomodulation, tissue transglutaminase inhibitors, HLA-DQ2 or HLA-DQ8 blockers, genetically modified gluten, and glutenase supplement diet could subjugate the onset of CD. These potential treatments for managing CDs are still in development and need more study (Figure 8).

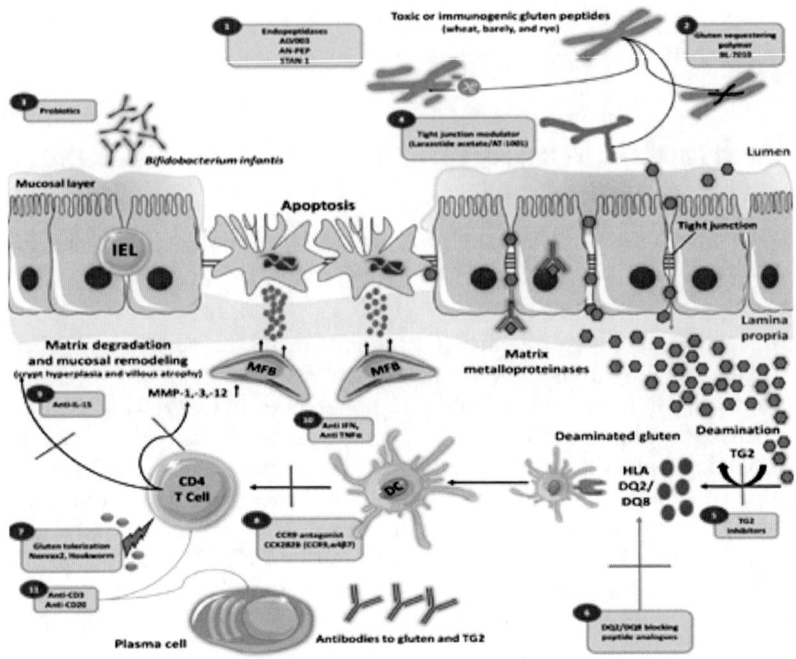

Figure 7. New non-dietary therapies for celiac disease. (1) Endopeptidases: Latiglutenase, STAN-1, and AN-PEP convert gluten into non-immunogenic fragments, reducing mucosal damage. (2) Gluten-sequestering polymer: BL-7010 binds gliadin to prevent breakdown into immunogenic peptides. (3) Probiotics: Bifidobacterium infantis protects epithelial cells by downregulating inflammation. (4) Tight junction modulator: Larazotide acetate inhibits gliadin-induced permeability. (5) TG2 inhibitor: Prevents conversion of gluten into more potent deamidated peptides. (6) DQ2/DQ8 blocking peptides: Block gliadin presentation to T cells. (7) Gluten tolerization: Nexvax2 and hookworm inoculation reduce immune response to gluten. (8) CCR9 antagonist: CCX282B blocks lymphocyte homing. (9) Anti-IL-15: Monoclonal antibody to prevent tissue destruction. (10) Anti-IFN-γ: Prevents inflammation. (11) Anti-CD3 and anti-CD20 antibodies: Suppress gluten-activated T cells and B cells.

Gluten Tolerance and Immunomodulation

Genetic predisposition and environmental factors combine to modify immunological tolerance and inflammation, which results in autoimmune diseases. Tolerance to dietary proteins depends on molecules like CD4, CD25, FOXP3, and Tregs. In CD, inflammatory cytokines including TNF-α, IFN-γ, IL10, and IL15 play a role in modulating immune response by involving both

T cells and Tregs (Hmida et al., 2012). It may be that the best treatment for CD involves preserving a reasonable balance between inflammation and tolerance, which can aid in "reorganizing" the immune system and ameliorating autoimmune illnesses (Veeraraghavan, Leffler, Kaswala, & Mukherjee, 2015).

HLA-DQ2 or HLA-DQ8 Blockers

The adaptive immune response in celiac patients with the HLA-DQ2 and HLA-DQ8 haplotypes is controlled by antigen-presenting cells (APCs). HLA-blocking drugs may be useful for immune activation in such circumstances (Xia et al., 2007; Xia, Siegel, Bergseng, Sollid, & Khosla, 2006). Numerous research teams have created inhibitors for particular HLA-DQ2 haplotypes. A few nonimmunogenic substances that inhibit gluten -mediated immune reactions have also been found. On the basis of structural scanning of a nonpeptide library to choose the most advantageous amino acid change that would increase binding, Juse and coworkers created high-affinity HLA-DQ2 binders (Jüse, van de Wal, Koning, Sollid, & Fleckenstein, 2010). Aldehyde-modified gluten peptide analogs were made using the crystallized HLA-DQ2 structure (Siegel et al., 2006). For HLA-DQ2 ligands and reversible TG2 inhibitors, these personalized peptides exhibit a high affinity and robust binding potential (Siegel & Khosla, 2007). The capacity of modified peptides to enter the lamina propria of the small intestine and to compete with immunogenic gluten peptides, however, are limitations of this therapeutic strategy (Veeraraghavan et al., 2015).

Genetically Modified Gluten

The use of genetically engineered low-gliadin wheat shown encouraging outcomes among the several gluten -targeted treatments (Gil-Humanes, Pistón, Tollefsen, Sollid, & Barro, 2010). Employing ribonucleic acid interference (RNAi) technology to attenuate gliadin expression in hexaploid wheat, Laursen et al., created transgenic lines that did not provoke T-cell responses, demonstrating the feasibility of producing wheat lines suitable for consumption by individuals with celiac disease. The transgenic lines exhibited an average of 7.8% of the poisonous gliadins typically present in wheat (Laursen, 2016).

A significant disadvantage of this method pertains to the rheological and technological characteristics of the flours derived from these down-regulated transgenic lines, as the equilibrium between glutenins and gliadins is essential for the proper development of the gluten network and its viscoelastic properties (Wrigley, Békés, & Bushuk, 2006). When evaluating bread volume, the loaf produced with transgenic line flour is around 30% smaller than that prepared with wild-type flour, and the rice-flour loaf is 57% smaller. The reduction in gliadin protein immunogenicity, while significantly influencing dough rheological characteristics, can nonetheless provide acceptable loaves with sensory attributes akin to those made from conventional wheat (Gil-Humanes et al., 2014). Future research aimed at optimizing the processing conditions of these changed goods may rectify certain existing technical deficiencies.

However, more potential issues emerge. Currently, it is evident that all kinds of gliadin and glutenin proteins might be detrimental to individuals with celiac disease (Camarca et al., 2009; J. A. Tye-Din et al., 2010). This technique fails to consider whether glutenin epitopes are immunostimulatory, necessitating updates to the RNAi constructs when additional hazardous epitopes are identified. Moreover, it has been demonstrated that the elimination of some gliadins and glutenins is frequently offset by the overexpression of the remaining storage proteins (Dumur et al., 2004). The absence of genetic stability over generations of transgenic wheat lines, together with the bureaucratic challenges and uncertainties surrounding genetically modified organisms (GMOs), may impede the acceptance of this method (Laursen, 2016).

A novel method for decreasing the gliadin content in wheat was recently reported (Sánchez-León et al., 2018). Sánchez-León et al., employed CRISPR/Cas9 gene editing technology to target conserved areas close to the coding sequence of the 33-mer inside the α-gliadin genes. Two individual guide RNAs (sgAlpha-1 and sgAlpha-2) were engineered, and mutations were added in particular gliadin genes to inhibit expression. This led to low-gliadin mutant lines exhibiting average decreases of 66.7% and 61.7% in R5 and G12 antibody reactivity, respectively, in sgAlpha-2 generated lines. CRISPR technology offers significant benefits over RNAi in this application, since it facilitates stable and heritable mutations without the need for transgene expression. This technique might provide alternative methods, such as replacing celiac-toxic fragments with non-toxic variants while preserving gluten functioning (Sánchez-León et al., 2018; Y. Zhang et al., 2016).

Additional investigation utilizing T-cell-based assays is necessary to acquire more accurate data regarding the immunostimulatory characteristics of these mutant lines in celiac patients. Despite the appeal of CRISPR gene editing as a method for gluten detoxification, fundamental issues akin to those encountered with RNAi down-regulated lines remain. The technical characteristics of the flours derived from these mutant lines have been examined. Initial findings using SDS sedimentation assessments indicated that more down-regulation of gliadins in edited lines correlated with reduced SDS values of flour, signifying a decline in quality (Sánchez-León et al., 2018). The SDS sedimentation findings were analogous to those reported by Gil-Humanes et al., (Gil-Humanes et al., 2010), and more research is required to thoroughly describe the technical features of these mutant lines. The hazardous epitopes from glutenins, the compensating effects of other gluten proteins, and the potential designation of the resultant wheat lines as GMOs are concerns that must be considered in determining future research routes.

Proteolysis of Immunodominant Peptides

Since the high proline and glutamine concentration of gluten proteins prevent them from being proteolyzed properly, they are only partially degraded by the pancreatic, intestinal, and gastric brush-border membrane proteases. Due to the persistence of large peptides in the intestinal lumen following gluten intake, immunostimulatory epitope survival and negative downstream effects are encouraged (Stepniak et al., 2008). In order to ensure thorough digestion of gluten proteins and lessen or even eliminate immunogenic peptides, proline and/or glutamine-specific proteases have been employed to treat gluten proteins before to ingestion of food (Brzozowski, 2016; Wolf et al., 2015), or even in co-administration with food (Rey et al., 2016; Tack et al., 2013). The drawback of processing wheat flour and gluten prior to consumption is that it causes the wheat dough to lose its original and distinctive viscoelasticity since the proteolysis of gluten will disrupt protein interactions and the creation of the gluten network (Wieser, 2007). Due to pepsin 's ability to break down the proteases that target gluten, the co-administration technique has several drawbacks (Stepniak et al., 2006) and/or chymotrypsin and trypsin when conjugated bile acids are present (Gass, Bethune, Siegel, Spencer, & Khosla, 2007). Fuller answers are needed for a few important concerns, such as how much gluten may be safely ingested by someone with celiac disease using this method and the quantity of gluten-targeted protease that would be required. In order to prevent intestinal injury, the function of these enzymes must be very strong to keep gluten concentrations below 10 mg (Catassi et al., 2007). In order to be effective, this prospective oral medication should ideally be able to operate in an acidic environment because toxic peptides trigger an immune reaction when they enter the duodenum and because the persistence of other proteins may inhibit its proteolytic action. In this context, Wolf et al., recently created a gliadin endopeptidase, Kuma030, supported by molecular modeling and computational design, which demonstrated a remarkable potential to effectively degrade immunogenic peptides obtained from wheat, rye, and barley and thereby limit their ability to stimulate a T-cell reaction. In a model of stomach digestion, this enzyme digested a gluten load that represented the consumption of 4–8 g in about 30 minutes (Wolf et al., 2015). These findings demonstrate the powerful potential of protein engineering in the creation of new enzymes with distinctive and advantageous properties, as well as the enormous promise of these designed proteases as an oral treatment for CD. The beginning of clinical trials is anticipated soon. One of the best-positioned strategies to target gluten is the proteolysis of immunodominant peptides. ALV003 in particular, which combines the prolyl endopeptidase from *Sphingomonas capsulate* with the glutamine endopeptidase from barley, reduced mucosal damage in people with celiac disease in promising clinical studies (Lähdeaho et al., 2014). However, these findings need to be cautiously interpreted. For instance, both the group receiving ALV003 and the group receiving a placebo medicine had some side effects. It should be highlighted that the major goal of this technology is not to permit unrestricted gluten eating, but rather to avoid uncomfortable symptoms and reduce harm to the small intestine from inadvertent gluten ingestion.

Transamidation of Glutamine Residues

Using microbial transglutaminase in the presence of particular amine nucleophiles like L-lysine, L-lysine methyl, or ethyl esters prior to consumption, glutamine residues found in gluten proteins are transamidation to block the immunogenicity of dietary gluten (Brzozowski, 2016; Heredia-Sandoval, Islas-Rubio, Cabrera-Chávez, & de la Barca, 2014). As a result, crucial processes in the pathogenesis of the celiac disease are stopped, including the identification of the glutamine residues and their deamidation via TG2 (Di Sabatino et al., 2012). Bread produced from formerly transamidated wheat flour was used in a randomized single-blind clinical investigation, together with microbial transglutaminase and lysine methyl ester as an amine nucleophile. This study demonstrated that the transamidation process at least partially achieved the goal of detoxifying the immunogenic proteins by lowering the incidence of clinical relapses in individuals with immune challenges. However, not all of the celiac disease patients analyzed had their gluten activity completely eliminated by this detoxification process (Mazzarella et al., 2012). Since it is yet unknown how many glutamine residues require to be changed in order to totally inhibit the immunogenic features of gluten, it may be desirable in this situation to investigate how to boost transamidation activity. The viscoelastic characteristics of the resultant wheat flours can also suffer from reactions utilizing L-lysine or its ester derivatives as amine nucleophiles because the gluten charge density is altered, which might affect the formation of hydrogen bonds between protein strands (Heredia-Sandoval et al., 2014; Ribeiro et al., 2015).

A chemo-enzymatic technology was recently published as a way to improve the transamidation activity while overcoming this detrimental impact on the dough's rheological qualities and ultimate technical value (Ribeiro et al., 2015). Reversed-phase high-performance liquid chromatography (RP-HPLC) was used to evaluate the change in the two-dimensional (2D) electrophoretic profile that occurred when microbial transglutaminase transamidated gluten proteins in the presence of *n*-butylamine under reducing circumstances. As a result, there are fewer immunostimulatory epitopes and improved technical qualities in the resulting wheat dough. Significant improvements have been made using this technique in comparison to the other studied approaches, which leads to the following findings. (I) It is preferable to have higher amine-nucleophile concentrations to prevent gluten protein cross-linking caused by transglutaminase. (II) Reducing circumstances can improve the transamidation reaction. (III) The effect of gluten on the rheological properties must be taken into account when choosing an amine nucleophile (for instance *n*-butylamine enhanced gluten hydrophobicity). Overall, this detoxification method demonstrated a significant improvement in the transamidation process while significantly reducing the cross-linking of gluten proteins. It has a definite favorable effect on the rheological characteristics, increasing the high resistance to extension (Ribeiro et al., 2015). This is crucial since every other detoxifying method that has been described has had a negative impact on the technical quality of wheat. Future research must examine the viability of employing various amine nucleophiles under the most advantageous transamidation conditions as an alternative treatment for celiac disease using pertinent *in vivo* models.

Sequestering of Gliadin Proteins

Sequestering gliadin proteins and stopping their deterioration into immunogenic peptides, hence preventing the detrimental downstream consequences, is another method of lowering gluten toxicity for celiac patients. A non-absorbable polymeric binder called poly (hydroxyethyl methacrylate-co-styrene sulfonate, or poly (HEMA-co-SS), BL-7010, which was formerly known as P(HEMA-co-SS), has demonstrated promising results because it can bind to α-gliadin with a high degree of efficiency in environments with pH levels that are comparable to those in the stomach and duodenum. HCD4/DQ8 and NOD-DQ8 mice have shown that it is effective in reversing the gluten-associated disease in a model of chronic gliadin-sensitization (McCarville et al., 2014; Pinier et al., 2009). The lack of systemic absorption suggests that long-term usage may be safe, and no interactions between BL-7010 and other vitamins or digestive enzymes such as pepsin and pancreatin were found. Phase I/II clinical studies are now being carried out to assess the safety and effectiveness of BL-7010 for celiac disease patients (McCarville et al., 2014). Recently, it was suggested that ascorbyl palmitate and zinc chloride might be utilized as food additives to bind to gliadins and inhibit TG2 action (Engstrom, Saenz-Méndez, Scheers, & Scheers, 2017). Engstrom et al., proved experimentally that ascorbyl palmitate combined with zinc chloride effectively lowered TG2 activity using computational methods including homology modeling and screening of substances for their affinities for a common TG2 binding motif of gliadins. Additional research is required to assess the stability of the ascorbyl palmitate and zinc chloride mixture under gastrointestinal circumstances, as well as its interaction with gluten proteins. It is unclear whether these ligands interfere with the digestion of gluten proteins and the transit of peptides through the lamina propria or function simply at the lamina propria level to inhibit TG2 activity, thus it is important to further research their precise involvement in the pathogenesis of CD. It is unknown how much gluten can be efficiently detoxified *in vivo* by a given amount of polymer or chemical, and the interactions with other gluten proteins, namely glutenins, have to be demonstrated in the sequestering method (Galipeau & Verdu, 2022). The nutritional value of flour that results from the sequestration of gluten proteins should also be the subject of further study, as should the effectiveness of supramolecular assemblies in the development of hypoallergenic flours via clinical trials involving gluten challenges.

Probiotics

Probiotics can enhance the function of the human digestive system through a number of mechanisms, including a) inhibiting pathogen growth by secreting chemicals like organic acids, bacteriocins, and hydrogen peroxide; b) competing with pathogens for nutritive materials; c) obstructing adhesion sites; d) modifying the immune system function; and e) disrupting toxin receptors (Sabahi, Abbasi, & Mortazavi, 2022; Wong & Yu, 2019). Additionally, they have therapeutic benefits on CD patients as well as preventive properties on epithelial cells versus harmful peptides produced from gliadin (Orlando et al., 2018). The most comprehensive *in vitro* and/or *in vivo* investigations on the effectiveness of the *Lactobacillus* and *Bifidobacterium* genera for the detoxification of gliadin-derived peptides (GDPs) have been conducted in this field. The right strains must be employed to detoxify hazardous peptides as the suppressive impact of these two genera is greatly reliant on the used strains.

Only a small number of strains, nevertheless, have a potent suppressive impact on GDPs. It is important to highlight that probiotics like *Lactobacillus* and *Bifidobacterium* can enhance the nonspecific cellular immune response by activating natural killer (NK) cells, macrophages, and T lymphocytes that are specific for antigens. As a result of probiotic type (e.g., strain, being Gram-positive or Gram-negative), concentration, and other factors, probiotics can also control the release of a variety of cytokines. Probiotics consumed through fermented foods may strengthen the gastrointestinal tract (GIT) mucosal immune response via increasing the number of IgA^+ and cytokine-producing cells in a particular section of the gut (Abbasi, Aghebati-Maleki, Yousefi, & Aghebati-Maleki, 2021; Ashraf & Shah, 2014; Nassiri, 2022). According to Haza et al., *L. salivarius* HA8 promoted the generation of proinflammatory cytokines TNF-α, IL-8, and IL-1β whether lipopolysaccharides (LPS) were present or not (Haza, Zabala, Arranz, & Morales, 2005). The best probiotic strains for treating CD patients and associated symptoms are covered in the following section.

Lactobacillus Species

The probiotic bacterial genus *Lactobacillus* is a member of the lactic acid bacteria (LAB) family. Gram-positive, facultative anaerobes or micro-aerophiles, nonsporulating *Lactobacillus* species can colonize the intestinal mucus layer and attach to it while secreting antimicrobial compounds such as organic acids and bacteriocins. Additionally, it was noted that some

Lactobacillus strains that were isolated from dairy products, such as *L. casei* ATCC 393, *L. paracasei* 34, and ATCC 27092, had some desirable traits, including high consistency versus bile and low pH, generation of H_2O_2, growth-inhibition of pathogenic organisms, and ability to adhere to the intestinal epithelium. The three strains indicated lacked drawbacks such as mucin breakdown and antibiotic resistance (Monteagudo-Mera et al., 2012). They are suitable for the human digestive system because of their intrinsic resilience to bile, acid, and restraint enzymes. *Lacticaseibacillus paracasei, L. casei, L. rhamnosus, L. brevis*, and *L. alimentarius* were among the *Lactobacillus* species that efficiently suppressed gliadin and its associated GDPs, according to the literature. In order to evaluate the effectiveness of the strains to detoxify the gluten, *L. alimentarius* and *L. brevis* were widely utilized in bread with various formulations based on wheat (Nazareth et al., 2015), rye (De Angelis, Coda, et al., 2006), and a mixture of buckwheat, millet, wheat, and oat flours. Di Cagno et al., showed that sourdough fermentation for 24 h by *L. alimentarius* 15M or *L. brevis* 14G could totally suppress peptide tryptic digest (PTG) of gliadin at the dosage of 0.875 g/L (the cell counts of probiotics nearly reached 10^9 CFU/g). They discovered that K 562 (S) cells, which are susceptible to gliadin and GDPs, could be totally agglutinated by PTG at a minimal concentration of 0.218 g/L. As a result, the latter probiotics' inoculation greatly enhanced the resistance against PTG (R. Di Cagno et al., 2004). Four probiotic strains—*L. hilgardii* 51B, *L. sanfranciscensis* 7A, *L. brevis* 14G, and *L. alimentarius* 15M—were examined by De Angelis et al., for their impact on rye flour's gliadin. They discovered that 0.52 g/L PTG was sufficient to totally agglutinate K 562 (S) cells, but that pre-incubation with these strains for a day at a concentration of 10^9 CFU/g (of each probiotic strain) at 37 °C may raise the required minimum concentration of PTG to 4.66 g/L (De Angelis, Coda, et al., 2006). Using *L. alimentarius* 15M, *L. hilgardii* 51B, *L. sanfranciscensis* 7A, and *L. brevis* 14G as fermentation species, Di Cagno, et al., proposed a gliadin-reduced sour dough formulation made from wheat (30%), oat (10%), millet (40%) and buckwheat (20%) flours. They discovered that the 24-hour fermentation completely damaged the structure of the wheat flour dough, therefore additional flours were added to the recipe to create the proper bread. After that, CD patients were given the bread to test how well it worked in contrast to bread produced with baker's yeast fermentation. When baker's yeast fermented bread was given to 13 CD patients, it changed their intestinal permeability, however, when sourdough fermented bread was ingested, it nearly did not change it at all (R. Di Cagno et al., 2002). The production process was relatively time-consuming, despite the fact that their innovative formulation demonstrated its effectiveness. In a different study, Greco et al., examined the symptoms of CD patients for a period of 60 days after consuming baked products (200 g/day), such as cakes and biscuits. The differences in formulations were caused by the types of wheat flour that were utilized, and they were grouped as follows: 1) natural wheat flour (contains about 80127 ppm gluten); 2) wheat flour fermented for 48 hours with a combination of three different types of *lactobacilli* (*L. hilgardii* 51B, *L. sanfranciscensis* 7A, *L. brevis* 14G, and *L. alimentarius* 15M) at a concentration of 5×10^8 CFU/g (contains about 2480 ppm gluten); and 3) formula 2 with 200 ppm of fungus proteases. Two of the six individuals who took the initial formulation were unable to complete the challenge because of discomforting symptoms including diarrhea and lethargy. Patients who took formulations 2 and 3 did not exhibit any symptoms, however, those who took formulation 2 after 60 days had subtotal atrophy and an increase in CD3 and γ-Δ intraepithelial cells (Greco et al., 2011).

The noteworthy GIT protective properties of *L. rhamnosus* include protection against cytokine-mediated gastrointestinal illnesses, antibiotic-associated diarrhea, and Crohn's disease recurrence (Yeo et al., 2020). Studies conducted *in vitro* (on Caco-2 cells) and *in vivo* (on Wistar rats) have shown that *L. rhamnosus* GG has both therapeutic and protective effects on CD patients (Orlando et al., 2018; Orlando, Linsalata, D'Attoma, & Russo, 2017). The intestinal barrier permeability brought on by PTG was reduced by *L. rhamnosus* GG, and changes in paracellular permeability were prevented. Additionally, Orlando et al., described how *L. rhamnosus* GG improved PTG-treated rats with damaged small intestinal villi. Additionally, it was claimed that administering PTG before *L. rhamnosus* GG was less effective than administering the probiotic concurrently with PTG (Orlando et al., 2018). Additionally, there is a connection between *L. rhamnosus* GG's capacity to maintain paracellular permeability and the existence of cellular polyamines such as spermidine, spermine, and putrescine (Orlando, Linsalata, Notarnicola, Tutino, & Russo, 2014). In cereal, pseudo-cereal, and leguminous substances, Kockova and Valik assessed the metabolic and growth characteristics of *L. rhamnosus* GG. At the end of the fermentation, the ultimate viable cell population of *L. rhamnosus* GG may reach 10^7 to 10^8 CFU/g on all substrates. The sensory evaluation revealed a substantial difference between freshly fermented items and those that had been stored due to the probiotic strain's metabolic activity throughout storage; the freshly fermented products exhibited more pleasing sensory qualities than the stored items (R D'arienzo et al., 2011; Kockova & Valík, 2014). D'Arienzo et al., examined the immunomodulatory effects of *L. casei* in mice with enteropathy brought on by gliadin. The cytokine pattern of the intestine, CD25+ cell density, weight loss, and the morphometry of the gut mucosa were all measured to confirm the effectiveness of *L. casei* ATCC 9595 inoculation for modifying the immune system of mice. In contrast to indomethacin (Indo) solely treated mice, it was shown that co-administration of gliadin and L. casei delayed the weight loss of mice by 5 days, and the morphometry was mostly unaltered in the probiotic-treated sample when compared to the normal gut mucosa. The mesenteric lymph node cells' release of cytokines was examined to evaluate changes in the intestine's immune response. In contrast to indo-treated mice, the level of TNF-α, IFN-γ, IL-10, and IL-4 remained consistent in the *L. casei* ATCC 9595 treated mice as compared to the control sample. However, compared to the control sample, the TNF-α level was lower in the mice treated with *L. casei* ATCC 9595. In samples treated with *L. casei* ATCC 9595, the density of CD25+ cells increased (R D'arienzo et al., 2011). According to D'Arienzo et al., *L. casei* could effectively prevent mice's mucosal injury. It is important to note that *L. casei* can grow an enlarged mucosal epithelium. By preventing gliadin from entering the epithelial cell, some probiotics can reduce the severity of enteropathy brought on by gliadin. P31-43 and P57-68, two undigested A-gliadin peptides that are important for the pathophysiology of celiac disease, may be successfully prevented from entering intestinal cells to a significant degree by *L. paracasei* CBA L74 (Rossana D'Arienzo, Maurano, Lavermicocca, Ricca, & Rossi, 2009; Rossana D'Arienzo et al., 2008). Additionally, it was shown that *L. paracasei* living cells and filtered supernatant both had the same impact on the inhibition of P31-43 and P57-68, indicating that the substance that caused the peptides' entry suppression originated from cell supernatant (Sarno et al., 2014).

Bifidobacterium Species

One of the most popular probiotics found in food goods, *Bifidobacteria*, has a number of health-improving benefits on the gastrointestinal system, including boosting the immune system and defending against pathogenic germs (Finamore et al., 2019). They are obligately anaerobic, Gram-positive, non-spore-forming bacilli. *Bifidobacterium* strains can attach to the mucous membrane of the intestine and establish colonies in order to maintain the hemostasis status of the body (Bhaskar, Sistla, & Kumaravel, 2017). Two species, *Bifidobacterium lacti0s* and *B. longum*, play a key part in the detoxification of gliadin.

The effects of administering PTG or PTG with B. lactis (10^5, 10^6, and 10^7 CFU/g) on Caco-2 cells were investigated by Lindfors et al., (Lindfors et al., 2008). They assessed three indicators, such as transepithelial resistance, which demonstrates epithelial permeability, membrane ruffle development, and tight junction (TJ) protein ZO-1 (zonula occludens-1) expression, in order to assess the effectiveness of *B. lactis*. The findings indicated that the effectiveness of gliadin detoxification was dose-dependent, and at the maximum concentration of *B. lactis* (10^7 CFU/g), epithelial cells' transepithelial resistance was comparable to control samples after 24 hours, in contrast to the PTG-administered sample. In comparison to PTG administration alone, which was similar to the control sample (11.3% for a sample to which nothing was added and 23.2% for a sample to which bovine serum albumin was added), co-administration of *B. lactis* and PTG to Caco-2 cells also diminished the generation of membrane ruffle from 51.5% to 25.7%. The TJs also seemed more conserved in the co-given sample than in the gliadin-only administered sample. These outcomes could be attributed to *B. lactis*' strong proteolytic activity, which degraded gliadin into safe amino acids and peptides. By assessing the mRNA expression of nuclear factor kappa-B (NF-κB), chemokine CXCR3 receptor, and TNF-α, Laparra and Sanz investigated the inhibiting effect of *B. longum* IATA-ES1 on the inflammatory response generated by digestions of gliadin peptide (0.25 mg protein/mL). Additionally, Caco-2 cells were shown to be producing pro-inflammatory markers such as TNF-α, IL-1, and NF-κB p50. They noticed that the gliadin sample inoculated with *B. longum* dramatically lowered the mRNA expression of CXCR3, NF-κB, and TNF-α. Additionally, compared to cells exposed to gliadin, *B. longum* inoculated Caco-2 cells produced fewer pro-inflammatory markers (Laparra & Sanz, 2010). In a rat enteropathy caused by gliadin, *B. longum* CECT 7347 was capable to significantly immunomodulate the immune system's reactions (Laparra, Olivares, Gallina, & Sanz, 2012).

Probiotics' Mechanisms for Reducing Gliadin Toxicity

Probiotics can reduce the toxicity of gliadin in various ways. Potential pathways for gliadin toxicity suppression include: I) the enzymatic breakdown of harmful peptides produced from gliadin, II) controlling intestinal permeability by regulating zonulin proliferation and tight junction (TJ) expression, III) enhancing the mucosal epithelium, IV) increasing the expression of cyclooxygenase (Cox)-1 in Caco-2 cells while simultaneously decreasing the expression of Cox-2, V) preventing the entry of toxic peptides into enterocytes, and VI) modulating the immune system through the expression of anti-inflammatory and pro-inflammatory cytokines (Orlando et al., 2014; Oscarsson, Håkansson, Andrén Aronsson, Molin, & Agardh, 2021). Although these strategies have been proposed and considered in several studies, there have been relatively few efforts in this area.

Due to the presence of several enzymes in their bacterium's cell wall and cytoplasm, practically all species of the *Lactobacillus* and *Bifidobacterium* genera were capable of gliadin and PTG enzymatic hydrolysis. Different probiotic species, however, differ in terms of the rate, kind, and variety of enzyme secretion. For example, *L. alimentarius* 15M and *L. brevis* 14G hydrolyzed PTG with a notable advantage over *L. hilgardii* 51B, and *L. sanfranciscensis* 7A (R. Di Cagno et al., 2002). Additionally, in a PTG culture inoculated with probiotics, a direct association between the kinds and quantities of free amino acids that were produced and the variety and activity of cell wall- and cytoplasmic enzymes was found. The presence of high proline levels in some gliadin components, such as the 31-43 and 62-75 segments of A-gliadin and the 33-mer peptide, makes them hazardous for CD patients. These components are resistant to the stomach and pancreatic enzymes (De Angelis, Rizzello, et al., 2006; R. Di Cagno et al., 2004). Therefore, the concentration of proline would noticeably increase in the detoxified PTG-probiotic suspension and may be utilized as a marker for gliadin suppression. Some probiotic strains, such as *L. rhamnosus* GG, have this capacity to offset damages brought on by gliadin through upregulating ZO-1 expression. TJs and adherent junctions (AJs) join intestinal epithelial cells and create a layer with selective permeability, both of which play a crucial role in maintaining the integrity of epithelial cells (Ciccocioppo et al., 2006). As a result, *L. rhamnosus* GG can control the expression of certain TJ proteins and prevent CD patients' ingestion of gluten from altering their intestinal permeability (Orlando et al., 2014).

Some probiotic strains, such as *B. lactis*, were able to hasten the release of mucus by intestinal enterocyte cells, leading to the establishment of mucosal epithelium enhancement and the formation of substantial membrane ruffles. This would prevent PTG from entering intestinal cells since the mucosal barrier on the surface of enterocytes would prevent it (Lindfors et al., 2008). Rats' CD4+ T cells would decrease and their CD4+/Foxp3+ T cells would rise when gliadin was added to their diet. However, the impact of gliadin was reversed when *B. longum* CECT 7347 was also administered. This might be because of a particular immunological activation brought on by the inclusion of *B. longum* CECT 7347 (Olivares, Laparra, & Sanz, 2012). As a result, the latter probiotic might successfully modify immunological reactions.

The Cox enzymes play a crucial part in preserving the health of the GIT. The production of "housekeeping" prostaglandins, which are essential for maintaining normal mucosal cohesiveness and controlling inflammation, is carried out by the two types of Cox enzymes, Cox-1 and Cox-2. On one extreme, the Cox-1 enzyme is in charge of preserving renal and gastrointestinal health. On the other hand, Cox-2 expression has the potential to cause inflammation. By enhancing the expression of the Cox-1 gene, *L. casei* ATCC 9595 may reduce the damage caused by gluten consumption to the intestinal villi of CD patients. Additionally, *L. casei* ATCC 9595 was shown to inhibit Cox-2, thereby reducing intestinal inflammation (R D'arienzo et al., 2011). Certain probiotics, such as *L. paracasei* CBA L74, prevent the entry of harmful peptides into enterocytes, thus decreasing the toxicity of gliadin and its associated PTG. The healing of the enterocytes' mucosal layer, along with the strengthening effect of probiotic bacteria on tight junctions (TJs) and adherens junctions (AJs), may contribute to the potential mechanism of this function. In other words, *L. paracasei* CBA L74 performs its function by restoring and assisting the enterocyte layer's barrier function (Sarno et al., 2014).

Overall, administering appropriate and effective probiotics to wheat-based goods (particularly in combination composition) would offer a potential celiac-therapy strategy, at least for reducing the manifestations of celiac disease. The mechanisms of probiotics should also be revealed by more clinical trials. It's also crucial to ascertain whether probiotics can reduce all celiac symptoms and keep working in cereal probiotic items even over extended periods of time at high storage temperatures. And last, there is a need for celiac disease associations and educational initiatives to tell patients about the advantages of probiotic cereal goods for their health.

Prebiotics

Prebiotics are food elements that are inedible but are chosen by the intestinal flora of the host (Ozma, Abbasi, et al., 2022). They are a major and contested factor in human health because they affect the growth and activity of a small number of beneficial bacteria, such as *Bifidobacterium* spp., *Anaerostipes* spp., *F. prausnitzii*, *Lactobacillus* spp., *Bilophila* spp. (Abbasi, Saadat, & Saadat, 2022; Karimi et al., 2020). The characteristics of a prebiotic energy source are as follows: I) the ability to ferment by gut microbiota; II) the ability to survive under the effect of gastric acidity and hydrolyzing enzymes in mammals; and III) the capacity to specifically reinforce the growth and activity of healthy bacteria for human health (Sarteshnizi, Hosseini, Bondarianzadeh, & Colmenero, 2015; Sarteshnizi et al., 2017). Inulin, galactooligosaccharides, and fructooligosaccharides are the most prevalent prebiotics (Haghshenas et al., 2014; Hurtado-Romero, Del Toro-Barbosa, Garcia-Amezquita, & García-Cayuela, 2020). Prebiotics' capacity to regulate the action of gut microbiota, i.e., promote the development and function of bacterial strains important for intestinal health, particularly *Lactobacillus* and *Bifidobacteria*, can be used to explain how CD symptoms and morphological damage can be improved. Therefore, a GFD including prebiotics is a simple and affordable adjuvant therapy among the emerging CD therapies. There have been few human studies looking at how prebiotics affect intestinal inflammation, particularly CD, and those that have been done frequently included probiotic formulations together with other drugs (Marasco et al., 2020). One of the initial investigations by Drabiska et al., on the effect of oligofructose-enriched inulin (Synergy 1) on the intestinal microbiota of individuals with CD on a GFD indicated that this substance produces a noticeable rise in *Bifidobacterium* and boosts SCFA concentrations, such as fecal acetate and butyrate, in the intestinal microbiota's metabolic process (Drabińska, Jarocka-Cyrta, Markiewicz, & Krupa-Kozak, 2018). Prebiotics are essential for the absorption of vitamins and minerals, which is an important issue of CD study. However, it is evident that vitamin D insufficiency and its clinical implications are more severe in adult CD patients given that there is evidence connecting vitamin D deficiency to an elevated risk of autoimmune diseases and that vitamin D levels diminish with age. According to research on the effects of oligofructose-enriched inulin on the number of fat-soluble vitamins and minerals in celiac children after a GFD, vitamin D and E serum levels increased but vitamin A concentrations remained the same in celiac kids taking prebiotics (Drabińska et al., 2018).

One of the most significant yet underutilized CD markers is amino acids. Under a prolonged GFD, the concentrations of essential amino acids in the biological fluids of CD patients may decline. They are essential for immune system function, maintaining the integrity of the intestinal barrier, and producing mucin and epithelial cells. For instance, amino acids are important building blocks for the creation of glutathione, a crucial mediator and antioxidant with anti-injury characteristics for epithelial cells. Prebiotics are crucial components with a reputation for assisting in the treatment of nutritional shortages. They are efficient in reducing CD signs and even the psychological harm that tryptophan and serotonin produce (Drabińska et al., 2018; Drabińska, Jarocka-Cyrta, Ratcliffe, & Krupa-Kozak, 2019).

Synbiotics

Prebiotics and probiotics work together synergistically to speed up the probiotic process in the large intestine. For this reason, the term "symbiotic" was created to describe a product in which the primary purpose of the prebiotic is to foster the development of the targeted probiotic (Homayouni Rad, Aghebati Maleki, Samadi Kafil, & Abbasi, 2021; H. Li et al., 2022). For instance, a synbiotic for people with ulcerative colitis was created as a result of research by Furrie et al., It mixed a probiotic, the *B. longum* from healthy rectal epithelium, with the prebiotic "Orafti®-Synergy1" to ensure optimum compliance and the development of symptoms in the severe phase (a preferential inulin-oligofructose growth substrate for the probiotic strain) (Furrie et al., 2005). Furthermore, a study by Adebola et al., investigated how three potential prebiotics, lactobionic acid, lactulose, and inulin may support the growth of five probiotic lactobacilli cultures while also protecting them against bile acid stress. Only *L. reuteri* NCIMB 11951, and *L. acidophilus* NCFM utilized lactulose out of the five probiotics investigated. Both *L. reuteri* NCIMB 1195, and *L. acidophilus* NCFM were capable of growing in synbiotic mixes containing lactulose (1%) or lactobionic acid and 2 mM cholic and taurocholic acid. A similar variation was found in the probiotics' resistance to bile acid stress (1%), which was influenced by prebiotics (Adebola, Corcoran, & Morgan, 2014). The combined benefits of probiotics and prebiotics inside the unique CD environment haven't been studied, though.

Postbiotics

Postbiotics are defined as deactivated microbial cellular components, cell fragments, and/or cell metabolites that are largely generated by fermentation in living probiotic cells (Abbasi, Rad, Maleki, Kafil, & Baghbanzadeh, 2023). Additionally, postbiotics are produced via laboratory procedures in pure form or as a response to environmental factors, and when consumed in sufficient quantities, they provide the host with a multitude of biological health benefits (Sabahi, Homayouni Rad, et al., 2022). Postbiotics provide benefits such as improved safety and stability. In the first scenario, the inactivity of the microbial cells may be attributed to their pathophysiology, and high levels of immunity can be associated with a lower risk of microbial transmission or infection as well as a milder inflammatory reaction in immunocompromised individuals (unbalanced or weak immunity) (Conte et al., 2021). According to research by Conte et al., *L. paracasei* CBA L74 postbiotic inhibited the synthesis of P31-43 and the function of gliadin in CD. The activation of the autophagy pathway, which requires the phosphorylation (virtual inactivation) of the mTOR, is required for maintaining cellular homeostasis, and the study found that *L. paracasei* postbiotic is capable of inhibiting this pathway's activation in Caco-2 cells (Conte et al., 2021). Postbiotics produced by *Bifidobacteria* spp. have lately been studied, which is an uncommon subject. Heat has an impact on the whole cell of the probiotic strain *B. longum* CECT-7347, resulting in the formation of a new postbiotic that is not viable. By triggering the innate immune system's processes, reducing the initial inflammatory response, and improving intestinal barrier integrity, this postbiotic prevents the colonization of pathogens. The findings also suggest HT-CECT-7347, a *Bifidobacterium longum* heat-treated strain, as a possible protection versus oxidative stress damage (Martorell et al., 2021). By lowering their regulation and boosting mucin expression while keeping its probiotic capacity, HM0539 postbiotic is efficient in preventing the gut from damage brought on by LPS and TNF-α (damage that results in reduced expression of cellular tight junction protein and mucus) (J. Gao et al., 2019). The core ideas in CD are the entry of immunogenic molecules into enterocytes and the stimulation of innate and specific immune pathways. Sarno and colleagues observed that the postbiotic impact of LP CBA L74 was similar in this manner in this case because postbiotic *L. paracasei* CBA L74 blocks the entrance of undigested peptides P31-43 and P57-68 into Caco-2 cells, which has a strong postbiotic influence on the pathogenesis of CD (Sarno et al., 2014). There are currently limited data on postbiotics' role in CD, and the findings of *in vitro* research are insufficient to make any judgments on the postbiotics' biological effects.

Viromebiotics

The human microbiome and the role of the corresponding dysbiota in particular chronic human illnesses have been extensively studied in the literature. An intriguing new field of study focuses on the function of the virome, a population of viruses found in the gastrointestinal system, in both health and sickness (Cao et al., 2022). There is very little understood about the ecology of intestinal viruses. Nevertheless, the ratio of intestinal viruses to bacteria is 10:1 (Mills et al., 2013). Without the gut phageome (a collection of bacteriophages), the microbiome cannot sustain a homeostatic balance.

The variety of gut bacteria varies during the human life cycle. The phage load declines as people age, while microbial community diversity and complexity rise substantially. The virome communities appear to suffer when gut bacterial diversity and composition increase (Vitetta, Vitetta, & Hall, 2018). It is not surprising that metagenomic investigation of children with CD revealed a statistically meaningful viral dysbiosis because viral dysbiosis in IBD has been documented in people. In this regard, it was recently discovered that viral dysbiosis occurred in kids who had just received a CD diagnosis prior to beginning the GFD (El Mouzan et al., 2022). The influence of the GFD on the characteristics of the gut virome is demonstrated by the fact that the lower initial variety of the human gut virome results in a more prominent impact of the GFD on its structure (Garmaeva et al., 2021). Clinical trials are being conducted on phages to demonstrate their safety, tolerability, and effectiveness as potential novel prebiotics. Phages did not significantly alter the microbiome in the short 28-day intervention. However, as more people from the butyrate-producing genera were present as a result of the intervention, certain populations changed. The authors came to the conclusion that bacteriophages might selectively kill off specific species without disrupting the whole gut microbiome (Febvre et al., 2019).

Phage treatment has been proposed as a potential new approach to treating CD in this direction. They might have a role in changing the luminal gluten load or the transglutaminase activity by choosing microorganisms that can digest gluten or lack the ability to produce glutenase. Different possible approaches have been outlined by Lerner et al., (Lerner, Ramesh, & Matthias, 2019). Studies using functional analysis to understand the interaction between bacteriophages and bacteria and the function of viruses in CD may result in the creation of new therapeutic alternatives. This route is being taken by a sponsored proof of concept research that aims to modify human gut microorganisms to treat gluten-related illnesses. The project's goals include creating bacteriophages with *Bifidobacterium* targets that can infect *B. longum* and produce a gluten-degrading enzyme from *Sphingomonas capsulata*, as well as introducing the glutenase-expressing phage into a *B. longum* within an *in-vitro* biofilm system (Wagh, Lammers, Padul, Rodriguez-Herrera, & Dodero, 2022). The technology readiness levels (TRLs) are a nine-stage system that has been proven to be effective in estimating technological maturity (Héder, 2017). Currently, the initial stage of the utilization of viruses for medical approaches in gastroenterology is being observed. Although the use of viruses in CD treatment in actual clinical settings is still relatively far off, it is nevertheless important to keep an eye on current developments and possible "viromebiotics" as they develop.

Polyphenols' Role in CD

Given that the gastrointestinal tract is the region where polyphenol concentrations may reach their peak and that Crohn's disease primarily impacts the small intestinal mucosa, polyphenols could represent a promising, safe, and natural approach to modulating essential regulatory pathways related to Crohn's disease. These encompass the digestion and bioavailability of gluten peptides at the intestinal level, oxidative stress and inflammation, the compromise of intestinal epithelial barrier integrity and function, dysbiosis of the intestinal microbiome, and an aberrant adaptive immune response to gluten. The subsequent sections will comprehensively examine these five aspects; however, it is crucial to emphasize that only a superficial understanding currently exists, necessitating further research to fully elucidate the molecular and cellular mechanisms underlying the therapeutic and colorectal cancer-preventive properties of dietary polyphenols.

Polyphenols' Impact on the Digestibility and Availability of Gluten Peptides

It is becoming evident that polyphenols exhibit several potential bioactivities in the human body, some of which are contingent upon their interactions with other macromolecules such as proteins, carbohydrates, and lipids (Jakobek, 2015). These interactions significantly influence the bioaccessibility, bioavailability, and biological effects of polyphenols (Dias, Oliveira, Fernandes, Simal-Gandara, & Perez-Gregorio, 2021). Conversely, by binding to proteins, particularly those rich in proline, polyphenols may hinder the availability of specific amino acids and impede the activity of digestive enzymes, thereby influencing the functionality, digestibility, and nutritional value of proteins (Cirkovic Velickovic & Stanic-Vucinic, 2018; de Freitas & Mateus, 2012). Van Buiten and colleagues have recently demonstrated, within a CD framework, that green tea catechins can inhibit gliadin digestion *in vitro* by engaging in physical interactions with gliadin proteins and by obstructing the activity of pepsin and trypsin (Van Buiten, Lambert, & Elias, 2018; Van

Buiten, Lambert, Sae-tan, & Elias, 2017). This led to less generation of low molecular weight gliadin peptides and a reduction in gliadin-induced elevations in intestinal permeability and inflammation.

The intraluminal confinement of gluten immunogenic peptides and proteins is being investigated as a potentially unique therapeutic strategy to prevent the onset of celiac disease symptoms and related immune responses, as T cell activation and mucosal inflammation persist only while gluten peptides are present in the intestinal mucosa. In 2017, Perot and colleagues established that polyphenol-rich extracts from artichoke leaves, cranberries, apples, and green tea leaves effectively modulate the immunogenicity and allergenicity of gluten proteins by interacting with gliadins, masking epitopes, and influencing basophil degranulation (Perot et al., 2017). Quercetin and anthocyanins (e.g., malvin and pelargonin) have demonstrated the ability to bind to and structurally alter gliadin proteins, therefore reducing their β-turn content and perhaps diminishing their immunoreactivity (Taddei, Zanna, & Tozzi, 2013; Q. Wang et al., 2020).

Prior studies have demonstrated the capacity of grape seed procyanidins (polymeric flavanols) to interact with gliadin-derived peptides through fluorescence quenching, dynamic light scattering, and mass spectrometry analyses (Dias, Perez-Gregorio, Mateus, & De Freitas, 2016; Dias, Perez-Gregorio, Mateus, & De Freitas, 2015). Nonetheless, the structural and thermodynamic foundations of polyphenol binding to CD-related peptides have remained inadequately elucidated. This subject has been explored exclusively in the last two years by several spectroscopic and in silico methodologies under near-physiological settings (Dias et al., 2018; Dias et al., 2019). Recent studies indicate that the total reactivity of polyphenols towards a 32-amino acid long CD peptide, the physiological version of the renowned 33-mer peptide, may be elucidated by a combination of structural and environmental variables. The binding of polyphenols to the 32-mer peptide mostly happens via an entropy-driven hydrophobic effect and is kinetically influenced by the substitution pattern and polymerization degree of the polyphenol molecules (Dias et al., 2018; Dias et al., 2019). The primary polyphenol-binding sites correspond to domains including leucine, tyrosine, and phenylalanine, situated inside four distinct yet almost identical hydrophobic clusters, evenly separated by non-polar proline residues. In addition to characterizing polyphenol binding to the 32-mer, their capacity to diminish the transepithelial transport of the 32-mer peptide across Caco-2 cell monolayers was also assessed (Dias et al., 2018; Dias et al., 2019). These trials demonstrated the capacity of dietary dosages of EGCG to effectively scavenge the 32-mer peptide under physiological settings, resulting in a significant decrease in the concentration of free peptide in the basolateral compartment. Likewise, substoichiometric quantities of procyanidin B3 and the trimer C2 were demonstrated to diminish the apical-to-basolateral translocation of the 32-mer peptide; however, this reduction did not seem to rely exclusively on their physical interaction but rather on other regulatory pathways that remain unexamined (Dias et al., 2019). The regulatory effects of particular food compositions and their interaction with the gut microbial ecosystem on the digestion and bioavailability of gluten peptides have yet to be elucidated, which would yield valuable insights into the impact of food matrix-polyphenol interactions on the release, transformation, availability, and activity of CD bioactive peptides.

Antioxidant and Anti-Inflammatory Properties of Polyphenols

Initially regarded merely as standard antioxidants, there is now a growing recognition that polyphenols and their metabolites play a significant role in cellular homeostasis by modulating critical signaling transduction pathways and gene transcription events, which are implicated in cell survival and apoptosis, some of which are associated with human diseases (X. Han, Shen, & Lou, 2007; Hae-Suk Kim, Quon, & Kim, 2014; Silva & Pogačnik, 2020; H. Zhang & Tsao, 2016). This encompasses the inhibition of reactive oxygen species generating enzymes, including xanthine oxidase (XO), NADPH oxidase (NOX), and inducible nitric oxide synthase (iNOS), as well as enzymes implicated in arachidonic acid metabolism, such as phospholipase A2 (PLA2), cyclooxygenase (COX), and lipoxygenase (LOX) (Hussain & Tan, 2016). Polyphenols have been demonstrated to modulate the NF-κB and MAPK inflammatory pathways and to upregulate phase II detoxifying and antioxidant enzymes such as heme oxygenase-1 (HO-1), glutathione peroxidase (GSH-Px), glutathione-S-transferase (GST), catalase, and superoxide dismutase (SOD) by targeting the common nuclear factor erythroid 2–related factor 2 (Nrf2). Polyphenols also promote the overexpression of Sirtuin 1 (SIRT1) across various models, thereby aiding in the protection of cells from oxidative stress, inflammation, and mitochondrial dysfunction through the deacetylation of transcription factors and proteins, including NF-κB, forkhead box class O (FOXO) 3, and PPAR-γ coactivator 1α (PGC-1α).

Given that oxidative stress facilitates the majority of cytotoxic effects caused by gluten peptides on intestinal epithelial cells, such as apoptosis, compromised cell proliferation, and disintegration of tight junctions, polyphenols may serve as inducers of the Nrf2 antioxidant system. They could assist in preserving the intestinal nucleophilic balance against the oxidative damage and inflammation induced by gluten proteins by providing cells with antioxidant enzymes and nucleophiles, specifically NADPH, glutathione, and thioredoxin (Qin & Hou, 2016). A recent investigation indicated that pre-treatment of hydrolyzed gliadins with decaffeinated green tea extract led to diminished inflammation (evidenced by lower production of IL-6 and IL-8) and decreased permeability of Caco-2 cell monolayers (Van Buiten et al., 2018).

Modulation of Intestinal Epithelial Barrier Integrity and Function

Like other intestinal disorders, CD is marked by heightened intestinal permeability and the disruption of epithelial tight junctions, resulting in impaired barrier function that facilitates the indiscriminate passage of gluten-derived peptides into the lamina propria, where they trigger an adaptive immune response through gluten-specific T cells (Cardoso-Silva et al., 2019). Individuals with Crohn's disease exhibit a reduced quantity of tight junction protein strands, characterized by an increase in pore-forming claudins such as claudin-2 and claudin-15, alongside a decrease in tightening claudins like claudin-3, claudin-5, and claudin-7. They also demonstrate diminished levels of the phosphorylated cytoplasmic scaffolding protein zonula occludens-1 (ZO-1), extensive phosphorylation of β-catenin, and altered localization and expression of proteins that regulate tight junction assembly, including the polarity complex protein Par-3 and the serine/threonine phosphatase PP-1 (Schumann et al., 2012). In 2005, Sanders and colleagues found that gliadin peptides induced a rearrangement of actin filaments and modified the expression of tight junction proteins occludin, claudin-3, claudin-4, ZO-1, and E-cadherin in differentiated Caco-2 cells (Sander, Cummins, & Powell, 2005). In 2008, it was discovered that certain gliadin peptides can bind to the chemokine receptor CXCR3 on intestinal epithelial cells, resulting in MyD88-dependent zonulin release and subsequent activation of the EGFR via proteinase-activated receptor-2 (PAR2) (Lammers et al., 2008). This compound then triggers an intracellular signaling cascade that leads to PCK-α-dependent breakdown of tight junctions and enhanced permeability (Sturgeon & Fasano, 2016).

Recent years have seen polyphenols get significant study attention for their possible involvement in modulating intestinal barrier integrity and function (Bernardi et al., 2019; G. Yang, Bibi, Du, Suzuki, & Zhu, 2017). The processes behind these biological impacts, however, remain unclear. The primary experimental evidence connecting polyphenols to regulatory mechanisms associated with intestinal permeability mostly derives from *in vitro* investigations, predominantly conducted on Caco-2 cells (Amasheh et al., 2008; Carrasco-Pozo, Morales, & Gotteland, 2013). Polyphenols, including EGCG, quercetin, berberine, theaflavins, resveratrol, anthocyanins, ellagic acid, procyanidins, curcumin, and polyphenol-rich red wine extract, along with certain microbial metabolites such as urolithin A, have demonstrated the capacity to enhance transepithelial electric resistance across cellular monolayers. They also promote the expression and cytoskeletal association of various tight junction proteins, including ZO proteins, occludin, and claudins, facilitate the restoration of ZO-1/occludin assembly, and inhibit several protein kinases, such as PI3K, PKC, MAPKs, and MLCK, which are involved in the phosphorylation of proteins that regulate intestinal permeability (Amasheh et al., 2010; Amasheh et al., 2008; Cremonini et al., 2017; Dryden, Bunch, Connors, Mehta, & Qazzaz, 2017; Iglesias, Cremonini, Fraga, & Oteiza, 2020; Lobo de Sá et al., 2019; Mayangsari & Suzuki, 2018; Nunes, Freitas, Almeida, & Laranjinha, 2019; H. Y. Park, Kunitake, Hirasaki, Tanaka, & Matsui, 2015; Wu et al., 2018). Recent findings indicate that urolithin A enhances intestinal barrier functions and inhibits inflammation by activating the aryl hydrocarbon receptor (AhR)-Nrf2-dependent pathway, which upregulates epithelial tight junction proteins (R. Singh et al., 2019). The results obtained from *in vitro* investigations are often consistent with those from animal experiments. The latter have emphasized the capacity of polyphenols to enhance intestinal permeability by augmenting the expression of tight junction proteins and modulating essential genes implicated in the inflammatory process, such as AMPK (AMP-activated protein kinase), ERK, and NF-κB. The polyphenols examined in these studies encompass berberine, epicatechin, and anthocyanins, in addition to polyphenol-rich extracts derived from raspberry, propolis, grape seeds, green tea, pomegranate, cinnamon bark, grape pomace, blueberry pomace, and loquat fruit, administered at doses ranging from nearly physiological to supraphysiological levels (Cheng et al., 2020; Cremonini et al., 2018; Zhipeng Gao et al., 2020; Gu et al., 2011; L. Li et al., 2014; W. Li et al., 2019; Van Hul et al., 2018; H. Wang et al., 2013; K. Wang et al., 2016; L. Zhang et al., 2020; Zhao et al., 2019). Human intervention studies, though limited, have reinforced the notion that polyphenols modulate intestinal cell function *in vivo* through various direct and indirect effects, including their influence on the gut microbial community and immune system (Bernardi et al., 2019).

Cross-Talk Between Polyphenols and the Gut Microbiota

Numerous pieces of evidence now indicate the essential role of the gut microbial ecosystem in the maturation, development, and functionality of the host immune system, which subsequently influences the microbial community and modulates immune responses to bacterial species on mucosal surfaces (Antonini, Lo Conte, Sorini, & Falcone, 2019). Most existing research on the composition and microbiota in pediatric and adult CD patients are notably varied and conflicting (Valitutti, Cucchiara, & Fasano, 2019). Numerous pre-clinical, cross-sectional, and prospective studies have indicated a correlation between altered microbiota and disease manifestation, pathogenesis, and risk; however, ascertaining whether intestinal dysbiosis is the cause or consequence of Crohn's disease presents a formidable challenge (Cenit, Olivares, Codoñer-Franch, & Sanz, 2015). Research indicates that representatives of Lactobacillus and Bifidobacterium are markedly reduced in active Crohn's disease, whereas Bacteroides, Staphylococcus, and E. coli exhibit considerable overabundance, with some displaying enhanced virulence characteristics. Notably, the host HLA-DQ genotype can independently affect gut microbial composition by selecting early gut colonizers in newborns at familial risk for celiac disease. This study indicates that infants with a high genetic predisposition for celiac disease (HLA-DQ2) exhibit elevated levels of Firmicutes (Clostridium spp) and Proteobacteria (Enterobacteriaceae), alongside diminished levels of Actinobacteria (including the genus Bifidobacterium), compared to those with a low genetic risk (non-HLA-DQ2/8 carriers) (Olivares et al., 2015).

Recent documentation indicates that polyphenol-rich meals can directly influence the composition and activity of gut microbiota (Kawabata, Yoshioka, & Terao, 2019). Once catabolized into bioactive and accessible molecules in the colon, polyphenols contribute to gut health and mitigate inflammation by inhibiting certain pathogenic groups and promoting the development of beneficial bacteria. The exact mechanisms require additional elucidation; however, they seem to rely on the prebiotic characteristics of polyphenols, their antimicrobial effects (either directly or by enhancing bacterial susceptibility to antibiotics), their influence on enzyme modulation, and their inhibition of bacterial quorum sensing (Kumar Singh et al., 2019). Recent studies have shown that the oral administration of wild blueberry procyanidins can restore colonic mucus thickness in mice fed a high-fat, high-sucrose diet by selectively promoting a prebiotic-like effect on the mucin-degrading Akkermansia muciniphila, thereby creating a more favorable ecological niche for mucosa-associated symbiotic bacteria(Rodríguez-Daza et al., 2020). In a separate study, Li and colleagues demonstrated that aging rats administered 20 mg.Kg-1.day-1 of bilberry anthocyanins exhibited a significant increase in the relative abundance of Lactobacillus and Bacteroides, while the proliferation of harmful bacteria (Verrucomicrobia and Euryarchaeota) was suppressed (J. Li et al., 2019). Green tea polyphenols were observed to influence the gut microbial ecosystem and intestinal inflammation in obese dogs by enhancing the bacterial population of Firmicutes while diminishing the relative abundance of Bacteroidetes and Fusobacteria, as well as decreasing the expression of pro-inflammatory cytokines such as TNF-α, IL-6, and IL-1β (Y. Li et al., 2020). Wang and colleagues proved that mice eating 300 mg.kg-1.day-1 of resveratrol exhibited significant alterations in their microbiota composition compared to standardly fed mice, characterized by a notable increase in the relative abundance of Bacteroidetes (primarily Bacteroides) and a reduction in Firmicutes (P. Wang et al., 2020). Interestingly, the transplantation of this bacterial population to mice on a high-fat diet resulted in several advantageous effects, including decreased body weight gain, reduced insulin resistance and inflammation, better lipid metabolism, and enhanced integrity and function of the intestinal barrier. Tea extracts abundant in polyphenols from Camellia sinensis and *Litsea coreana* exhibited a prebiotic-like effect in a mouse model of dextran sulfate sodium (DSS)-induced colitis, enhancing the relative abundance of beneficial bacteria such as Faecalibaculum and Bifidobacterium, and reinstating the generation of short-chain fatty acids (SCFAs), such as butyrate (Y. Liu et al., 2020).

Collectively, our experimental data reinforces the modulatory capacity of polyphenols in influencing gut microbiota composition and function, hence suggesting their potential use in alleviating symptoms or mitigating the risk of Crohn's disease. This subject remains predominantly unexamined and need to be prioritized in the forthcoming years.

Immunomodulatory Role of Polyphenols

Both *in vitro* and *in vivo* research have demonstrated that polyphenols can regulate immunological responses in several aspects (Ding, Jiang, & Fang, 2018). *In vitro* studies utilizing various cell types demonstrated that curcumin (along with other monoketone analogs), quercetin, kaempferol, myricetin, resveratrol, genistein, and EGCG inhibited the expression of several pro-inflammatory cytokines (e.g., IL-12, TNF-α, and IL-6)(Francisco, Costa, Neves, Cruz, & Batista, 2018; H. Khan et al., 2019; Olivera et al., 2012) and the activity of the enzymes COX-2 and iNOS, which are frequently overexpressed in autoimmune disorders(Cuevas, Saavedra, Salazar, &

Abdalla, 2013). Furthermore, in LPS-stimulated murine bone marrow-derived dendritic cells (BMDCs), these polyphenols can diminish the expression of immunomodulatory molecules, including the adhesion and co-stimulatory markers CD40, CD80, CD86, MHC-I, and MHC-II, which are essential for T cell activation (Ding et al., 2018; Francisco et al., 2018).

Mouse models of autoimmune illnesses have demonstrated their use in examining the impact of polyphenols on disease outcomes. In this context, a mouse model of lupus (SNF1 mice) demonstrated that the flavonoid apigenin effectively inhibited many inflammatory pathways, including auto-antigen presentation and the generation of IL-6 and COX-2(Kang, Ecklund, Liu, & Datta, 2009). In another research, apigenin, in conjunction with curcumin and a procyanidin-rich extract, alleviated the clinical manifestations of a murine model of multiple sclerosis (MS) by eliciting several anti-inflammatory responses (Brück et al., 2017; Miyake et al., 2006). The promising outcomes observed in these and other animal models have motivated researchers to conduct multiple clinical trials in humans suffering from various diseases, including multiple sclerosis, lupus, rheumatoid arthritis, Type 1 diabetes, and ulcerative colitis, utilizing polyphenols or polyphenol-rich extracts as immunomodulatory agents (Khan et al., 2019). The oral use of curcumin capsules (3 g/day for 1 month) by individuals with ulcerative colitis was associated with disease remission (A. Lang et al., 2015). In another clinical trial, quercetin (4 x 500 mg within 24 hours) demonstrated a reduction in inflammatory and oxidative stress markers in sarcoidosis, a multisystem inflammatory disease. *In vitro,* quercetin was shown to reduce the expression of iNOS and COX-2 genes and proteins in RAW 264 macrophages activated by gliadin and IFN-γ, through a mechanism involving the transcription factors NF-κB, signal transducer and activator of transcription-1α (STAT-1α), and interferon regulatory factor-1 (IRF-1) (De Stefano et al., 2007).

Numerous research on chronic illnesses indicates a strong correlation between inflammation and oxidative stress, since both phenomena can activate the NF-κB signaling pathway (Biswas, 2016). In Crohn's disease, the sequence of events initiated by the NF-κB transcription factor leads to the upregulation of many immunological stimuli, including cytokine production that maintains an inflammatory milieu (Ferretti, Bacchetti, Masciangelo, & Saturni, 2012). This insight is crucial for investigating the pathways via which polyphenols may confer protection in CD, since they might avert oxidative damage while modulating gene expression, for instance, by inhibiting the cascade of events triggered by NF-κB activation (Ferretti et al., 2012; H. Zhang & Tsao, 2016).

Epigenetic regulatory mechanisms, including histone modifications, DNA methylation, and microRNA expression, do not alter an individual's DNA sequence but can modify gene expression in response to environmental and lifestyle variables, such as food (Allis & Jenuwein, 2016). In this context, dietary polyphenols have been demonstrated to influence many signaling transcription factors, such as NF-κB, and to counteract harmful epigenetic alterations via diverse regulatory pathways (Cuevas et al., 2013). The flavonol fisetin can inhibit the NF-κB transcription factor in monocytes subjected to elevated glucose levels by deacetylating the p65 subunit, leading to a reduction in NF-κB transcriptional activity (H. J. Kim, Kim, & Yun, 2012). Drugs targeting epigenetic variables are now employed in several clinical studies to mitigate the symptoms of different autoimmune illnesses (Zhernakova, Withoff, & Wijmenga, 2013). Consequently, with polyphenols recognized as possible epigenetic regulators, their prospects as novel therapeutic agents in Crohn's disease are undeniably attractive (Remely et al., 2015).

Gluten Vaccination

Nexvax2, a desensitizing or therapeutic vaccination for CD patients, was created by Immusan T in Cambridge, Massachusetts, USA. By promoting immunological tolerance for gluten and aiding in the digestion of foods containing gluten, the peptide-based immunotherapy vaccination was able to change the T-cell response from one that was proinflammatory to one that was regulatory (Keijzer, Zee, Eden, & Broere, 2013). These peptides enhanced gluten tolerance and increased the expression of Tregs in HLA-DQ2 transgenic mice by suppressing $CD4^+$ T-cell proliferation and lowering IFN-γ and IL-2 production (Veeraraghavan et al., 2015).

Fecal Microbiota Transplantation

Fecal microbiota transplantation (FMT) is the process of moving feces and, in principle, intestinal microbiota from a normal donor gastrointestinal tract to a recipient patient whose condition is dysbiotically influenced (Ghaffari et al., 2022). This approach seeks to normalize the gut microbiota and, in certain situations, aims to treat the disease. Treatment utilizing the FMT mechanism is based on clinical experiences gathered from the treatment of *Clostridioides difficile* infectious disease (Baunwall et al., 2020). FMT has been used to successfully treat inflammatory bowel disease, intestinal barrier integrity, pathogen inhibition, and immunogenicity modulation caused by changed gut microbiota composition (Littmann et al., 2021). The study is currently underway since there aren't enough convincing arguments in favor of applying this strategy to the treatment of CD or other gastrointestinal disorders (Akobeng, Singh, Kumar, & Al Khodor, 2020). For instance, according to one research, a 68-year-old lady with refractory CD demonstrated symptoms including malnutrition and intestinal villi shrinkage following FMT treatment (Malamut & Cellier, 2019; van Beurden et al., 2016).

Tissue Transglutaminase Inhibitors

Breaking intermolecular isopeptide connections between glutamine and lysine, which might result in immunogenic peptides, is one of the numerous functions of the TG2 protein (Siegel & Khosla, 2007). In CD patients, TG2 deaminates the glutamine residues in gluten peptides to produce an effective T-cell epitope (Sollid & Jabri, 2011). An increase in autoantigens is caused as a result of the crosslinking that TG2 causes between the gluten peptides and the matrix protein. Therefore, creating TG2 inhibitors as prospective CD treatment targets may be beneficial (Makharia, 2014; Sollid & Jabri, 2011).

It was long believed that TG2 inhibition would prevent gluten peptides from interacting with HLA-DQ8 and HLA-DQ2 (Xia et al., 2006). Along with KCC009, an irreversible inhibitor that enhances TG2 affinity, competitive inhibitors such as cystamine, which can inhibit the growth of gluten-reactive T cells, were also developed concurrently (Choi et al., 2005). These inhibitors are effective oral alternatives with minimal toxicity and a short serum half-life, capable of blocking TG2 in the small intestine. Therefore, it was concluded that TG2 inhibition could be useful for inhibiting the innate immune response both *in vitro* and *ex vivo*, as well as for preventing gliadin-induced adaptive immune responses (Büchold et al., 2022; Jabri, 2021; Verdu & Schuppan, 2021).

Oral Enzyme Strategy

It has been discovered that fungi, bacteria, plants, and insects all have gluten -degrading enzymes (K. A. Scherf et al., 2018). Though fascinating exopeptidases have also been identified, these enzymes, usually referred to as glutenases, are mostly endopeptidases (Krishnareddy, Stier, Recanati, Lebwohl, & Green, 2017). Depending on their catalytic mechanism, endopeptidases are further categorized into threonine endopeptidases, metalloendopeptidases, aspartic endopeptidases, cysteine endopeptidases, and serine endopeptidases (de Lourdes Moreno et al., 2021). Prolyl endopeptidases (PEPs), a subclass of serine endopeptidases, are extremely impressive in breaking down peptide bonds on the carboxyl face of internal proline residues in gluten-derived oligopeptides (Shan, Marti, Sollid, Gray, & Khosla, 2004). Peptides with less than 30 residues can be hydrolyzed by PEPs (Polgar, 2002). Despite the characterization of membrane-bound PEPs, cytosolic PEPs are often reported (Rea & Fülöp, 2006). The enzymes now on the market that are labeled as digestive assistance for GFD are capable of breaking down gluten, but they are largely useless with gluten peptides that are immunogenic (Janssen et al., 2015). Therefore, randomized, placebo-controlled trials examining the impact of glutenases on the signs and biomarkers in CD patients are required; however, this is not as simple as it may appear (Krishnareddy et al., 2017; Ozma, Abbasi, & Sabahi, 2022).

Sources of Gluten - Degrading Enzymes

Bacterial Peptidases

Different enzymatic pathways have been used to identify bacteria that can degrade gluten in a variety of environmental settings. To be taken into consideration as potential CD treatments, three bacterial PEPs from *Flavobacterium meningosepticum*, *Myxococcus xanthus*, and *Sphingomonas capsulata* were thoroughly described and recombinantly generated in *Escherichia coli* (Pyle et al., 2005; Shan et al., 2004). Despite the three enzymes' varying degrees of specificity based on the length of the gluten peptide chain, they all displayed extremely specific activity when tested against standard chromogenic reagents (Shan et al., 2004). The 33-mer was cleaved preferentially by PEP from *F. meningosepticum*, while PEPs from *M. xanthus* and *S. capsulata* were more selective for shorter peptides like PQPQLPYPQPQLP. All enzymes have shown modest persistence with pancreatic proteases and remained active in the small intestine's mildly acidic environment. Pepsin, on the other hand, fully rendered these enzymes inactive, indicating that they need to be shielded from both stomach acid and pepsin (Hausch, Shan, Santiago, Gray, & Khosla, 2002; Piper, Gray, & Khosla, 2004). Additional research has shown that these enzymes are resistant to being inactivated by brush boundary membrane peptidases (Wei, Helmerhorst,

Darwish, Blumenkranz, & Schuppan, 2020). Gliadin was hydrolyzed by an aciduric bacterial enzyme from *Pseudomonas aeruginosa* known as pseudolysin or lasB. This pseudolysin is a –X↓L– peptide bond-specific zinc metalloprotease that is active at pH 2-4. Further research is necessary to determine whether it is effective in eliminating other CD-active epitopes (Wei et al., 2015). Numerous investigations have also shown that certain *Bacillus* strains are capable of hydrolyzing gluten. Wheat gliadin might be hydrolyzed by the bacterial enzymes subtilisin and thermolysin, respectively, from *Bacillus licheniformis* and *Bacillus thermoproteolyticus*. However, it is yet unknown if these enzymes can completely eliminate CD immunoreactivity (Socha, Mickowska, Urminská, & Kačmárová, 2021). The peptidase S9 family member gliadinase from *Bacillus tequilensis* fully hydrolyzes gliadin polypeptides after 180 minutes of incubation. This enzyme was also evaluated *in vivo*, demonstrating its activity in the presence of bile salts and intestinal proteases such as trypsin, chymotrypsin, or pepsin (Wagh, Gadge, & Padul, 2018). The ability of a newly discovered enzyme to cleave Y↓P, L↓Q, Q↓P, and Q↓L in *Bacillus subtilis* spp. GS 188 was demonstrated to be effective in designing gluten-reduced wheat food items for CD (Rashmi et al., 2020). Recently, PEP 2RA3 from *Chryseobacterium taeanense*, a novel microbial PEP that breaks down gluten, was identified, cloned, and produced in *E. coli*. When the enzyme targeted immunogenic gluten domains in gliadin and beer samples, it displayed interesting specificities. Nevertheless, in order to be acceptable and safe for CD patients, it must be used with other particular enzymes to eradicate GIP (Maria de Lourdes Moreno Amador, Arevalo-Rodriguez, Durán, Martinez Reyes, & Sousa Martin, 2019). Contrarily, the new glutenase E40 from the soil actinomycete *Actinoallomurus* A8 was initially demonstrated and its recombinant active form was recombinantly synthesized in *Streptomyces lividans* TK24. It is a member of the serine-carboxyl peptidase S53 family. Pepsin and trypsin have no effect on E40, which is active in the pH range of 3-6. Along with other gliadin proteins, this enzyme effectively broke down the 33-mer, which is the most immunogenic. E40 showed a significantly reduced or nonexistent generation of interferon-γ when exposed to gluten in experiments involving T cells from duodenal biopsies of CD patients (Cavaletti et al., 2019). It has also been shown that bacteria from dental plaque and human saliva are capable of breaking down gluten. Gluten immunogenic epitopes were broken and eliminated by the serine protease subtilisin generated by *Rothia aeria* and *Rothia mucilaginosa*, demonstrating its significant potential for CD treatment (Zamakhchari et al., 2011). These bacterial enzymes were able to break down the 33-mer peptide and wheat gliadins after surviving the gastric transit and become reactivated in the duodenum at alkaline pH levels. Their enzymatic end-products were not well detected by sandwich, competitive, or TG2 enzyme-linked immunosorbent tests (Tian, Wei, Schuppan, & Helmerhorst, 2014).

Fungal Peptidases

Aspergillus peptidases are often utilized in the processing of food and feed because they are typically regarded as safe by the Food and Drug Administration (K. A. Scherf et al., 2018). The PEP produced by *Aspergillus niger*, also known as AN-PEP, is well-known for its pH range of 2 to 8, optimal pH of 4, and resistance to pepsin digestion. In addition to degrading GIP, intact α- and γ-gliadins, as well as LMW and HMW glutenin subunits, AN-PEP also demonstrates post-proline cleavage activity (Stepniak et al., 2006). In a study by Mitea and colleagues, T-cell stimulatory activity completely vanished from a gastrointestinal model system when AN-PEP was added to a bread slice and a fast-food meal. This peptidase has formerly been utilized to hydrolyze the gluten found in rye flour, sourdough, beer, bread drink, and wheat bran (Guerdrum & Bamforth, 2012; Walter, Wieser, & Koehler, 2015). 14 CD patients were randomly assigned by Tack et al., to consume 7 g of gluten per day along with either AN-PEP or a placebo over the course of two weeks. The effect of the enzyme on clinical signs and symptoms, however, could not be demonstrated because this level of gluten did not cause clinical worsening in the placebo group (Tack et al., 2013). Tolerase G, an AN-PEP-based product, was tested in a clinical investigation, and the results showed that it significantly decreased the quantity of gluten introduced to the duodenum even though it did not entirely degrade the gluten (Salden et al., 2015). Aspergillopepsin (ASP) is a different *A. niger* enzyme with gluten-degrading activity. This enzyme proved less effective and substrate selective than AN-PEP since the 33-mer peptide was unaltered after being added to the entire gluten. As a result, ASP may be administered in addition to other enzymes that break down gluten. *Aspergillus oryzae*'s extracellular dipeptidyl peptidase IV (AO-DPP-IV) is an exopeptidase that preferentially cleaves NH_2-XP↓X- peptide bonds while releasing an N-terminal dipeptide from polypeptides (Ehren et al., 2009). However, AO-DPP-IV was incapable of hydrolyzing the 33-mer peptide and was ineffective in the degradation of gluten (Janssen et al., 2015).

Plant Peptidases

In order to provide the growing embryo with amino acids and nitrogen, gluten proteins are broken down during germination. Up to 90% of the overall degradation is accounted for by cysteine endopeptidases, with metalloendopeptidases coming in second at 7% and serine and aspartic endopeptidases coming in third. Exopeptidases further degrade the resultant peptides into amino acids (Simpson, 2001). Intriguingly, these circumstances are comparable to those seen in the stomach and the cysteine endopeptidase EP-B2 from barley is released as a proenzyme into the acidic endosperm of germination seeds, where it is activated to its mature form. After glutamine, EP-B2 cleaves peptide bonds, frequently with proline at the P2 position (Q↓XP), although it can also break Q↓XX motifs (Bethune, Strop, Tang, Sollid, & Khosla, 2006). The activity of mature EP-B2 has also been verified *in vivo*, and it is resistant to pepsin and chymotrypsin but vulnerable to trypsin at physiological doses. Mature EP-B2 is effective versus 33-mer and some other immunogenic peptides throughout a wide range of acidic pH values (Bethune, Ribka, Khosla, & Sestak, 2008). From the latex of the *Carica papaya*, another cysteine endoprotease known as caricain (GluteGuard) has been discovered. Once the latex is taken from the plant, this enzyme is transformed from its inactive zymogen form, which it first synthesizes, to its active form Caricain cleaves immunogenic peptides into 33-mers on the N-terminal position of proline residues and operates most effectively at pH 6.8 (Bethune et al., 2008; Siegel et al., 2006). Twenty CD patients in clinical remission participated in a randomized, placebo-controlled experiment to examine GluteGuard. Treatment with this enzyme considerably reduced the patients' unpleasant symptoms when they were given a daily gluten challenge of 1 g, and mucosal injury was not made worse. Contrarily, four of the six participants taking a placebo experienced severe sign within the first two weeks of the experiment and were forced to stop participating in future gluten challenges. At pH ranges of 3.0-6.5, the wheat cysteine endopeptidase triticain also displayed hydrolysis of CD-active gluten peptides. The glutenins and α-, γ-, and ω-gliadins were broken down by the recombinant triticain-α. This enzyme prefers proline in the P2 and/or P2′ positions, acting either before or after glutamine (Savvateeva et al., 2015). Recently, the ability to break down gluten was investigated in the papain-like C1A family cysteine protease HvPap-6 from *Hordeum vulgare*. Wheat gliadins were shown to be hydrolyzed after one hour of incubation. However, complete disintegration was shown to have occurred after 12 hours of incubation (Martinez et al., 2019).

Insect Peptidases

Due to their diet of cereals, insects, particularly grain pests, possess endogenous enzymes that may degrade gluten. Two serine endopeptidases and one carboxypeptidase from the beetle *Rhyzopertha dominica* were studied for their significant gluten breakdown capabilities. High prolyl-specific peptidase activity was confirmed, with the major cleavage site occurring after proline. A breakdown percentage of up to 65% for the α-gliadin peptide was achieved using peptides from the α-gliadin fraction and another from a hordein fraction high in proline (Mika, Zorn, & Rühl, 2015). A proline-specific metallopeptidase was purified and characterized from the midgut of *Tenebrio molitor* larvae. The prolidase was inhibited by Z-Pro and had an optimal pH of 7.5, suggesting it is a type I prolidase. This enzyme, which hydrolyzes imidodipeptides in the cytoplasm of midgut epithelial cells, appears to be crucial for the later stages of digestion of dietary gliadins rich in proline (Tereshchenkova et al., 2017).

Human Peptidases

Human feces include proteins that may particularly break down gluten. Different enzymes from healthy individuals and CD patients have previously been discovered, isolated, and described. The gliadin peptides 13-mer and 19-mer, as well as a 33-mer, were completely degraded by the digestive enzymes elastase 3B, 2A, and A1 (Gutiérrez et al., 2017).

Enzymatic Cocktails with Gluten Hydrolysis Activities

It's possible that a combination of gluten -degrading enzymes with different cleavage specificities and preferred pH levels will work together to more efficiently reduce the antigenicity of digested gluten fragments. *A. niger* 's ASP and *A. oryzae* 's DPP-IV effectively metabolized a modest quantity of gluten *in vitro* (Ehren et al., 2009). Both enzymes are often utilized as nutritional supplements in the food and feed sectors. Similar to this, when DPP-IV from *A. oryzae* and AN-PEP from *A. niger* were combined and taken internally as STAN1, modest quantities of gluten were successfully degraded. Due to the nonspecificity of AN-PEP and the extremely modest proteolytic impact of DPP-IV, this effect seems to be subdued. There were no serological changes between the treated patients and the placebo group in a trial that looked at the impact of STAN1 on CD patients who continued to test positive for gluten despite following a GFD and were told to consume 1 g of the protein daily for 12 weeks (Kivelä et al., 2021; Korponay-Szabo et al., 2010). It is well known that the cysteine endoproteases EP-B2 and PEP from *F.*

meningosepticum work well together when it comes to digesting gluten. While PEP typically cleaves targets of 30 amino acids, EP-B2 favors intact proteins and cuts at glutamine residues. Although it has been demonstrated that this enzyme combination can detoxify gluten proteins, major attempts have been made to strengthen their thermostability so that they may be used in industrial settings (Osorio, Mejías, & Rustgi, 2019). ALV003, also known as latiglutenase, is one of the most well-known enzymatic concoctions. It is a 1:1 mixture of cysteine endoprotease derived from barley, EP-B2 (ALV001), and PEP derived from *S. capsulata* (ALV002). In a gluten challenge trial, latiglutenase reduced the mucosal damage caused by gluten in CD patients. However, further clinical research (phase 2b) in CD patients in which latiglutenase was given together with 2 g of gluten over the course of 6 weeks failed to provide unambiguous proof of latiglutenase-stimulated mucosal healing as the main objective. In a later large dose-ranging study with 500 CD patients, analysis of the symptoms and QOL data supporting secondary endpoints revealed that there was statistically and clinically meaningful proof of latiglutenase-stimulated reduction of several main signs associated with gluten ingestion, as well as a correlation with QOL improvement, for seropositive patients (Sartor & Wu, 2017; Syage, Murray, Green, & Khosla, 2017). As a result, ALV003's efficacy has not yet been determined (Syage et al., 2019).

Molecular Modeling and Engineered Gluten -Degrading Enzymes

Molecules with perfect enzymatic activity under certain circumstances and against particular substrates have been created using molecular modeling and engineering. For instance, it was discovered that altering the catalytically active site of the acidic serine endopeptidase kumamolisin-As from *Alicyclobacillus sendaiensis* will change its cleavage specificity from -P↓R- or -P↓K- to -P↓Q-, a pattern that occurs often in CD peptides. The KumaMax-designed recombinant peptidase produced a 116-fold increase in hydrolytic efficiency on the target PQPQLP with an 877-fold improvement in substrate specificity (Gordon et al., 2012). The variation Kuma030 was created by further optimizing KumaMax and introducing six-point mutations that permitted the breakdown of CD-active peptides, such as the 33-mer. After 30 minutes under simulated gastrointestinal circumstances, Kuma030 had broken down 99.97% of a whole wheat bread's gluten load. Therefore, using Kuma030 to eliminate gluten from food during processing may also be appropriate (Wolf et al., 2015). In order to boost the degree of thermostability, mutations were recently introduced into the PEP from *F. meningosepticum* and EP-B2 using a sequence-guided site-saturation mutagenesis strategy. Although PEP with thermostability up to 90°C and an EP-B2 variant with thermostability up to 60°C were found, this was insufficient. Enzymes that can withstand temperatures of less than 100°C are continually being sought after in new tests to enable their use in the food industries (Osorio et al., 2020).

Technological Advancements in Gluten -Degrading Enzymes

The fact that gluten -degrading enzymes are less effective in acidic environments, such as the stomach, is one of their most prevalent drawbacks. As a result, technological advancement could increase the effectiveness of enzyme delivery. PEGylation is the process of attaching polyethylene glycol (PEG) either covalently or noncovalently to a target protein. This increases the protein's stability *in vivo* by improving its resistance to proteolytic destruction and fast excretion (Suk, Xu, Kim, Hanes, & Ensign, 2016). Microencapsulation, on the other hand, is a process that offers an enteric coating, creates microparticles that partially resist enteric breakdown, and permits the distal administration of pharmaceutical agents (Abedi, Rismanchi, Shahdoostkhany, Mohammadi, & Hosseini, 2016). As an illustration, the PEGylation modification and microencapsulation of the gluten-degrading enzyme subtilisin-A from *B. licheniformis* dramatically boosted its protection against acid exposure. This was shown *in vitro*, and the efficacy was validated *in vivo* (Darwish, Helmerhorst, Schuppan, Oppenheim, & Wei, 2019).

Larazotide Acetate: Tight Junction Modulator

The sequence of larazotide acetate (also known as AT-1001), a synthetic octapeptide, was chosen because it resembles the zonula occludens toxin released by *Vibrio cholerae*. By lowering gliadin-induced permeability and tight junction integrity, larazotide acetate lowers small intestine inflammation. Larazotide acetate clinical studies in both phases I and II have been finished. Larazotide acetate was proven to be safe, well tolerated, and reduce diarrhea following gluten exposure in phase I, a double-blind, randomized, placebo-controlled safety investigation. However, permeability and the generation of proinflammatory cytokines did not vary statistically (Paterson, Lammers, Arrieta, Fasano, & Meddings, 2007). Larazotide acetate was shown to be well tolerated and to stop the progression of gastrointestinal symptoms brought on by the gluten challenge, according to a phase II, placebo-controlled research (Leffler et al., 2012). According to a recently ended phase II clinical research, larazotide acetate 0.5 mg given three times daily alleviated CD patients' symptoms more effectively than a GFD alone. Larazotide was successfully tested in this research as a potential treatment drug for CD patients who continue to have symptoms while receiving a GFD (Leffler et al., 2015). Additionally, it was shown that larazotide acetate, which was typically well tolerated, decreased gluten-induced immunological reactivity (i.e., tTG response) and signs in CD patients who underwent gluten challenge (Kelly et al., 2013). The lack of data on histologic alteration despite symptom improvement is a limitation of this research, which has uncertain consequences even though the findings are encouraging in terms of symptom improvement.

Zamaglutenase

Zamaglutenase, previously referred to as TAK-062, is a very powerful endopeptidase that has been computationally developed and derived from the precursor Kuma030. Researchers at PvP Biologics developed TAK-062 to enhance proteolytic activity and to specifically target proline-glutamine dipeptide motifs, which are abundant in the immunogenic sections of gliadin peptides. This may confer an advantage to TAK-062 compared to latiglutenase, which only targets a single amino acid (proline or glutamine). Moreover, TAK-062 was engineered to preserve proteolytic activity throughout a spectrum of physiologically pertinent pH values in the gastrointestinal system (pH 2.5-6.0) and to exhibit resistance to the gastric and intestinal proteases pepsin and trypsin.

TAK-062's efficacy in degrading ingested gluten was recently evaluated in healthy subjects (Pultz et al., 2021). This Phase I trial (NCT03701555) involved healthy participants consuming TAK-062 prior to a complicated meal comprising 1–6 g of gluten. The oral administration of TAK-062 was well tolerated and achieved a median gluten breakdown rate between 97% and over 99% in complicated meals comprising 1–6 g of gluten at 20–65 minutes post-dose. The medication is presently undergoing evaluation in an extensive Phase II trial with 377 individuals with active celiac disease who are undertaking a gluten-free diet (NCT05353985). The study aims to replicate unintentional gluten exposures through the use of gluten-containing bars.

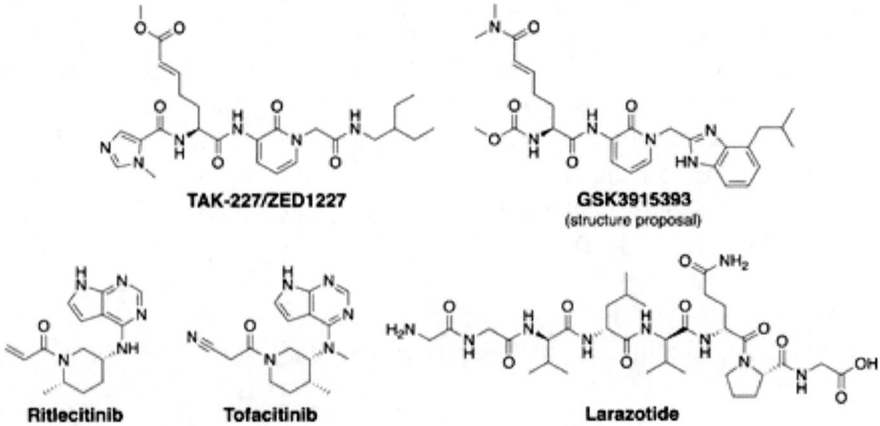

Figure 8. Chemical structures of potential oral small-molecule therapies for celiac disease as discussed in the respective chapters.

ZED1227/TAK-227

ZED1227 is an orally bioavailable, intestinal TG2-specific small molecule inhibitor that covalently binds to the TG2 active site, effectively inhibiting TG2 with great specificity. By doing so, it inhibits the synthesis of deamidated gluten and, presumably, the preliminary stages of gluten-induced T-cell activation.at Phase I clinical trials (EudraCT 2014-003044-13 and 2015-00528342) involving 108 healthy subjects, ZED1227 was provided at dosages up to 500 mg, exhibiting an acceptable safety profile and good tolerability. A Phase II proof-of-concept trial (EudraCT 2017-002241-30) shown that ZED1227 significantly mitigated intestinal mucosal damage in individuals with CeD subjected to a modest daily gluten intake (3 g/day) for a duration of 6 weeks. ZED1227 therapy preserved transcriptome markers associated with mucosal shape, inflammation, cell differentiation, and nutrient absorption at levels akin to those in the GFD group. A Phase IIb research is now underway for individuals with celiac disease who exhibit symptoms while adhering to a gluten-free diet (EudraCT 2020-004612-97).

AGY 010

AGY 010, an oral egg yolk antigliadin antibody designed to neutralize gluten, has demonstrated safety and possible symptom improvement in a 6-week, open-label, single-arm research including 10 patients with celiac disease (CeD). 40 Phase II research (NCT03707730) further evaluated it in individuals with symptomatic CeD who were adhering to a GFD. No data had been disseminated at the time of composing this book.

GSK3915393

GSK3915393, an irreversible TG2 inhibitor (as depicted in Figure 8 of US11548892), underwent clinical evaluation, with GSK concluding a Phase I study (NCT04604795) involving healthy volunteers. However, the clinical development of this compound for CD was halted in February 2023, and there are no intentions to further pursue CD (Buriánek, Gege, & Marinković, 2024).

TAK-101

TAK-101 (formerly CNP-101 or TIMP-GLIA) is a biodegradable, negatively charged 500-nm poly (DL-lactide-co-glycolic acid) nanoparticle that encapsulates gliadin protein. TAK-101 is administered intravenously, allowing it to reach the liver and spleen, where it is absorbed and processed by antigen-presenting cells (APCs). This method elicited gliadin tolerance and reduced inflammation and enteropathy markers in a CeD animal model (Freitag et al., 2020). Recent early clinical studies shown that TAK-101 was well tolerated in individuals with CeD and effectively reduced immune activation and small intestine mucosal damage following gluten exposure. No indication of systemic immune suppression was detected (NCT03486990 and NCT03738475). (p48) A Phase II trial is under underway to evaluate the effectiveness and safety of TAK-101 in preventing gluten-specific T-cell activation in patients with celiac disease on a gluten-free diet (NCT04530123).

KAN-101

KAN-101 is an experimental liver-targeted treatment aimed at inducing tolerance and inhibiting T-cell activation following gluten intake in individuals with celiac disease, via intravenous delivery of deaminated gliadin peptides linked to a liver-targeting glycosylation signature.50 In a first-in-human trial, KAN-101 demonstrated a satisfactory safety profile in individuals with CeD, with no dose-limiting toxicities or maximum tolerated dosage identified. Additionally, KAN-101 demonstrated the capacity to promote gluten tolerance by attenuating the inflammatory response of gliadin-specific CD4+ and gut-homing CD8+ T cells following gluten exposure (NCT04248855). (p50) KAN-101 is presently undergoing assessment in Phase Ib/II and Phase II trials (NCT05574010, NCT06001177).

TPM502

TPM502 is a nanoparticle-based method involving polymer-coated superparamagnetic iron oxide particles coupled with peptides pertinent to CD. The objective is for the nanoparticles to be internalized by liver sinusoidal endothelial cells, which possess immune-tolerogenic properties. (p49) TPM502 is presently undergoing evaluation in a Phase IIa trial including individuals diagnosed with CeD (NCT05660109). This placebo-controlled trial aims to assess the safety and tolerability of two infusions of increasing doses of TPM502 in patients with well-managed celiac disease on a gluten - free diet for at least six months. The study will assess alterations in markers that may signify the induction of gluten tolerance following gluten exposure.

PRV-015

PRV-015 (formerly AMG 714), a completely human immunoglobulin monoclonal antibody (IgG1j), obstructs IL-15-mediated T-cell proliferation by binding to and blocking the activity of IL-15 in all its forms [cis, trans, and soluble or associated with the IL-15 receptor subunit alpha (IL-15RA)]. (p44) In a Phase IIa gluten challenge study of PRV-015 (NCT02637141 and EudraCT, 2015-003647-19), the primary endpoint, the alteration in the villous height-to-crypt depth ratio from baseline to week 12 of treatment, did not reveal a significant difference between the 150 mg or 300 mg doses of PRV-015 and the placebo. Nevertheless, the elevated 300 mg dosage suggested the possibility of alleviating the adverse effects of gluten, as demonstrated by a decrease in IEL density, enhanced patient-reported outcomes, and a diminished occurrence of diarrhea. The 300 mg dosage was determined to be well tolerated by patients. (p44) PRV-015 was further evaluated in a Phase IIa trial with individuals with type 2 RCD. The primary outcome, the alteration in the proportion of aberrant IELs from baseline to week 12, was not achieved.

Notable advantages were observed in IEL T-cell receptor clonality and in the decrease of diarrhea. (p52) A Phase IIb research (NCT04424927) is in underway involving adult patients with refractory celiac disease adhering to a gluten-free diet.

CALY-002

In 2017, Vicari and colleagues identified a novel humanized anti-IL-15 monoclonal antibody, designated CALY-002, which inhibits IL-15 activity by obstructing its interaction with the IL-15 receptor subunit beta (IL-15Rb). (53) CALY-002 was been evaluated in a Phase I trial including healthy individuals and patients with celiac disease and eosinophilic esophagitis (NCT04593251). Patients with CD were administered varying dosages of CALY-002 or a placebo, in addition to 3 g of gluten daily for a duration of 8 weeks. CALY-002 demonstrated safety and tolerability while effectively mitigating gluten-induced mucosal damage (54).

TEV-53408

TEV-53408, an IL-15 antibody, is presently undergoing evaluation in a Phase Ib trial. The TEV-CD research seeks to determine the safety and tolerability of a single injection of the study medicine in people with CD, in comparison to a placebo, both before to and following the ingestion of gluten -containing snacks (55).

EQ102

EQ102 is a peptide that specifically inhibits the binding of IL-15 and IL-21 to the common γc receptor and is designed for subcutaneous delivery. Increased concentrations of IL-15 and IL-21 in the duodenal tissue of individuals with untreated celiac disease synergistically stimulate intestinal intraepithelial cytotoxic T lymphocytes, seemingly enhancing their transcriptional activity, proliferation, and cytolytic function. The peptide EQ102 is formulated to mitigate these effects and may be used to prevent T-cell-mediated tissue damage. Phase I research was recently conducted on healthy individuals (56). Although EQ102 was generally well tolerated and shown pharmacodynamic action in both the single- and multiple-ascending-dose segments of the research, the bioavailability of this first formulation was less than anticipated. Consequently, additional clinical research is scheduled for EQ302 rather than EQ102, a second-generation, orally administered stapled peptide targeting IL-15 and IL-21, as a prospective therapy for individuals with gastrointestinal and dermatological disorders (57).

DONQ52

DONQ52 is a multi-specific antibody targeting a combination of HLADQ2.5 and gluten peptides. It directly obstructs gluten-dependent T-cell activation through the neutralizing interaction of the T-cell receptor (TCR) with HLA-DQ2 .5/gluten peptide complexes. (58) DONQ52 was recently evaluated in HLA-DQ2.5+ individuals with celiac disease (N = 44) who participated in a 3-day grain challenge using either 12 g of wheat gluten, 6 g of barley hordein, or 5.8 g of rye secalin, with blood samples collected before to and 6 days following the initiation of the challenge. Peripheral blood mononuclear cells (PBMCs) were extracted and evaluated by an IFN-γ enzyme-linked immunosorbent spot (ELISpot) test to assess responses to gluten peptides including several immunodominant T-cell epitopes. The inhibitory effects of DONQ52 (at doses of 4 or 40 μg/mL) were assessed and contrasted with the effects of pan-HLA-DQ blocking. DONQ52 suppressed the T-cell response specific to wheat gluten and diminished the T-cell responses to barley hordein and rye secalin. (p. 59) DONQ52 is presently being evaluation in a Phase I trial including well-managed individuals with CD (NCT05425446).

Lymphocyte Trafficking

An alternate method for immunological regulation is the suppression of lymphocyte migration and localization to the intestinal mucosa. PTG-100, an oral selective α4β7 integrin antagonist peptide, was evaluated in a Phase IIa trial for ulcerative colitis (NCT02895100) and subsequently investigated in a Phase Ib study (NCT04524221) including patients with celiac disease undertaking a gluten challenge. No statistics on CD were published at the time of this book's composition.

Janus Kinase (JAK) Inhibition

The JAK family consists of four receptor-associated tyrosine kinases: JAK1, JAK2, JAK3, and TYK2. These enzymes phosphorylate tyrosine residues on proteins, often activating them, although they may also inhibit them, frequently within a signaling cascade. All JAKs often operate with type I and II cytokine receptors, which are essential for immune responses. Consequently, the inhibition of JAKs presents potential for modulating excessive or abnormal immunological activation (p60).

Pan-JAK Inhibitor

Tofacitinib (Xeljanz®) is a broad-spectrum JAK inhibitor authorized for the management of rheumatic disorders, including rheumatoid arthritis and ankylosing spondylitis, in addition to ulcerative colitis. RCDII is propelled by the clonal proliferation of IELs, which frequently possess gain-of-function mutations in JAK1. A previous *in vitro* investigation shown that tofacitinib might modulate the activity of an aberrant IEL population. In an open-label Phase II study [Eudra clinical trials number (EudraCT): 2018-001678-10] involving six patients with RCD II (four patients treated per protocol, two patients treated off protocol), a 12-week regimen of tofacitinib resulted in the resolution of diarrhea/loose stool within 2–14 days, alleviation of abdominal pain, and an increase in weight. One patient was able to cease parenteral feeding at week 9. The main immunologic objective, an absolute reduction of about 20% in aberrant IELs (of the total IELs) from baseline to week 12, was not achieved. Mucosal enhancement, as the secondary objective, was noted in four out of six individuals. All patients had a swift resurgence of symptoms, including weight loss, following the cessation of treatment; however, the reinstatement of medication resulted in a rapid and full remission once more (62).

Modulation of the Immune System and Gluten Tolerance

Infection with Hookworms (Necator americanus)

It is believed that intestinal parasite infections assist in immune system regulation and guard against autoimmune and allergy disorders. The absence of early childhood contact with intestinal parasites, according to the "hygiene theory," has led to a susceptibility to develop autoimmune illnesses in industrialized nations (Bach, 2002). The impact of hookworm infection on the gluten challenge in CD was investigated in a randomized, double-blind, placebo-controlled experiment. After a 5-day gluten challenge, there was no statistically significant difference between the hookworm *Necator americanus* -inoculated patients and the control group in terms of the histological damage and stimulation of IFN-γ producing cells in the peripheral blood (Daveson et al., 2011). The gluten challenge was extended for an additional 12 weeks in the trial. The study's findings have not yet been published (NCT01661933). Another study used increasing gluten challenges on CD patients to explore the role of simulated hookworm infection in reducing intestinal harm and signs. Within a 52-week period, 12 CD individuals on a gluten-free diet were inoculated with *N. americanus* larvae and given increasing amounts of gluten. After the gluten challenge, the median villous height-to-crypt depth ratios did not drop as expected, the quality of life indices increased, and the mean tTG-IgA titers decreased despite the increasing gluten dosages (Croese et al., 2015). These results lead us to assume that *N. americanus* infection can be used to increase immunological control and gluten tolerance in CD. It is difficult to envision the routine therapeutic usage of *N. americanus* in the treatment of CD given the nature of this innovative therapy.

Cathepsin S Inhibitor

Lysosomal cysteine protease known as cathepsin plays a part in the antigen presentation to MHC class II. A cathepsin S competitive inhibitor that is taken orally is called RO5459072 (Theron et al., 2017). a phase 1 randomized, double-blind, multiple-dose, placebo-controlled trial to examine the tolerability, safety, pharmacodynamics, and pharmacokinetics of RO5459072 in patients with well-controlled CD. The proportion of individuals that responded to the gluten challenge served as the major metric for this study's result. The investigation is concluded, and we anticipate the results' publication (NCT02679014).

Nanoparticle

A nanoparticle-based experimental therapy called TIMP-GLIA (Cour Pharmaceuticals, Northbrook, IL) claims to induce immunological tolerance to gluten consumption by non-inflammatory antigen presentation. The product has received Fast Track Designation from the Food and Drug Administration, and a phase I trial is now being conducted to define its tolerability and safety when either 1 or 2 intravenous doses are administered to participants with CD (NCT03486990).

Nexvax2

Nexvax2 is a peptide-based, epitope-specific gluten -tolerizing drug that works similarly to desensitization techniques for allergic disorders while employing immunotherapy principles. Antigenic peptides identified by CD4+ T cells in CD may be safely delivered to patients at high maintenance dosage levels without immunological activation if preceded by slow dose escalation, according to a randomized, double-blind, placebo-controlled phase I research (Goel et al., 2017). The maximal tolerable dose of Nexvax2 (150 mg), administered intradermally twice weekly for eight weeks, changed the immunological response to Nexvax2 peptides without impairing the duodenal histology, according to two randomized, double-blind, placebo-controlled phase I investigations. The gastrointestinal signs that appeared after the vaccine's initial intradermal delivery mimicked those brought on by an oral gluten challenge (Goel et al., 2017). We think that gastrointestinal symptoms brought on by taking Nexvax2 signify intestinal immune activation akin to taking gluten orally. The safety profile of Nexvax2 was deemed to be satisfactory overall. To ascertain its function in CD management, more information is needed.

Immune Cell–Targeted Therapies

IL-10 Agonists

When exposed to modest levels of gluten, the immune-modulating factor IL-10, which is released by T regulatory cells, may play a protective function in CD. It has only been researched thus far in RCD patients. Its function in the management of CD is not yet known.

IL-15 Antagonists

A cytokine called IL-15 controls the growth and activation of natural killer cells and T lymphocytes. IEL counts rise as a result of IL-15 overexpression, a CD-specific observation. IL-15 possesses antiapoptotic effects. IL-15 inhibits a number of antiapoptotic pathways, including Bcl-2 or Bcl-XL, JAK 1, and JAK 3. A pan-JAK inhibitor called tofacitinib disables 1L-15 signaling. The FDA has given it the go-ahead for the management of rheumatoid arthritis. In a mouse transgenic model of CD where human IL-15 is overexpressed, tofacitinib has proved successful. Pathologic signs were permanently reversed as a result of tofacitinib treatment (Yokoyama, Perera, Waldmann, Hiroi, & Perera, 2013). Tofacitinib is now being thought about for potential usage in celiac disease patients with RCD. Human monoclonal IL-15 antibody AMG 714 is an additional promising substance. Three phases II clinical studies testing this medication on individuals with RCD and nonresponsive CD are now under progress (NCT03439475, NCT02633020, and NCT02637141). Additionally, a phase I clinical trial including Hu-Mik-β-1, a monoclonal antibody that inhibits IL-2 and IL-15, is being conducted in RCD patients (NCT01893775).

CCR9 Antagonist

Chemokine receptor CCR9 is well recognized for being necessary for lymphocyte transit into the gut. A CCR9 receptor antagonist called CCX282-B has been investigated as a potential treatment for inflammatory bowel disease and CD. To assess the impact of CCX282-B on the villous height/crypt depth ratio of small intestine biopsy specimens before and after the gluten challenge, patients with CD who adhered to a rigorous GFD for at least 24 months participated in phase II clinical research. Although this study is finished, the findings have not yet been made public (NCT00540657). There have been worries that this kind of drug might increase the risk of infection, particularly gastrointestinal infections because the cell-homing mechanism involving CCR9 is not antigen-specific. These medications' safety is still unknown.

Anti-CD3 and Anti-CD20

The T cell receptor complex, which assists in activating both cytotoxic T cells, and T helper cells contains the CD3 antigen. Theoretically, anti-CD3 antibody treatment might decrease gluten -activated T cells and hence lessen CD inflammation. Studies have shown that anti-CD3 antibodies can stimulate T regulatory cells *in vitro*, which may support CD tolerance to gluten.55 However, there is a dearth of published data to back the efficacy of anti-CD3 in CD. Additionally, B cells' generation of different antibodies plays a significant part in the pathogenesis of CD. Numerous monoclonal antibodies target the B-cell marker CD20. However, it is understood that CD20 antagonists do not completely stop the production of IgA plasmablasts in the gut mucosa (Mei et al., 2010). As a result, CD20 antagonists might not be useful in the management of CD. Although various monoclonal antibodies directed toward CD20 have already received clinical approval, it is yet unknown how they will be used to treat CD.

Chapter 8

Challenges and Unmet Needs in Celiac Disease Treatment

Abstract

Despite significant advancements in celiac disease (CD) diagnosis and treatment, many challenges remain. This chapter identifies key unmet needs, including the difficulty in managing non-responsive or refractory CD, the lack of effective treatments beyond the gluten-free diet, and the psychological and socioeconomic impact of the disease on patients. It also addresses the need for better diagnostic tools to detect CD early and prevent long-term complications. The chapter calls for more research to address these gaps and improve the quality of life for individuals living with CD.

Non-Responsive/Refractory CD

Refractory celiac disease (RCD) and non-responsive celiac disease (NRCD) are two crucial clinical categories to recognize and differentiate. Up to 20% of people who are diagnosed with CD may have NRCD, which is defined as persisting signs, symptoms, or test abnormalities associated with the illness after reporting strict compliance with a GFD for six to twelve months (Leffler et al., 2007). Up to 36% of patients with non-responsive CD are believed to have unintentionally consumed gluten; however, microscopic colitis, irritable bowel syndrome (IBS), pancreatic insufficiency, small intestinal bacterial overgrowth (SIBO), lactose intolerance, and refractory RCD is also thought to be contributing factors (Hujoel & Murray, 2020). A diagnosis of really "refractory" CD may be considered once the aforementioned disease entities have been assessed and treated, particularly nutritional examination for exposures or a lack of compliance with a GFD, and repeat small intestine histology and serologies have confirmed the CD diagnosis. Only 1% to 2% of CD patients have RCD (Roshan et al., 2011). The intraepithelial lymphocyte population in type 1 RCD is frequently similar to that in CD, but the T cell population in type 2 RCD is typically phenotypically aberrant and has a poorer prognosis. Systemic steroid treatment and immunosuppressive drugs may be used in addition to normal care for CD patients, however, there is a lack of evidence to support their efficacy (Green, Paski, Ko, & Rubio-Tapia, 2022).

Differentiation From Exercise-Induced Wheat-Dependent Asthma/Wheat Allergy

Only up to 0.5% of the total population suffers from a wheat allergy, which is rare but clinically different. Nevertheless, the omega-5 gliadin component is the most frequent allergen linked to food-dependent exercise-stimulated asthma. Clinical signs of wheat allergy, which might include urticaria, eczema, diarrhea, vomiting, or anaphylaxis, are thought to be largely IgE-mediated (Burkhardt, Chapa-Rodriguez, & Bahna, 2018). Adults seem to have a higher prevalence of wheat-dependent exercise-stimulated asthma, whereas children only have IgE-mediated wheat allergy. Although the majority of kids overcome their wheat allergy (Burkhardt et al., 2018), a small European study found that kids with severe food sensitivities may actually have a five times higher chance of developing CD (Pillon et al., 2015). The most often used diagnostic tests are still allergic skin screening or IgE-specific antigen serologies, and therapy is centered on avoiding exposures (Burkhardt et al., 2018).

Eosinophilic Esophagitis and CD

Eosinophilic esophagitis (EoE) and CD are two conditions that have both gotten significantly more attention in the literature than they have individually. Unfortunately, it is difficult to draw any firm conclusions from the available research, and further research is required. In a previous retrospective cohort research, 595 children had EoE and 546 had CD; the probability of developing EoE was not elevated in relation to the presence of CD (OR 0.29, 95% CI 0.154 to 0.545). Over 10,000 children had undergone at least one endoscopy in the study. In a meta-analysis, the same authors found 45 instances of concurrent EoE and CD, with comparable outcomes (OR 0.525, 95% CI 0.364 to 0.797) (Hommeida et al., 2017). Prior to this, a number of cohort studies and cross-sectional research with both children and adults seemed to indicate a relationship between EoE and CD (Jensen, Eluri, Lebwohl, Genta, & Dellon, 2015; Johnson, Boynton, & Peterson, 2016). The diagnosis of EoE, however, is one that often necessitates a number of endoscopies over time, so it is crucial to keep this in mind. Given that EoE is only one of many factors that contribute to esophageal eosinophilia, it is possible that these studies demonstrate a relationship between esophageal eosinophilia and not only EoE. Moreover, the resolution of eosinophilia in at least two experiments (Ari et al., 2017) that looked at multiple endoscopies over time in CD patients with the implementation of a GFD raises the possibility that some patients may be misdiagnosed as having EoE when, in reality, their esophageal eosinophilia is linked to their CD rather than having concomitant EoE.

Atopic Disease and CD

The literature is replete with reports of connections between CD and a number of other autoimmune diseases, such as autoimmune hepatitis, autoimmune thyroid disease, type 1 diabetes mellitus, and Sjogren's syndrome (Denham & Hill, 2013). It appears that there is a connection between cutaneous atopy and CD according to the data linking atopic illness to CD. Atopic dermatitis or chronic urticaria has been mentioned in the literature in several case reports and small studies as symptoms that people with CD come with (Enroth, Dahlbom, Hansson, Johansson, & Gyllensten, 2013; Ress et al., 2014). At the time of CD diagnosis for allergies, a sizable sample of celiac patients, their family members, and their spouses were polled. The further screening included total and antigen-specific IgE in addition to PRICK assessment in some of those who reported allergy symptoms. The presence of allergies, asthma, food allergies, rhinitis, conjunctivitis, sporadic urticaria, and atopic dermatitis were all compared by the authors. The only condition associated with a significantly higher risk was atopic dermatitis, which affected 3.8% of CD individuals, 2.3% of their family members, and 1.3% of their spouses (Ciacci et al., 2004). More recently, in line with earlier studies, sizable population research found an elevated incidence of asthma in CD patients (OR 1.5), but less so than thyroid illness (OR 1.8), and type 1 diabetes mellitus (OR 5.5) (Assa, Frenkel-Nir, Tzur, Katz, & Shamir, 2017). According to further population-based cohort research, CD increases the chance of developing asthma by 1.6 times (Ludvigsson, Hemminki, Wahlström, & Almqvist, 2011). Clearly, some atopic illness seems to be linked to CD, but these connections need to be clarified.

Malignancy

In individuals with celiac disease, there is a known elevated risk for lymphoproliferative malignancies, notably enteropathy-associated T-cell lymphoma and other non-Hodgkin lymphomas (Smedby et al., 2005). However, this risk appears to be much smaller today than it was originally claimed (Ilus, Kaukinen, Virta, Pukkala, & Collin, 2014). The burden of this link may also fall on patients with prolonged villous atrophy and persistently positive celiac serologies, while individuals with really latent CD and mucosal repair may be spared a substantial association, according to current findings (Lebwohl et al., 2013).

Pregnancy

When compared with the general population, women with CD seem to have comparable overall fertility rates (Dhalwani, West, Sultan, Ban, & Tata, 2014; Zugna, Richiardi, Akre, Stephansson, & Ludvigsson, 2010). However, there is some proof that they have their children later in life (Tata et al., 2005) and that individuals with CD may have diminished fertility up to two years before their diagnosis, which suggests that extremely high disease activity may foretell a worse prognosis with regard to fertility (Zugna et al., 2010).

Follow-Up

The rigorous adherence to a GFD as recommended and regular clinical follow-up visits with a doctor and a certified dietician/nutritionist are the cornerstones of celiac disease care. Seroconversion following a GFD should be observed and reaches 95% in patients with systematic 5-year follow-up, as well as clinical response to a GFD and growth in children (Zanini et al., 2010). As mucosal regeneration may take two to three years, endoscopic follow-up is advised beginning about two years following the commencement of a GFD (Rubio-Tapia et al., 2010; Wahab, Meijer, & Mulder, 2002). The monitoring of poor density of bone minerals and dietary deficits is maybe the most crucial extra factor for these individuals. With untreated CD, both are visible. The former appears to become better if a GFD is started, however, the improvement is slow and bone mineral density might not fully return to normal

(Kalayci, Kansu, Girgin, Kucuk, & Aras, 2001). zinc, copper, carnitine, vitamin D, vitamins B_{12} and B_6, folic acid, and iron are a few examples of micronutrients that might be deficient. For people with CD who can tolerate oats, adding oats may help to alleviate some of the vitamin deficits that have been linked to a GFD (TA Kemppainen, Heikkinen, Ristikankare, Kosma, & Julkunen, 2010).

Chapter 9

Animal Models in Unravelling Therapeutic Targets in Celiac Disease

Abstract

Animal models play a crucial role in advancing the understanding of celiac disease (CD) and identifying potential therapeutic targets. This section reviews various animal models used to study CD pathogenesis, focusing on their ability to replicate human-like immune responses to gluten. By using these models, researchers can investigate mechanisms of immune activation, tissue damage, and therapeutic interventions. The chapter explores how these models have contributed to developing novel treatments, such as HLA-DQ2 blockers and immune modulation strategies, providing valuable insights for future therapeutic development in CD management.

Overview of Existing Animal Models

Spontaneous models of gliadin-dependent enteropathy have been documented in rhesus macaques and Irish setters. Both species exhibit characteristics of celiac disease, including partial villus atrophy, elevated intraepithelial lymphocytes, and anti-tissue transglutaminase antibodies (present just in macaques). A recent study reported the emergence of spontaneous inflammatory small bowel illness in horses with partial villus atrophy, which improved following six months of a gluten -free diet. Subsequent to gluten sensitization, alternative animal species, specifically mice and rats, are employed to investigate gluten-dependent enteropathies. Rodent models can be classified as HLA-independent or HLA-dependent. An HLA-independent model was established using the T-cell transfer colitis model, originally designed to study chronic inflammatory bowel disease in the colon (Freitag et al., 2009; Powrie et al., 1994). The adoptive transfer of *in vitro* gliadin-primed CD4+CD45RBlowCD25- T cells into RAG1-/- mice resulted in crypt hyperplasia and villus atrophy following an oral gluten challenge (Freitag et al., 2009). Additionally, Wistar rats administered gluten with intraperitoneal injections of IFN-γ exhibited reduced villus height, elevated TNF-α levels, and increased cellular infiltrates in the small intestine lamina propria (Laparra et al., 2012). This model has not investigated the formation of anti-gliadin or anti-TG2 antibodies. Significantly, HLA-independent models do not facilitate the examination of the involvement of the CD-associated risk alleles HLA-DQ2 and -DQ8, which are present in 90% and 10% of CD patients, respectively.

To achieve this goal, HLA-dependent models have been established. HLA-DQ8 transgenic mice were created by crossing mice expressing human DQ8 with MHCII -/- mice resulting in thymic selection of DQ8 reactive T cells only (Black, Murray, & David, 2002). In these mice, injection of crude gliadin with complete Freund's adjuvant (CFA) in the tail and footpad followed by three weeks of gluten gavage leads to T-cell proliferation, IEL accumulation and anti-gliadin antibodies but no villus atrophy (Black et al., 2002; Verdu et al., 2008). An alternative model was developed by crossing DQ8 mice with NOD mice, conferring them a predisposition to autoimmune diseases (Galipeau et al., 2011). After sensitization by weekly gavage with pepsin trypsin (PT)-digested gliadin and cholera toxin, NOD-DQ8 mice develop a decreased villus/crypt ratio, impaired epithelial barrier, a modest accumulation of IEL at the tip of the villus, and for some mice anti-gliadin (4 out of 11 mice) and anti-TG2 antibodies (3 out of 11 mice) (Galipeau et al., 2011).

Two models featuring mice that express the predominant HLA-DQ2 risk allele have been developed through backcrossing mice that express either DR3-DQ2 genes and human CD4 or DQ2.5 genes on MHCIID/D mice, in conjunction with gliadin-TCRxMHCIID/D transgenic mice, wherein all CD4+ T cells possess a humanized DQ2.5-glia-γ1-specific T-cell receptor (de Kauwe et al., 2009; Du Pré et al., 2011) or DQ2.TCR specific to 5-glia-α2(de Kauwe et al., 2009). Significantly, in these animals, the gliadin-TCR transgenic T cells exhibit proliferation in response to gliadin. Despite the production of anti-gliadin antibodies and T-cell proliferation following oral exposure to chymotrypsin -digested gluten, these mice do not exhibit small intestine enteropathy; instead, they demonstrate tolerance to gliadin (de Kauwe et al., 2009; Du Pré et al., 2011).

Considering the hypothesized function of IL-15 in CD, murine models have been established to examine its participation. In one experiment, DQ8 mice were mated with mice that overexpress IL-15 regulated by the ubiquitous H2-Dd promoter (H2-Dd-IL-15Tg animals) and administered gliadin bi-daily for 10 days (DePaolo et al., 2011). Mice exhibited no intestinal damage; however, they showed elevated serum antigliadin and anti-TG2 antibodies, a heightened frequency of IFN-γ-producing T cells in mesenteric lymph nodes (MLN) and lamina propria, an increase in intraepithelial lymphocytes (IEL), and a compromised generation of Foxp3+ regulatory T cells (Treg) (DePaolo et al., 2011). These modifications were proposed to replicate latent celiac disease, which may occur prior to villous atrophy and manifest celiac disease. The brief exposure of mice to gluten and the absence of IL-15 production in the gut epithelium in this paradigm may elucidate why the animals did not exhibit epithelial damage. This theory is corroborated by data acquired from a second model that is further removed from CD. This model involved crossing OTII mice, which contain ovalbumin (OVA)-specific CD4+ T cells, with mice that produce a soluble version of human IL-15 regulated by a promoter specific to enterocytes (hIL-15Tge mice) (Korneychuk et al., 2014). Chronic exposure to an OVA-containing diet resulted in a significant proportion of OTII+/- hIL-15Tge+ mice exhibiting growth retardation, villus atrophy, and a marked increase of granzyme B-expressing CD8+ T cells in the duodenal mucosa by three months of age, several months prior to the spontaneous enteropathy seen in older IL-15Tge mice (Korneychuk et al., 2014). This model demonstrated that cytokine production by OVA-activated cells synergizes with IL-15 to promote the proliferation of non-cognate cytotoxic CD8+ T cells and the onset of tissue damage (Korneychuk et al., 2014).

Therapeutic Approaches

Avoidance of Immunogenic Encounters

The elevated proline residue abundance in gluten -derived proteins hinders effective breakdown by luminal enzymes, which predominantly lack prolyl-endopeptidase activity. Consequently, to remove substantial immunogenic particles that may migrate from the intestinal lumen to the intestinal lamina propria and provoke the anti-gluten response, oral administration of exogenous prolyl-endopeptidases is a promising strategy (Cerf-Bensussan, Matysiak-Budnik, Cellier, & Heyman, 2007). This was initially evaluated in macaques with gluten-sensitive enteropathy (H. Xu et al., 2013). The oral delivery of the glutamine-specific cysteine endoprotease EP-B2, which effectively degrades gluten *in vitro,* inhibits illness recurrence with the reinstatement of a gluten-containing diet. No clinical relapse occurred over the eight-week study period. However, the macaque produced IgG against gliadin as well as against TG2, an unexpected outcome considering the absence of anti-TG2 antibodies prior to treatment (Bethune et al., 2008). These results constituted the initial indication that oral administration of glutenase might provide therapeutic advantages in gluten-dependent enteropathies. However, investigations of human celiac disease biopsies indicated that EP-B2 did not breakdown gluten fast enough in the duodenal lumen to prevent transepithelial transit of immunogenic peptides (Matysiak–Budnik et al., 2005). To enhance potency, EP-B2 was amalgamated with a prolyl-endopeptidase derived from Sphingomonas capsulate (Gass et al., 2007). In a recent phase two experiment, the glutenase cocktail ALV003 mitigated gluten-induced small intestine mucosal damage in celiac disease patients adhering to a gluten-free diet with daily gluten intake of up to 2 g (Lähdeaho et al., 2014).

The new proposal involves the utilization of non-absorbable polymers that can trap gluten inside the intestinal lumen to inhibit the transfer of immunogenic peptides formed from gluten. BL-7010, a polymer with a strong affinity for gliadin, improved the villus/crypt ratio and reduced the formation of intraepithelial lymphocytes (IEL) in NOD-DQ8 mice that were orally sensitized with a combination of PT-digested gliadin and cholera toxin, followed by four weeks of oral gluten treatment (McCarville et al., 2014). In HLA-DQ8 transgenic mice that were mucosally sensitized with gluten and cholera toxin, and then orally challenged with gluten, the copolymer P(HEMA-co-SS) largely reinstated the intestinal architecture and reduced the production of pro-inflammatory cytokines (Liang, Pinier, Leroux, & Subirade, 2009; Pinier et al., 2012). P(HEMA-co-SS) notably restricted the elevation in intestinal permeability seen in sensitized HLA-DQ8 transgenic mice following gluten exposure (Pinier et al., 2012).

Patients with celiac disease have gluten -induced heightened intestinal permeability, perhaps enabling the transfer of gliadin peptides to the lamina propria (Heyman, Abed, Lebreton, & Cerf-Bensussan, 2012). Inhibiting intestinal permeability may thereby restrict the early exposure of immunogenic peptides to the immune system. Larazotide acetate, a peptide capable of enhancing tight junction construction both *in vitro* and *in vivo,* was evaluated in HLA-DQ8 mice. Mice sensitized intraperitoneally with gliadin and CFA, followed by bi-weekly oral challenges with gliadin for seven weeks, exhibited normalized tissue conductance and improved tight junction structure after treatment with Larazotide acetate (Gopalakrishnan et al., 2012). In asymptomatic celiac disease patients on a gluten-free diet undertaking a gluten challenge, Larazotide acetate shown no significant advantage over placebo

(Kelly et al., 2013; Leffler et al., 2012). In individuals with CD who continue to exhibit symptoms while adhering to a GFD, a 0.5 mg dosage of Larazotide acetate decreased the frequency of symptomatic days, intensity of stomach discomfort, and extraintestinal symptoms relative to placebo (Leffler et al., 2015). The efficacy of fortifying tight junctions in preventing the flow of gluten peptides remains inadequately proved. Other investigations indicate a primary transepithelial transport of gluten peptides (as discussed in Ref. (Heyman et al., 2012). Furthermore, in active celiac disease, fast apico-to-basal transepithelial transport of intact gluten peptides bound to particular secretory IgA has been shown. These complexes bind to the ectopically produced CD71 receptor at the apex of enterocytes and are swiftly transported into the lamina propria (Lebreton et al., 2012; Matysiak-Budnik et al., 2008).

A novel strategy involves using wheat genotypes with less immunogenic properties. Ancient wheat varieties induce reduced proliferation in T-cell clones derived from celiac disease patients compared to contemporary wheat varieties (Øyvind Molberg et al., 2005; Spaenij–Dekking et al., 2005). Consequently, the genetic alteration of wheat strains to produce non-immunogenic wheat is proposed (Anderson, van Heel, Tye-Din, Jewell, & Hill, 2006; Mitea et al., 2010). The removal of the immunogenic a-peptide in Chinese spring wheat (van den Broeck et al., 2009), together with the recent use of RNA interference (Gil-Humanes et al., 2010), resulted in a reduction in T-cell activating epitopes. The diversity of wheat epitopes and the significant variability of the T-cell response to these epitopes challenge the production of non-immunogenic wheat variants. The expansion of polyclonal T-cell lines and T-cell clones derived from CD patients serves as an effective method for assessing reactivity; nevertheless, the cellular specificity may be biased towards immunodominant epitopes, hindering definitive findings about the non-toxicity of ancient wheat strains (Šuligoj, Gregorini, Colomba, Ellis, & Ciclitira, 2013).

Utilizing animal models serves as a valuable method for investigating the toxicity of wheat products. DQ8 transgenic mice were recently employed to assess the safety of non-wheat grain diet in celiac disease patients. Following mucosal vaccination with PT-digested gliadin, the responsiveness of mesenteric lymph node and spleen cells to non-wheat grains was assessed to eliminate stimulatory epitopes (Bergamo et al., 2011).

The potential safety of germinated rye sourdough for ingestion by celiac disease patients was examined in an HLA-independent mouse model of gluten -sensitive enteropathy, wherein memory CD4+ T cells were extracted from C57BL/6 donor mice sensitized at the tail base with secalin in CFA.

Subsequent to the adoptive transfer of secalin-sensitized memory T cells, RAG-/- mice subjected to oral challenges with germinated rye sourdough exhibited comparable duodenitis scores to those challenged with native rye sourdoughs, despite manifesting reduced titers of anti-secalin IgG(Freitag et al., 2014), thereby contesting the incorporation of germinated rye sourdough in products intended for celiac disease patients. This model's value is in facilitating a polyclonal T-cell response, encompassing a broad spectrum of epitopes; nevertheless, it neglects the significance of interactions among gliadin peptides, HLA molecules, and TCR in the pathogenic T-cell response in celiac disease. It would be optimal to replicate this work in an HLA-dependent setting to facilitate the observation of a polyclonal HLA-restricted T-cell response. This is presently achievable just in HLA-DQ8xMHCIID/D transgenic mice, where murine CD4 T cells chosen on human HLA-DQ8 multiply in reaction to gluten. In HLA-DQ2x MHCIID/D transgenic mice, murine CD4+ T cells chosen on human DQ2 do not undergo proliferation until transduced with a human gliadin-specific TCR (de Kauwe et al., 2009).

TG2 as a Therapeutic Target

The deamidation of gliadin peptides by TG2 enhances their binding affinity to HLA-DQ2 and HLA-DQ8, making TG2 a promising therapeutic target. Numerous TG2 inhibitors have been formulated, which are expected to obstruct deamidation, hence diminishing antigen presentation and gliadin-induced T-cell proliferation. The many biological roles of TG2 in cell adhesion, apoptosis, cell differentiation, matrix stability, and transmembrane signaling necessitate comprehensive evaluation to identify potential off-target effects (de Kauwe et al., 2009). TG2-deficient animals exhibit few phenotypic alterations, and continuous administration of dihydroisoxazole inhibitors is non-toxic, suggesting that TG2 activity is non-essential under steady-state circumstances (Sarang et al., 2009). Extracellular TG2 is catalytically inactive in healthy tissues (Siegel et al., 2008), but intraperitoneal administration of TLR3 Poly (I:C) induces enzyme activation in murine small intestine tissue damage (Siegel et al., 2008). At present, TG2 inhibitors have demonstrated the ability to obstruct gliadin-induced proliferation of patient T cells and to inhibit gliadin-induced T-cell activation in tissue segment cultures. Ultimately, assessing the ramifications of these TG2 inhibitors need animal models of tissue damage. At now, only a limited number of models facilitate such evaluations.

Ideally, pharmacodynamic investigations are conducted in a model exhibiting TG2 activation in the upper small intestine following tissue damage (R. Zhou, Wei, Sun, & Tian, 2007). The intraperitoneal injection of Poly (I:C) induces a temporary yet highly repeatable villus atrophy and TG2 activation, and this paradigm has been modified for this purpose (Dafik, Albertelli, Stamnaes, Sollid, & Khosla, 2012). In C57BL/6 mice, efficient suppression of TG2 by the TG2 inhibitor ERW1041E was demonstrated following intraperitoneal administration of 15 and 20 mg/kg Poly (I:C) (Dafik et al., 2012). Treatment with ERW1041E or genetic deletion of the enzyme in mice did not mitigate villus atrophy (Dafik et al., 2012).

The activation of TG2 with *in vivo* gliadin deamidation was examined using HLA-DQ2 -transgenic mice (Du Pré et al., 2011). In this animal, neither Poly (I:C) therapy nor methotrexate stimulated T-cell proliferation in response to gavaged non-deamidated chymotrypsin -digested gluten, while both treatments resulted in villus atrophy (Du Pré et al., 2011). Immunohistochemical staining following the injection of 5-biotinamidopentyl amine (5BP) verified TG2 activation in the small intestine (Du Pré et al., 2011), indicating that the regimens employed with Poly (I:C) and methotrexate therapy may not provoke enough gliadin deamidation to stimulate observable T-cell proliferation (Du Pré et al., 2011). Conversely, intramuscular injection of non-deamidated gliadin effectively stimulated T-cell proliferation, indicating *in situ* deamidation at the injection site (Du Pré et al., 2011). Intramuscular injection caused TG2 activation, as shown by 5BP (Du Pré et al., 2011). Collectively, our results establish a paradigm for testing gliadin deamidation inhibitors by intramuscular injection, utilizing the following proliferation of gliadin-TCRtg T cells *in vivo* as a readout (Du Pré et al., 2011).

It was recently observed that the serine protease inhibitor Elafin inhibited the kinetics of deamidation of the 33-mer gliadin peptide *in vitro* (Galipeau et al., 2014). The potential advantageous effects of Elafin were evaluated *in vivo* in NOD-DQ8 mice (Galipeau et al., 2011). Mice were sensitized through weekly gavage of PT-digested gliadin and cholera toxin for three weeks, followed by a weekly gliadin challenge for two weeks, resulting in moderate enteropathy characterized by diminished barrier function, a reduced villus/crypt ratio, and an increased population of CD3+ IEL at the villi tips (Galipeau et al., 2011). The administration of recombinant Elafin via Lactococcus lactis 24 hours post-oral sensitization mitigated intestinal barrier failure and maintained zonula occludens protein-1 expression (Galipeau et al., 2014). This intriguing technique has yet to provide data on the activational state of TG2 *in situ* or demonstrate if Elafin inhibits gliadin 33-mer deamidation *in vivo*.

Targeting the Innate Arm of the Immune System and APC

After gliadin peptides penetrate the lamina propria and undergo deamidation, their absorption by HLA-expressing antigen-presenting cells is a critical step in initiating the immunological cascade that leads to celiac disease. Inhibiting HLA molecules is a compelling strategy for avoiding the start of CD. Prototypical HLA-DQ2 inhibitors, developed from the structure of the immunogenic 33-mer gliadin peptide, effectively restrict the gliadin-induced proliferation of T-cell clones derived from celiac disease patients (Xia et al., 2007; Xia et al., 2006). So far, these inhibitors have only been examined using *in vitro* systems, measuring the proliferation of T-cell clones derived from CD patients or lymph node T cells of gliadin-sensitized HLA-DQ8 mice (Black et al., 2002). To consider these compounds as viable therapies, their safety and efficacy must be evaluated *in vivo,* and both HLA-DQ2 and -DQ8 transgenic mice may serve as appropriate models for this purpose.

Besides their function in antigen presentation, antigen-presenting cells (APCs) guide the T-cell response to gliadin by supplying costimulatory cytokines that promote the development of pathogenic T cells. Gliadin induces proinflammatory cytokine production by monocyte-derived dendritic cells (DC) from celiac disease patients and murine bone marrow-derived DC (De Palma et al., 2012; Di Sabatino et al., 2007; Maiuri et al., 2003; Palová-Jelínková et al., 2013). The actual role of gliadin in stimulating proinflammatory cytokine production by antigen-presenting cells is contentious, as the purity of gliadin preparations does not eliminate the possibility of endotoxin contamination, which may explain the induction of proinflammatory cytokines. Nonetheless, the activation of antigen-presenting cells correlates with pathogenic T-cell activation in individuals with Crohn's disease, suggesting that inhibiting APC activation or enhancing their regulatory function may effectively prevent disease development. Cyclooxygenase-2 (Cox-2), an enzyme produced by dendritic cells (DCs), appears to play a role in maintaining small intestine homeostasis in response to dietary antigens (Newberry, Stenson, & Lorenz, 1999). In transgenic mice with T cells expressing a TCR specific for hen egg white lysozyme (HEL), inhibition of Cox-2 through indomethacin treatment induced small intestinal pathology, including crypt hyperplasia and villus blunting, following HEL administration. This phenomenon was similarly observed in HLA-DQ8 mice after the intragastric delivery of chymotrypsin-digested gliadin (D'Arienzo et al., 2009).

To effectively target APC in CD, it is essential to identify the specific APC responsible for the digestion and presentation of gliadin to T cells. Macrophages possess superior breakdown capacity relative to dendritic cells; yet, dendritic cells have demonstrated exceptional efficacy in delivering peptides to T cells. Macrophages expressing CX3CR1 have lately been recognized as the lamina propria population capable of absorbing ovalbumin (OVA)(Mazzini, Massimiliano, Penna, & Rescigno, 2014). The presentation of OVA to T lymphocytes was subsequently conducted by CD103+ dendritic cells following the transfer of the OVA peptide by CX3CR1 macrophages (Mazzini et al., 2014). This work was conducted in a situation of preserved epithelial barrier function with an intraluminal peptide. In celiac disease, the compromised epithelial barrier permits gliadin fragments to migrate to the lamina propria, where both macrophages and dendritic cells are located. Therefore, these findings cannot be generalized to gliadin, and investigations conducted in gluten -dependent enteropathies, ideally in an HLA-dependent manner, are necessary to address this inquiry.

Re-Establishment of Tolerance to Gliadin

The violation of tolerance to gliadin results in the phenotypic characteristics of celiac disease. Comprehending how persons with HLA-DQ2 and HLA-DQ8 develop tolerance to gliadin is crucial for reinstating tolerance to gliadin in patients. In the 1970s, it was proven that a single administration of gliadins to mice raised on a gluten -free diet is sufficient to suppress immunization-induced immunoglobulin G antibody responses and systemic delayed-type hypersensitivity (Troncone & Ferguson, 1991). Recent patient research sought to tolerate newborns at risk for celiac disease with a daily dose of 100 mg of gluten administered between 16 and 24 weeks of life (Vriezinga et al., 2014). The introduction of little amounts of gluten did not diminish the likelihood of celiac disease by the age of three. Regrettably, due to the absence of immunological measures indicative of active oral tolerance development, this study cannot now ascertain whether the introduction of gluten had advantageous immunological consequences. This instance illustrates the necessity for biological markers that indicate active oral tolerance induction to gluten, with animal models serving as a crucial instrument to meet this requirement.

In the small intestine, Treg and CD4$^+$ Foxp3neg IL-10 secreting CD4$^+$ T cells (Tr1-like cells) are the two principal subpopulations of suppressive CD4$^+$ T cells that contribute to the maintenance of local homeostasis. Both cell types provide evidence for a potential function in oral tolerance to gluten. In NOD-DQ8 mice, partial Treg depletion with anti-CD25 therapy before sensitization did not exacerbate intestinal disease despite inducing diabetes (Galipeau et al., 2011). The temporary and inadequate nature of Treg depletion precludes the conclusion that Treg are not implicated in oral tolerance to gliadin. In contrast, augmenting Treg populations in a model utilizing L. lactis for oral gliadin delivery in NOD-DQ8 mice resulted in systemic hypo-responsiveness to gliadin delayed-type hypersensitivity, diminished antigen-specific proliferation of lamina propria lymphocytes, and elevated Treg frequency in the spleen and mesenteric lymph nodes (Huibregtse et al., 2009). Furthermore, the inhibition of proliferation seems to rely on IL-10 and TGF-β (Huibregtse et al., 2009). Given that the majority of trials in this investigation utilized non-purified cells and lacked cellular depletions, the protective function of Treg or Tr1-like cells has to be clarified.

Targeting IL-15: Reducing Epithelial Damage and IEL Infiltration

IL-15 is believed to synergize with gluten -specific T cells to enhance the survival, proliferation, and activation of cytotoxic intraepithelial lymphocytes (IEL) that target and lyse epithelial cells, while also promoting the formation of lymphoma from IEL. Two animal models have been established to examine the interaction between CD4+ T cells and IL-15: hIL-15Tge mice and H2-Dd-IL-15Tg mice. Only H2-Dd-IL-15Tg mice allow the examination of the response to gluten. In these animals, oral administration of gluten does not provoke enteropathy but results in an enhanced T helper-1 response to gluten, indicating compromised oral tolerance to gluten (DePaolo et al., 2011). These animals may thus be useful for assessing the feasibility of re-inducing tolerance through IL-15 overexpression. IL-15 transgenic mice are valuable for evaluating therapeutic interventions aimed at preventing the growth of intraepithelial lymphocytes, particularly malignant IELs invading the gut epithelium in patients with type II refractory celiac disease (CD). This serious consequence of CD is characterized by the proliferation of clonal IELs, which initially manifests as a low-grade intraepithelial lymphoma but can progress into invasive lymphoma (Malamut, Meresse, Cellier, & Cerf-Bensussan, 2012). The spontaneous emergence of NK or CD8+ leukemias in H2-Dd-IL-15Tg mice clearly suggests a causal role for IL-15 (Fehniger et al., 2001). Methods to inhibit human IL-15 signaling have been evaluated in hIL-15Tge mice. These animals have significant intestinal CD8+ T cell infiltration, particularly in the epithelium, and ultimately, with age, manifest epithelial lesions and villus sloughing. Treatment of hIL-15Tge mice with antibodies that inhibit human IL-15, the β chain of its receptor, or with Tofacitinib, a Janus kinase 3 inhibitor, eliminated CD8 infiltration and facilitated epithelial recovery, thereby justifying the application of IL-15 blocking drugs in type II refractory CD (Malamut et al., 2012).

Chapter 10

Food and Gluten-Free Product Development

Abstract

The gluten-free market has seen significant growth, with new innovations in gluten-free foods aimed at improving nutritional quality and taste. This chapter explores the role of food hydrocolloids and alternative cereal flours in gluten-free baking. It also discusses the nutritional challenges of gluten-free products, including the risk of nutrient deficiencies. Additionally, the chapter addresses the economic aspects of gluten-free food production, compliance with regulatory guidelines, and the growing demand for gluten-free products that meet the dietary needs of individuals with celiac disease.

Gluten Replacement in Baked Foods: Food Hydrocolloids

The increasing prevalence of CD, the expense of refined wheat flour, and consumers' pursuit of health-enhancing foods have compelled the food industry to create gluten -free (GF) goods (Irondi, Imam, & Ajani, 2022; Ronie, Mamat, Abdul Aziz, & Zainol, 2023). CD is a chronic immunoglobulin E-mediated enteropathy triggered by the ingestion of gluten-containing foods in genetically predisposed individuals (Mir, Shah, Naik, & Zargar, 2016; Theodoridis et al., 2019). The sole recognized effective treatment for CD is a lifelong, stringent avoidance of gluten-containing foods (Lamacchia, Camarca, Picascia, Di Luccia, & Gianfrani, 2014). Conversely, GF goods are deemed safe for those with CD (Cristina M Rosell, Barro, Sousa, & Mena, 2014). In the formulation of GF products, various substances, including food hydrocolloids (FHs), are utilized as alternatives for gluten to replicate its viscoelastic properties. The Codex Alimentarius Commission (Commission, 2008) classified GF products as "food products containing less than 20 mg/kg of gluten." GF goods were originally designed for individuals with gluten-related diseases, including CD, wheat allergies, non-celiac gluten sensitivity, gluten ataxia, and exercise-induced anaphylaxis (Khairuddin & Lasekan, 2021). Nonetheless, due to the escalating price of wheat, the prevalence of other nutrition -related non-communicable diseases, and consumer demand for healthier meals, GF products are now extensively adopted (Irondi et al., 2022; Parenti, Guerrini, & Zanoni, 2020). Nonetheless, the creation of high-quality GF-baked goods presents a considerable barrier to the food industry, owing to the lack of gluten, which imparts distinctive viscoelastic qualities to the dough (Mir et al., 2016). Diverse components, including GF cereal flours and additives that replicate the viscoelastic qualities of gluten, such as hydrocolloids, are used to address this difficulty in the manufacture of GF products (Filipčev, Pojić, Šimurina, Mišan, & Mandić, 2021; Mir et al., 2016).

Food hydrocolloids, sometimes referred to as gums, are a category of high-molecular-weight polysaccharides and proteins that function as ingredients in the food business, altering the rheological and textural characteristics of food. They serve as stabilizers, viscosity modifiers, gelling agents, water binders, fibers, and ice crystal inhibitors in food products (Filipčev et al., 2021; Horstmann, Axel, & Arendt, 2018; Manzoor, Singh, Bandral, Gani, & Shams, 2020; Mir et al., 2016). Examples of FHs used as gluten substitutes in baked goods include agar, acacia, locust bean gum, guar gum, pectin, tara, xanthan gum, and carboxymethylcellulose. The effects of FHs on the quality of gluten-free (GF) baked goods vary depending on factors such as the FH's charge, molecular weight, and concentration. Horstmann et al., (2018) utilized six different hydrocolloids - guar gum, locust bean gum, hydroxypropyl methylcellulose, pectin, xanthan gum, and sodium alginate - under optimal conditions as gluten substitutes in potato starch-based gluten-free bread. The researchers observed an increase in bread volume, which was attributed to the incorporation of negatively charged FHs, including pectin and sodium alginate. They proposed that these negatively charged FHs create repulsive forces with the negatively charged phosphate groups of potato starch, thereby inhibiting the pasting and gelatinization of the starch granules. This effect reduces starch viscosity, leading to increased bread volume due to enhanced gas cell expansion. Conversely, high-molecular-weight FHs with a neutral charge, such as locust bean and guar gums, do not generate such repulsive forces. The authors (Horstmann et al., 2018) posited that the reduced bread volume associated with the incorporation of these neutrally-charged high-molecular weight FHs was due to the formation of many hydrogen bonds with leached amylose, leading to elevated viscosity values. As a result, the dough's flexibility was diminished due to elevated viscosity levels, restricting gas cell expansion and thus resulting in a reduced bread volume. The incorporation of FHs as a substitute for gluten in food systems imparts various health benefits, including the reduction of postprandial blood glucose and plasma cholesterol levels, prevention of colon cancer, and modification of intestinal transit and satiety (Fratelli et al., 2021; Irondi et al., 2022; Manzoor et al., 2020). These advantages are essential in light of the rising incidence of nutrition -related non-communicable diseases, attributed to nutritional transition among other variables (Ford, Patel, & Narayan, 2017; Raj, 2020). The nutrition transition delineates the progression from natural foods to highly processed, energy-dense foods (Ford et al., 2017; Islam et al., 2021).

Cereal Flours in Baked Foods: Wheat versus GF Cereals

Refined wheat flour is the benchmark for manufacturing baked goods like bread and biscuits. Nonetheless, these foods are generally energy-dense, containing minimal critical nutrients and health-enhancing bioactive compounds (Irondi et al., 2022; Parenti et al., 2020). Refined flour is created by grinding solely the starchy endosperm, after the removal of the bran, which contains a high concentration of phytochemicals, and the germ. The functional superiority of refined wheat flour compared to gluten -free cereal flours in baked goods is ascribed to gluten (Irondi et al., 2022; Parenti et al., 2020). Moreover, aside from inducing CD in predisposed individuals, the sustainability of utilizing refined wheat for baking is compromised by its elevated cost in nations reliant on wheat imports for their baking sector. A recent analysis by Qu (Dongyu, 2022) indicates that the price of wheat surged by 31% as a result of COVID-19-related variables, including heightened demand, elevated shipping costs, and port interruptions. The economic strain from elevated wheat prices has intensified recently due to the Ukraine-Russian conflict, as Ukraine constitutes approximately 12% of world wheat exports (T. Lang & McKee, 2022).

To create gluten -free items with health-enhancing attributes, numerous studies have concentrated on developing baked goods using gluten-free cereal flour (X. Z. Hu et al., 2011; Irondi et al., 2022; Pessanha et al., 2021; Santos, Aguiar, Rosell, & Capriles, 2021). Various gluten-free cereals utilized for this purpose comprise sorghum (*Sorghum bicolor* (L.) *Moench*), maize (*Zea mays* L.), rice (*Oryza sativa* L.), millets, teff, and several pseudocereals, including amaranth, quinoa, and buckwheat (Aguiar, Santos, Centeno, & Capriles, 2022; Khairuddin & Lasekan, 2021). Several studies have identified oats as a gluten-free cereal (I. S. Cohen, Day, & Shaoul, 2019; El Khoury, Balfour-Ducharme, & Joye, 2018; Fajardo et al., 2020), although the Codex Alimentarius categorizes them as a gluten-containing cereal (Rai, Kaur, & Chopra, 2018).

The flours from these gluten-free cereals are utilized either independently or in combination for the production of gluten-free baked goods (Aguiar et al., 2022). Nonetheless, the manufacture of high-quality gluten-free goods from these gluten-free grains presents a significant challenge to the food industry, owing to the lack of gluten (Mir et al., 2016). The proteins in the flours of these gluten-free cereals are incapable of forming a network, thereby failing to satisfy the baking quality standards (Salehi, 2019). As a result, their GF products exhibit a compact and arid structure, minimal volume, subpar mouthfeel and flavor, and elevated crumb hardness, culminating in an overall worse quality (Zoghi, Mirmahdi, & Mohammadi, 2021).

The Role of Gluten in Baked Foods

Gluten is the primary structural protein found in wheat, barley, and rye, imparting viscoelastic characteristics to dough and enabling the retention of gas generated by yeast fermentation, facilitating oven rise during baking (Houben, Höchstötter, & Becker, 2012; Salehi, 2019). It also influences the final baked products' appearance and crumb structure (Zoghi et al., 2021). Gliadins and glutenins constitute the two categories of gluten. The former is a monomeric protein, while the latter is a polymeric protein. The principal function of gluten in baking is to provide a viscoelastic characteristic to the dough, mostly facilitated by the action of gliadins (Espinosa-Ramirez, Garzon, Serna-Saldivar, & Rosell, 2018). It has been recorded that the gluten network is established in the presence of water and through mechanical action, facilitated by the interaction of gliadin and glutenin proteins in wheat (Rai et al., 2018).

Gluten facilitates the proofing of baked goods, such as bread loaves, and enhances the quality of baked items (Skendi, Papageorgiou, & Varzakas, 2021). During baking, refined wheat flour is moistened, resulting in the development of a viscous mass due to its gluten content. This imparts viscosity, structure, mixing tolerance, dough consistency, and gas retention during leavening (Morreale, Garzón, & Rosell, 2018). Gluten can encapsulate flour components, including fibers and starch granules, through the created structure (Gallagher, Gormley, & Arendt, 2004). Consequently, the absence of gluten adversely affects the rheology of the dough and the quality of the final result, as gluten-free doughs exhibit diminished elasticity and cohesiveness compared to wheat dough (Cappelli, Oliva, & Cini, 2020). The color, texture, alveolar structure, and crumb of baked goods are predominantly influenced by the presence and strength of gluten (Laignier et al., 2022; Lamacchia et al., 2014).

Food Hydrocolloids as Gluten Replacement in GF-Baked Foods

Hydrocolloids are a type of polysaccharides (either water-soluble, food-grade, or modified) or proteins with diverse chemical structures, which account for their functional properties, capacity to form gels when dispersed in water, and applications in the food business (J. M. Li & Nie, 2016; Nautiyal, 2011; Cristina M Rosell, Collar, & Haros, 2007). Numerous roles have been ascribed to FHs as gluten substitutes in the food business, either independently or in combination with other food components. These encompass thickening, gelling, emulsifying, dispersing, and stabilizing actions (X. Yang, Li, Li, Sun, & Guo, 2020). In addition to serving as a gluten alternative, they can also function as food additives to enhance qualities such as shelf-life and flavor (Nautiyal, 2011; Saha & Bhattacharya, 2010). Seisun & Zalesny (Seisun & Zalesny, 2021) recently characterized hydrocolloids as "essential and critical ingredients in food" due to their varied functions in food systems. Incorporating FHs is the most straightforward method to enhance the nutritional fiber content in GF goods.

The principal food hydrocolloids include alginates, agar, acacia, cassia tora, gelatin, carrageenan, gellan, locust bean gum, guar gum, pectin, tara, starches, xanthan, carboxymethylcellulose, methyl cellulose/hydroxypropyl methyl cellulose (MC/HPMC), and microcrystalline cellulose (MCC). Alongside these principal food hydrocolloids, karaya, tragacanth, konjac, pullulan, tamarind, and scleroglucan are some of the less prevalent food hydrocolloids (Seisun & Zalesny, 2021). Numerous studies discuss the use of these functional hydrocolloids as gluten substitutes, including xanthan gum, guar gum, hydroxypropyl methyl cellulose (HPMC), carrageenan, agar, and alginate (Rhein-Knudsen & Meyer, 2021). The exact intrinsic processes governing the interactions between functional hydrocolloids (FHs) and other dietary ingredients, as well as among different FHs, remain insufficiently understood (Zhiming Gao et al., 2017; Lu, Nishinari, Matsukawa, & Fang, 2020). Naji-Tabasi and Mohebbi (2015) suggested that FHs enhance the cohesiveness of starch granules, thereby facilitating the production of gluten-free baked goods, such as bread.

Natural Food Hydrocolloids Used in GF-Baked Foods

Natural flavoring agents have been extensively employed in the food sector to enhance the functionality of items such as confectionery, beverages, meat and poultry, sauces, and dressings (Yemenicioglu, Farris, Turkyilmaz, & Gulec, 2020). The categorization of natural FHs is predicated on their chemical structures, behaviors, and origins (Salehi, 2019). Natural food hydrocolloids originate from several sources, including microbial (e.g., xanthan gum), plant (e.g., starch, pectin, locust bean gum, and carrageenan), and animal (e.g., chitosan) (Irondi, Imam, Ajani, & Alamu). They are categorized into many categories based on the source, including microbial gums, seed gums, exudate gums, seaweed gums, mucilage gums, and tuber gums, among others (Barak, Mudgil, & Taneja, 2020). Nonetheless, plant materials constitute the primary and more economical sources of natural FHs (Irondi, Imam, & Ajani, 2021; Yemenicioglu et al., 2020).

Natural FHs were regarded as a more economical substitute for gluten compared to modified FHs, due to their availability and cost-effectiveness (Irondi et al., 2021). In this regard, several studies have explored their use as a gluten substitute in baked goods. Soulef et al., (Benkadri, Salvador, Zidoune, & Sanz, 2018) documented the use of xanthan gum to create a gluten-free biscuit from a rice-chickpea flour mixture. Naji-Tabasi and Mohebbi (Naji-Tabasi & Mohebbi, 2015) also produced gluten-free bread using a blend of rice flour, maize flour, and corn starch, supplemented with cress seed gum and xanthan gum at a concentration of 1% (W/W). Irondi et al., (Irondi et al., 2021) presented a trial in which gluten-free bread was prepared using a mixture of whole pearl millet flour and Brachystegia eurycoma flour. In a corresponding study, Irondi et al., (Irondi et al., 2022) made gluten-free bread utilizing sweet detar (Detarium microcarpum) and whole pearl millet flour. Filipčev et al., (Filipčev et al., 2021) additionally documented the use of psyllium in gluten-free buckwheat/carob bread. Psyllium was also used with chickpea in the manufacture of gluten-free bread by Santos et al., (Santos et al., 2021), in combination with cassava starch and rice flour. Okra powder, known for its mucilage content, primarily pectin (dos Santos, de Figueirêdo, Queiroz, de Lima, & Moreira, 2019), has also been utilized in the production of gluten-free bread (Tufaro, Bassoli, & Cappa, 2022).

Reports have also highlighted the use of natural animal-derived FHs in baking. Lieke et al., (van Riemsdijk, van der Goot, Hamer, & Boom, 2011) and Marina et al., (Komeroski et al., 2021) indicated that whey protein was used in gluten-free bread. A mixture of various natural food hydrocolloids (guar gum, gum acacia, gum tragacanth, and xanthan) incorporated into buckwheat flour was utilized in the preparation of a gluten-free biscuit, as noted by Maninder et al., (Kaur, Sandhu, Arora, & Sharma, 2015). Additionally, Ejet et al., (Andrade et al., 2018) prepared a gluten-free cake using fava bean, galactomannan, and xanthan gum. An infant biscuit was made from rice-chickpea flour by integrating locust bean and xanthan gum (Benkadri, Salvador, Sanz, & Nasreddine Zidoune, 2020).

Modified Food Hydrocolloids Used in GF-Baked Foods

Modified food hydrocolloids represent an alternative category of FHs employed as gluten substitutes in GF baked products. They are generated either via natural hydrocolloid derivatization and selective chemical modification (Milani & Maleki, 2012) or through physical and enzymatic treatments (Seisun & Zalesny, 2021). The most often utilized modified FHs comprise methylcellulose (MC), carboxymethylcellulose, hydroxypropyl methylcellulose, and hydroxyethyl cellulose (HEC) (Milani & Maleki, 2012). They are cellulose derivatives (cellulose ethers) produced through chemical modification (Irondi et al.; Milani & Maleki, 2012). Among these modified FHs, HPMC is the most utilized and is recognized as the most advantageous hydrocolloid in GF bread production (Cappelli et al., 2020). It is synthesized via the reaction of methyl chloride and propylene oxide with alkali cellulose (BeMiller, 2018).

Several obstacles, including cost (Ohimain, 2014), manufacturing process (Adedeji, Alakali, Adewale, & Ngadi, 2012), and availability and demand (Nwokocha & Williams, 2012), restrict the application of modified FHs in the baking process. Nevertheless, akin to natural FHs, numerous researchers have utilized modified FHs as a gluten alternative in baked goods. Tabrizi et al., (Nwokocha & Williams, 2012). recently employed HPMC in the baking of GF bread. Additionally, Sadeghnia et al., (Sadegh Nia, Azizi, Seyedin Ardebili, & Mohammadi, 2016). employed CMC to manufacture GF bread. In a separate investigation, sodium-CMC was combined with whole pearl millet flour at two ratios (1.5% and 3% by weight) to generate GF bread (Irondi et al., 2021, 2022). Baldino et al., (Baldino, Laitano, Lupi, Curcio, & Gabriele, 2018). utilized HPMC and CMC to prepare gluten-free bread from rice and buckwheat. Additional research that documented the application of modified FHs in baked products encompass Hager & Arendt (Hager & Arendt, 2013),

Ronda et al., (Hager & Arendt, 2013). Liu et al., (X. Liu et al., 2019). and Belorio & Gomez (Belorio & Gómez, 2020).

Functional Benefits of Natural and Modified Hydrocolloids in GF-Baked Foods

The functional advantages, encompassing physicochemical, nutraceutical, and sensory significance, of natural and modified hydrocolloids in gluten -free baked goods are detailed in the subsequent sections.

Physicochemical Importance of Natural and Modified Hydrocolloids in GF-Baked Foods

The incorporation of FHs (natural and modified) in baked GF products has been documented as significant in terms of physicochemical properties. The FHs, by emulating the viscoelastic characteristics of gluten, influence the physicochemical properties of GF flours and their derivatives, including bread (Irondi et al., 2021, 2022), cake (Andrade et al., 2018), and biscuits (Irondi et al.). The use of Brachystegia eurycoma and Detarium microcarpum flour, both underutilized legume sources of hydrocolloids, into pearl millet flour has been shown to enhance the physicochemical and pasting qualities of the resultant gluten-free flour (Irondi et al., 2021, 2022). FHs enhance dough stability by augmenting viscosity, coalescence, and flocculation (Dickinson, 2010). The ability of FHs to enhance viscosity is recognized for its potential to improve dough development, gas retention, and the quality of GF bread (Capriles & Arêas, 2014).

In the research conducted by Mariotti et al., (Mariotti, Pagani, & Lucisano, 2013). The presence of HPMC restricted water loss in the bread crumb, as well as the diffusion and interactions of starch and protein macromolecules. It also diminished the staling kinetics of the GF bread during storage. Additional research has demonstrated that FHs are essential in the formulation of GF-baked items throughout dough preparation, battering, baking, or in the final products. Additional functional significance encompasses altering dough behavior, enhancing internal structure, augmenting porosity, and diminishing the strength and extensibility of the 3D network in the baked product (Baldino et al., 2018). They also enhance the water absorption of GF dough and goods (Correa, Añon, Perez, & Ferrero, 2010; X. Liu et al., 2018), potentially attributable to the hydroxyl groups in the structures of functional hydrocolloids (Cristima M Rosell, Rojas, & De Barber, 2001). Nevertheless, certain research confirmed that the incorporation of FHs enhanced the hardness of GF products. Shahzad et al., (Shahzad et al., 2020). determined that both commercial and unconventional food hydrocolloids (xanthan gum, gum Arabic, fenugreek, cress seed, okra, and flaxseed) enhanced the hardness of gluten -free cookies produced from Turkish bean and sorghum flours. Furthermore, two other investigations (Devisetti, Ravi, & Bhattacharya, 2015; Gül, Hayit, Acun, & Tekeli, 2018) indicated that the incorporation of guar and xanthan gums in millet flour, as well as xanthan gum in GF flour, resulted in enhanced hardness. The augmented hardness of the GF product resulting from the incorporation of FHs has been attributed to the hydrocolloids' ability to retain significant amounts of free water (Shahzad et al., 2020). Gul et al., (Gül et al., 2018). ascribed the enhanced hardness of the GF product resulting from xanthan gum incorporation to the "highly branched structure of xanthan," which facilitates its interaction with other components to form associations. Moreover, Shahzad et al., (Shahzad et al., 2020). shown that using non-conventional (fenugreek, cress seed, okra, flaxseed) and commercial (xanthan gum) functional hydrocolloids led to a reduction in the pasting temperature of blends based on Turkish bean flour and sorghum flour. The study concluded that the water activity, moisture, and fiber content of GF crackers produced from hydrocolloid-substituted blends increased.

Certain research has indicated that the incorporation of FHs reduces the specific volume of GF-baked goods, including cookies, cakes, and breads. Ostermann-Porcel et al., (Ostermann-Porcel, Quiroga-Panelo, Rinaldoni, & Campderrós, 2017). reported that the specific volume of gluten -free cookies diminished with an increase in the substitution amount of okara flour. Yildiz & Dogan (Yildiz & Dogan, 2014) documented a reduction in the specific volume of GF cake made with a combination of chestnut flour and potato starch in another trial. The reduction in specific volume is ascribed to the fibers' ability to affect gas retention and structure, thereby impeding the dough (Mohammadi, Khorshidian, Yousefi, & Khaneghah, 2022). Moreover, the incorporation of xanthan gum led to a reduction in the volume of GF bread (Hager & Arendt, 2013) and GF flatbread (Mohammadi, Sadeghnia, Azizi, Neyestani, & Mortazavian, 2014). The reduction in GF breads was attributed to the thickening action of xanthan gum, which diminished gas diffusion in air cells during baking, thereby hindering gas expansion (Noorlaila, Hasanah, Asmeda, & Yusoff, 2020).

Additionally, the anti-staling properties of hydrocolloids in GF baked goods have been documented. Filipcev and his colleagues (Filipčev et al., 2021) confirmed that the incorporation of psyllium exhibited a significant anti-staling effect on gluten -free bread made with a composite of buckwheat and carob flour. A comparable study indicated that using psyllium husk powder at doses of 2.86%, 7.14%, and 17.14% in rice flour-based GF bread formulations delayed bread staling (Fratelli et al., 2021). The researchers noted that the integration of 17.14% psyllium husk powder resulted in the most prolonged delay in bread staling and enhanced the bread's structure. Wronkowska et al., (Wronkowska, Haros, & Soral-Śmietana, 2013). observed a delayed staling of GF bread when buckwheat was augmented with commercial maize starch, potato starch, and pectin. The delay in staling was attributed to the development of complexes between the emulsifiers and amylose, which restricted the swelling, leaching, and subsequent retrogradation of starch (Wronkowska et al., 2013). The anti-staling properties of hydrocolloids are attributed to their ability to hold water, hence restricting water redistribution within starchy matrices (Sozer, Bruins, Dietzel, Franke, & Kokini, 2011). Some researchers have asserted that the impact of psyllium on the quality of GF bread is contingent upon the water content, the interaction between psyllium and water, and its significant potential to form complexes with proteins through ionic and non-ionic bonding. Consequently, the strength of GF bread dough and the quality of its crumb are influenced (Filipčev et al., 2021; Santos, Aguiar, Centeno, Rosell, & Capriles, 2020; Wronkowska et al., 2013).

Nutraceutical Benefits of Natural and Modified Food Hydrocolloids in GF-Baked Foods

In addition to their physicochemical significance, FHs impart nutraceutical and health-enhancing attributes to GF-baked products (Goff & Guo, 2019). The health-promoting attributes encompass immunological modulation, weight management, reduction of postprandial blood glucose and plasma cholesterol levels, colon cancer prevention, and cardiovascular disease protection. Additional health benefits linked to FHs include insulin and glycemic regulation in type 2 diabetes, decreased risk of osteoporosis, and modulation of intestinal transit and satiety (Bosscher, Van Loo, & Franck,

2006; Fratelli et al., 2021; Irondi et al., 2022; J. M. Li & Nie, 2016; Manzoor et al., 2020). The nutraceutical advantages of FHs are mostly ascribed to their chemical composition (Manzoor et al., 2020). Irondi et al., (2022) showed that including sweet detar flour (a natural hydrocolloid) at a concentration of 1.5% in whole pearl millet GF flour significantly enhanced the inhibition of starch-digesting enzymes (α-amylase and α-glucosidase) activity compared to the native pearl millet flour. Liu et al., (2018) found that the incorporation of HPMC, CMC, xanthan gum, and apple pectin substantially reduced the levels of rapidly digested starch and the estimated glycemic index of potato flour-based GF bread compared to control bread. The ability of hydrocolloids to reduce the glycemic index of GF food is attributed to their tendency to form a barrier around starch granules, which subsequently slows their hydrolysis by starch-hydrolyzing enzymes (α-amylase and α-glucosidase). As a result, this reduces the quantity of absorbable monosaccharides (Chung HyunJung, Liu Qiang, & Lim SeungTaik, 2007; X. Liu et al., 2018).

The nutraceutical advantages of FHs in GF-baked goods extend beyond the aforementioned studies, as their incorporation also influences further health-enhancing attributes of the GF products. Shahzad et al., (Shahzad et al., 2020). demonstrated that using cress seed gum enhanced the antioxidant activity in GF cookies produced from Turkish bean and sorghum flours. A unique GF bread including maize starch, pectin, and potato starch, enhanced with flaxseed oil cake extract, demonstrated superior antioxidant capacity compared to the control (Krupa-Kozak, Bączek, Capriles, & Łopusiewicz, 2022). Mishra et al., (S. Mishra, Sinha, Dey, & Sen, 2014). showed that the use of psyllium gum in GF bread, owing to its bulking properties, produced a laxative effect. This may mitigate the risk of osteoporosis, enhance bowel function (Bárcenas & Rosell, 2006), avoid colon cancer, coronary heart disease, type 2 diabetes (X. Z. Hu et al., 2011), and alleviate constipation.

FHs provide dietary fiber in GF products (BeMiller, 2018). A recent investigation by Ronie et al., (Ronie et al., 2023). demonstrated that Bario rice (red-pigmented) flour-based GF bread with 30% potato starch had a greater fiber content than its wheat bread counterpart. The elevated dietary fiber content and their function as prebiotics in GF baked goods foster a healthy gastrointestinal system. The consumption of specific functional foods may augment the proliferation of beneficial bacteria like lactobacillus and bifidobacterium, therefore modulating the makeup of gut microbiota. The simultaneous rise in the fermentative activity of intestinal bacterial flora and the synthesis of short-chain fatty acids (Viebke, Al-Assaf, & Phillips, 2014) may enhance their related effects on cell proliferation, angiogenesis, and apoptosis modulation (J. M. Li & Nie, 2016).

Sensorial Importance of Natural and Modified Hydrocolloids in GF-Baked Foods

By altering their rheological properties, FHs enhance the sensory attributes of baked goods (J. M. Li & Nie, 2016). Moreover, the interaction between protein and sugar during baking induces the Maillard reaction and the creation of its products, accompanied by a color shift (Mohammadi et al., 2022). Consequently, attaining an optimal sensory acceptability poses a significant difficulty in the development of GF baked products (J. Xu, Zhang, Wang, & Li, 2020). Nonetheless, although consumers choose refined wheat products (Parenti et al., 2020), their adoption of GF items derived from GF cereals has been associated with the health advantages attributed to GF products (Irondi et al., 2022). Several research investigations have reported the impact of FHs on the sensory attributes of baked goods. Thejasri et al., (Irondi et al., 2022) examined the sensory attributes of gluten-free (GF) biscuits made with foxtail millet (*Setaria italica*) and quinoa (*Chenopodium quinoa* Willd.), supplemented with guar and xanthan gums. The researchers found that the incorporation of 1% guar and xanthan gums significantly enhanced the sensory qualities of both foxtail millet and quinoa biscuits (Irondi et al., 2022). Kaur et al., (Kaur et al., 2015) discovered that adding xanthan gum to buckwheat flour biscuits notably improved their color, texture, flavor, and overall acceptability. Additionally, the inclusion of galactomannan and xanthan gum improved the sensory attributes of GF cakes made from fava (*Phaseolus lunatus*) beans (Andrade et al., 2018). Furthermore, flours from *Detarium microcarpum* and *Brachystegia eurycoma* have been shown to enhance the sensory characteristics of GF bread made from whole pearl millet (Irondi et al., 2021, 2022).

A GF bread made with rice flour instead of sweet potato flour and 2% CMC had sensory attributes that were on par with those made without CMC (Franco, Garcia, & SILVA, 2020). A separate study indicated that substituting 6% of rice flour and starch with amaranth in rice flour: corn starch and rice flour: tapioca-based flatbread enhanced the bread's color (Piga et al., 2021). Additionally, Shahzad et al., (Shahzad et al., 2020). examined the effects of various non-conventional (fenugreek, cress seed, okra, flaxseed) and commercial (xanthan gum and gum Arabic) hydrocolloids on the sensory attributes of GF cookies formulated with Turkish beans and sorghum. They established that cookies using okra and gum Arabic at a 5% replacement level had an acceptability score comparable to the control (plain flour of Turkish beans and sorghum). A GF bread composed of 70% Bario rice flour (red-pigmented) and 30% potato starch received high sensory evaluations in color, flavor, texture, and overall acceptability (Ronie et al., 2023).

Food hydrocolloids are widely utilized as substitutes for gluten in GF baked goods, aimed at those with gluten allergies, owing to their ability to replicate gluten's viscoelastic properties. They originate from botanical, zoological, and microbiological sources and can be utilized in either natural or altered forms. Food hydrocolloids enhance the textural, rheological, and dough handling capabilities, as well as gas retention of GF dough, prolong shelf-life, and improve the overall quality of GF baked goods. They also provide nutraceutical advantages, including antioxidant properties, reduction of postprandial blood glucose and plasma cholesterol levels, regulation of intestinal transit and satiety, support for a healthy gastrointestinal system through the promotion of beneficial bacteria, and prevention of colon cancer. Gluten-free baked items are considered to possess significantly inferior nutritional quality due to the absence of some key elements, including minerals and vitamins (Culetu, Duta, Papageorgiou, & Varzakas, 2021). Consequently, next study may focus on enhancing the nutritional content of gluten-free goods, potentially through the utilization of GF legume flour, either alone or in conjunction with cereal or pseudo-cereal flour. The formulation of GF products can be enhanced with product development software, such as Design Expert. Moreover, numerous projections and market analyses suggest that the value of FHs in the worldwide FHs market will rise by 50% over the next decade (Yemenicioglu et al., 2020). This is anticipated to elevate the prices of FHs and GF-baked items, potentially intensified by the elevated costs associated with creating modified FHs. Consequently, research initiatives can be augmented to investigate the more accessible and economical natural FHs in the formulation of GF baked goods, to mitigate the impact of a potential price increase on the food sector and consumers of GF baked items.

Considerations for Development of Gluten-Free Foods

To far, the sole treatment for individuals afflicted with CD is adherence to a GFD (Rubio-Tapia et al., 2013). Complete abstinence from gluten facilitates intestinal healing and alleviates nutritional shortages and associated symptoms (Dhankhar & Tech, 2013). Strict adherence to a GFD diminishes the risk of acquiring numerous severe long-term consequences associated with untreated CD. Adhering to a GFD may appear straightforward, yet it is challenging, as it necessitates the exclusion of gluten-containing grains and all associated products, demanding continuous vigilance. Additionally, it entails a sense of social isolation and pressure throughout the process (Bauman, 2008). The avoidance of wheat-based products such as bread, biscuits, pasta, cakes, cookies, breakfast cereals, bagels, and soups necessitate a comprehensive lifestyle alteration that may not be attainable for everyone. Consequently, the demand for GF products is currently increasing.

The production of gluten -free food poses significant challenges for manufacturers, namely in identifying appropriate substitutes for gluten (Gallagher et al., 2004). The primary protein portions of gluten, glutenin and gliadin, are crucial for baking quality attributes, since they govern water absorption capability, cohesiveness, viscosity, and dough elasticity (Wieser, 2007). Consequently, the elimination of gluten poses significant challenges for bakers regarding quality (Gallagher et al., 2004). In addition to this, developers encounter problems related to product safety, acceptability, price, and compliance with FDA (Food and Drug Administration) rules. Therefore, manufacturers must adhere to numerous concerns while manufacturing GF products.

Avoidance of Gluten-Containing Sources

The first consideration in the preparation of gluten -free product includes the exclusion of any food or food ingredient that contains gluten, as celiac disease is triggered by the ingestion of gluten or its protein fraction i.e., gliadin in wheat, hordeins in barley, secalins in rye and avenins in oats (María de Lourdes Moreno Amador, Comino Montilla, & Sousa Martín, 2014). Among these, according to European standards oats have been placed in the list of gluten-free foodstuffs; nonetheless, their safety when consumed by celiac patients remains contested (Comino, de Lourdes Moreno, & Sousa, 2015). Therefore, it would be prudent to avoid oats for development of goods. In case of wheat, all of its forms such as wheatstarch, wheat bran, wheat germ, durum, emmer, einkorn, faro, farina, gliadin, semolina, spelt, matzo, cracked wheat and graham flour must be avoided (Kerr & Cherney, 2015).

Alternate Sources

The avoidance of gluten -containing cereals necessitates the elimination of significant food items that serve as primary protein sources in the diet. The protein concentration in wheat ranges from 10% to 12%, and the complete removal of wheat from the diet of a celiac patient would result in the absence of a significant protein source. Consequently, the protein composition of the alternative source must be taken into account. In addition to these, alternative gluten-free materials suitable for creating food products for people who have CD encompass nuts (almonds, hazelnuts, walnuts, chestnuts, cashews), seeds (flax seeds, chia seeds, pumpkin seeds), and tubers (arrowroot, tapioca, jicama, taro, potatoes, etc.) (Green & Cellier, 2007). So far, several researchers have made multiple attempts to create and develop gluten-free cuisine for celiac patients utilizing certain cereals, pulses, and nuts.

Ensure Sensory Characteristics

Gluten is the primary structural protein in flour, responsible for the elasticity of dough and contributing to the look and crumb structure of various baked goods (Gallagher et al., 2004). One of the primary problems in developing gluten -free products is ensuring that the product possesses the correct texture and mouthfeel comparable to gluten-containing products. Numerous authors have reported technical challenges, including the dry, gritty, and crumbly texture of gluten-free bread and pasta (Ahlborn, Pike, Hendrix, Hess, & Huber, 2005; Malcolmson, Matsuo, & Balshaw, 1993; Sanchez, Osella, & De La Torre, 2002; Ylimaki, Hawrysh, Hardin, & Thomson, 1991). Ahlborn et al., (Ahlborn et al., 2005). showed that gluten-free bread exhibits a greater staling propensity than its gluten-containing counterpart. A suitable gluten substitute is also necessary to provide the right texture, mouthfeel, and color of the product. Rotsch (Rotsch, 1954) indicated that gluten-free bread dough can only retain gas if an alternative gel-like material substitutes for gluten. Numerous experiments have been undertaken to enhance the textural attributes of gluten-free products by utilizing gluten substitutes, including starch, plant proteins (Sanchez et al., 2002), animal proteins (Toufeili et al., 1994), and hydrocolloids such as gums, pectins, hydroxy methylcellulose (Moreira, Chenlo, & Torres, 2013), and xanthan gums (Mahmoud, Yousif, Gadallah, & Alawneh, 2013).

Nutritional Value of Gluten-Free Products

Research indicates that patients adhering to a stringent GFD frequently experience multiple nutritional deficits. Hallert et al., (Hallert et al., 2002). documented indications of vitamin insufficiency in celiac patients on a GFD. Ciacci et al., (Ciacci, Cirillo, Cavallaro, & Mazzacca, 2002). demonstrated that persons with CD adhering to a stringent GFD exhibit significantly reduced weight, body mass index, fat mass, and lean body mass compared to control patients. Additionally, it was revealed that the diet of these patients was imbalanced, with a larger proportion of calories derived from fat and a lower proportion from carbs. The scientists ascribed the insufficiency of the GFD to dietary practices and food items. Strict compliance with a GFD also diminishes fiber intake in celiac patients (Grehn, Fridell, Lilliecreutz, & Hallert, 2001; Lohiniemi, Mäki, Kaukinen, Laippala, & Collin, 2000). Gluten-free cereal products, made from refined gluten-free flour or starch that is neither enhanced nor fortified, are primarily high in carbohydrates and lipids (María de Lourdes Moreno Amador et al., 2014). Additionally, mechanical and sensory challenges must be addressed in the preparation of these products, as gluten-free dough tends to have a fragile structure, is technologically difficult to manipulate, and often exhibits a suboptimal mouthfeel (Matos & Rosell, 2015). To optimize sensory attributes, various flours and starches, along with numerous ingredients (enzymes, proteins, hydrocolloids), are used to replicate the viscoelastic characteristics of gluten, enhance the structural integrity of gluten-free products (Marco & Rosell, 2008), and improve the nutritional profile of gluten-free foods (Matos & Rosell, 2015). A gluten-free product should not only be free from gluten but also match the nutritional profile of gluten-containing products. Numerous researchers have worked to develop gluten-free products with an improved nutritional profile.

To Meet Recommended Dietary Allowance (RDA) Requirements

The Recommended Dietary Allowance (RDA) is defined as the average daily intake of nutrients adequate to satisfy the requirements of about 97%–98% of healthy persons within a specific age group (Shrilakshmi, 2012). The Indian Council of Medical Research (ICMR) has established the RDA for certain nutrients across different age groups of the Indian population. Meeting the

RDA ensures the provision of essential nutrients to the body and aids in the prevention of diet-related chronic diseases in adults, including cardiovascular disease, cancer, and osteoporosis (Story & Stang, 2005). GFD therapy frequently exhibits low levels of vitamins and minerals, including vitamins B and D, calcium, iron, zinc, magnesium, and fiber, indicating that the Recommended Dietary Allowance for certain nutrients is commonly unmet. Miranda et al., (Miranda, Lasa, Bustamante, Churruca, & Simon, 2014). analyzed the nutritional composition of 206 gluten -free products predominantly consumed in Spain, comparing them to 289 equivalent gluten-containing food items, and highlighted the disparities in calories, macronutrients, fiber, sodium, salt, and cholesterol content between the two categories. They also indicated that gluten-free (GF) products may cause a nutritional imbalance for both CD patients and non-celiacs adhering to a diet rich in GF processed foods. A recent study by Missbach et al., (2015) in an Austrian supermarket revealed that GF products contained significantly lower levels of essential nutrients, such as proteins, while exhibiting comparatively higher levels of total fat and saturated fat than their gluten-containing counterparts. Consequently, a critical criterion in the formulation of GF foods is to maintain their nutritional profile at a level that does not compromise the individual's recommended dietary allowance.

Economics

Numerous studies and market surveys indicate that following a GFD imposes a lifelong financial burden on people, primarily due to the significantly higher prices of GF products (L. Castillo & Rivas, 2008; Lee, Ng, Zivin, & Green, 2007; Stevens & Rashid, 2008) compared to their non-gluten -free counterparts, as well as their limited availability in the market (J. Singh & Whelan, 2011). A comparative study in Chile revealed an 89% increase in the feeding costs for CD patients regarding gluten-free food products (L. Castillo & Rivas, 2008). Conversely, a study in Atlantic Canada indicated that GF products were 242% more expensive than their gluten-containing counterparts (Stevens & Rashid, 2008). Nascimento et al., (Bagolin do Nascimento, Medeiros Rataichesck Fiates, dos Anjos, & Teixeira, 2014). assessed the availability, pricing, and nutritional composition of gluten-free items in retail establishments within a Brazilian capital and found that the availability and diversity of such products were constrained, while costs were elevated. Missbach et al., (Missbach et al., 2015). conducted the research in an Austrian supermarket, demonstrating that many GF goods were significantly deficient in essential nutrients such as proteins compared to their gluten-containing counterparts, although their prices remained elevated relative to the latter. A recent study by Lambert and Ficken (Lambert & Ficken, 2016) in Australia assessed the cost and affordability of a GF healthy food basket for four reference families, revealing that the GF basket was significantly more expensive than the gluten-containing counterpart for all family types examined. To prevent imposing an economic burden on patients, the cost of developing any GF food product must be taken into account.

Compliance with the FDA Guidelines

Adhering to the norms and regulations established by numerous national and international organizations is crucial when designing goods for celiac sufferers. The Codex Standard for GF foods was established by the Codex Alimentarius Commission (CODEX) of the World Health Organization (WHO) and the Food and Agricultural Organization (FAO) in 1976(Arendt & Moore, 2006; Gallagher et al., 2004; Saturni, Ferretti, & Bacchetti, 2010). The criteria were amended in 1981 and again in 2000, defining gluten -free products as "gluten-free foods," which can be characterized as:

a. Composed solely of ingredients devoid of prolamins from wheat or any Triticum species, including spelt, kamut, or durum wheat, as well as rye, barley, oats, or their hybrid variants, with a gluten concentration not surpassing 20 ppm (Arendt & Moore, 2006; Gallagher et al., 2004; Saturni et al., 2010).
b. Comprising components derived from wheat, rye, barley, oats, spelt, or their hybrid types, which have been processed to eliminate gluten; with a gluten concentration not surpassing 200 ppm (Arendt & Moore, 2006; Gallagher et al., 2004; Saturni et al., 2010).
c. Any combination of the two substances specified in (a) and (b) with a concentration not above 200 ppm (Arendt & Moore, 2006; Gallagher et al., 2004; Saturni et al., 2010).

In August 2013, the U.S. Food and Drug Administration (FDA) released a regulation that delineated the phrase "gluten -free" for food labeling purposes. The FDA permits various labeling methods for gluten-free foods.

- "Gluten-free"
- "Free of gluten"
- "No gluten"
- "Without gluten"

Labeling is essential for enabling consumers to make informed decisions regarding foods with improved health benefits (Zou & Hobbs, 2010), and in the context of celiac disease, it assures them that the product they are consuming is safe.

Consequently, CD impacts roughly 1% of the global population and is significantly on the rise due to underdiagnosis of the disorder. The sole treatment for individuals with CD is lifelong adherence to a GFD. Adhering to a lifelong GFD may result in nutritional imbalances in patients. Avoiding gluten -containing foods necessitates the exclusion of primary protein sources from the diet, resulting in a reliance on a high-carbohydrate diet. Consequently, there is a significant necessity to create GF products that are both highly nutritional and cost-effective. Nevertheless, various factors must be considered prior to designing products for those with celiac disease. Considerations encompass the elimination of all potential gluten-containing raw materials, the selection of an alternative flour source, the acceptable texture and color of the product, the increase of the product's nutritional content, as well as product safety and labeling. These factors will assist in creating nutritionally comprehensive and safe GF health foods for those with CD.

Chapter 11

The Role of Technology and Artificial Intelligence in Celiac Disease

Abstract

Technology and artificial intelligence (AI) are transforming the field of celiac disease diagnosis and management. This chapter explores the use of AI in predicting and diagnosing CD, as well as in personalized treatment planning. It also reviews the applications of wireless capsule endoscopy, electronic medical records, and diagnostic tools like serology and genome analysis. The chapter highlights how technological advancements are improving the accuracy of CD diagnosis and the efficiency of patient care, while also pointing to future possibilities in the management of CD.

Artificial Intelligence in Celiac Disease

In recent years, medical data utilized for clinical practice has been widely accessible in electronic format. This data guides physicians' decision-making in patient care, aiming to customize each patient's assessment and strategy to the person. The objective of "precision medicine" is to leverage many data modalities, such as genomic data, electronic medical records (EMR), textual data (e.g., unstructured patient notes), and imaging data (e.g., CT scans, MRI, endoscopy), to enhance and individualize patient care (Bray et al., 2016).

To analyze this vast dataset, practitioners have utilized algorithmic methods from machine learning (ML), a comprehensive domain of artificial intelligence (AI) that fundamentally aims to correlate a set of inputs with a set of outputs through an algorithmically derived function from an extensive collection of examples. Historically, ML methodologies depended on specialized domain knowledge and manually designed features (Cui, Luo, Tseng, Ten Haken, & El Naqa, 2019); however, deep learning (DL) techniques have gained prominence in recent times (Kan et al., 2019).

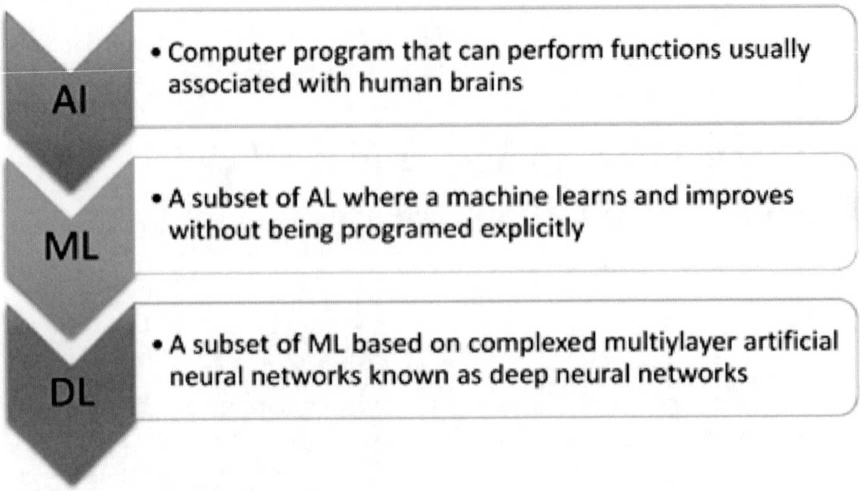

Figure 9. Artificial intelligence and its subsets. AI, artificial intelligence; ML, machine learning; DL, deep learning methodologies, including enhanced computational capacity through superior hardware and greater data accessibility (Min, Lee, & Yoon, 2017).

Deep learning, a subset of ML (Figure 9), is a type of representation learning in which an algorithm receives raw data as input and generates representations utilized for pattern identification. These representations, essentially automatically-derived "features," are generated through multiple "layers," each functioning as a non-linear transformation. The aggregation of these non-linear functions across numerous layers is termed a "neural network" (Figure 10). Numerous advancements have facilitated the swift advancement of deep learning methodologies, including enhanced computational capacity through superior hardware and greater data accessibility (Min, Lee, & Yoon, 2017).

DL is increasingly becoming the standard in this day. Today, we have already observed its implementation in autonomous vehicles, facial recognition technologies, and deepfake applications, among others. In 2011, International Business Machines (IBM) launched Watson, a computer system capable of responding to natural language. It was originally designed to compete in Jeopardy and triumphed in the 2011 tournament (Rachlin, 2012). Subsequently, it was declared that Watson will be employed in the management decisions about cancer cases at a hospital in New York (Hamilton et al., 2019). In 2018, the United States Food and Drug Administration (FDA) sanctioned an AI-based device known as IDx-DR (W.

H. Yang et al., 2019). This technology assists in screening decisions for diabetic retinopathy by utilizing uploaded retinal scans. The true potential of AI remains largely unexplored.

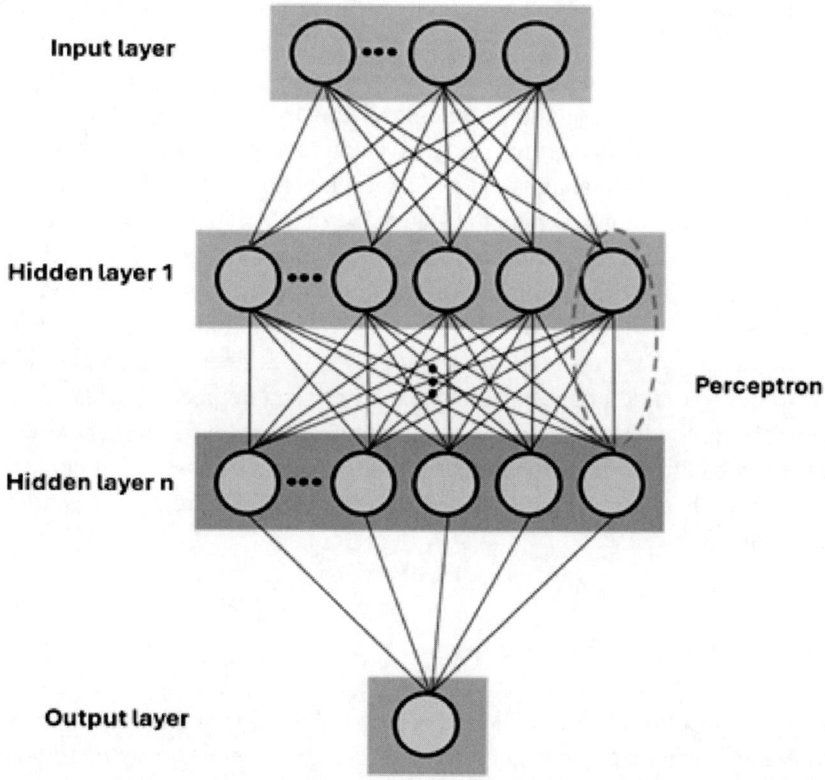

Figure 10. A basic overview of the Artificial Neural Network (ANN). A perceptron here is analogous to a neuron of the human brain. ANN can have *n* number of hidden layers. When the training dataset is provided, the weights of perceptrons are adjusted with each input until optimization is achieved. The new sample then is classified according to the weights of perceptrons.

Healthcare can be significantly enhanced by the application of MLtechnology (J. Holmes, Sacchi, & Bellazzi, 2004). A fundamental prerequisite of any ML-based model is the capacity to integrate substantial volumes of data. Electronic medical records (EMR) provide a vast and expanding repository that assists physicians in diagnosis, management, and personalized recommendations (Golden, 2017). The recruitment process for clinical trials is laborious and monotonous; however, a ML algorithm may efficiently identify potential applicants within minutes to hours by analyzing EMR data (Harrer, Shah, Antony, & Hu, 2019). While ML methodologies in healthcare exhibit significant potential, there are specific limitations and constraints that practitioners must recognize.

The diverse manifestations, inadequate response to GFD, substantial follow-up demands, recurrent testing, and the chronic character of this disease necessitate the advancement of innovative diagnostic techniques, therapeutic interventions, and management strategies. ML can be advantageous in CD and analogous disorders that require extensive and repetitive testing for diagnosis, therapy, and patient management, thereby alleviating the strain of clinicians. Figure 11 illustrates a fundamental schematic of a ML model. The majority of these investigations concentrated on clinical data obtained from electronic medical records and imaging data from endoscopies. A study utilized Field Asymmetric Ion Mobility Spectrometry (FAIMS), biomarker assays, single nucleotide polymorphisms (SNPs), endomysium antibody (EMA) tests, and histopathology slide images as inputs. A significant degree of variation in the materials, procedures, and quality parameters employed may complicate future systematic reviews in comparing the results. The absence of consensus and standardization in methodologies for doing ML-related research is presumably the cause.

Wireless Capsule Endoscopy

Wireless capsule endoscopy (WCE) is frequently utilized for individuals who are either unsuitable for traditional endoscopy or reluctant to undergo the treatment repeatedly. The analysis of the recording is particularly burdensome for clinicians due to its extensive duration and the suboptimal yield resulting from the capsule's spontaneous movement within the intestine. Recent advancements indicate that real-time localization of wireless capsule endoscopy will enable the recording to be confined to the specific region of the gastrointestinal tract (Than, Alici, Zhou, & Li, 2012). Ciaccio et al., (Ciaccio, Tennyson, Bhagat, Lewis, & Green, 2010) utilized images from wireless capsule endoscopy (WCE) as input data to train their model, achieving 80% sensitivity (SN) and 96% specificity (SP) with a threshold classifier. This method involved selecting three optimal features through threshold learning, where each pixel is replaced with a black pixel if its intensity exceeds a predetermined constant (referred to as the 'threshold') and a white pixel if it falls below that threshold. The study achieved an SN of 88%

and an SP of 80% using an incremental classifier, which employs the three most significant features through incremental learning. This method continuously incorporates new input to further train the model without requiring a complete retraining from the testing dataset to predict celiac disease (CD) versus control. The study concluded that the quantitative markers from WCE can be used for screening for CD and assessing the extent and severity of small bowel involvement.

A primary weakness of the study was the aggregation of data from all small bowel regions instead of analyzing specific areas, such as the duodenal bulb, jejunum, and ileum. Eleven volunteers were recruited to provide WCE video clips for the training dataset, although data from only ten participants were used for model testing. An expanded cohort could allow for sub-analysis of various regions of the small intestine and help corroborate the findings of this research.

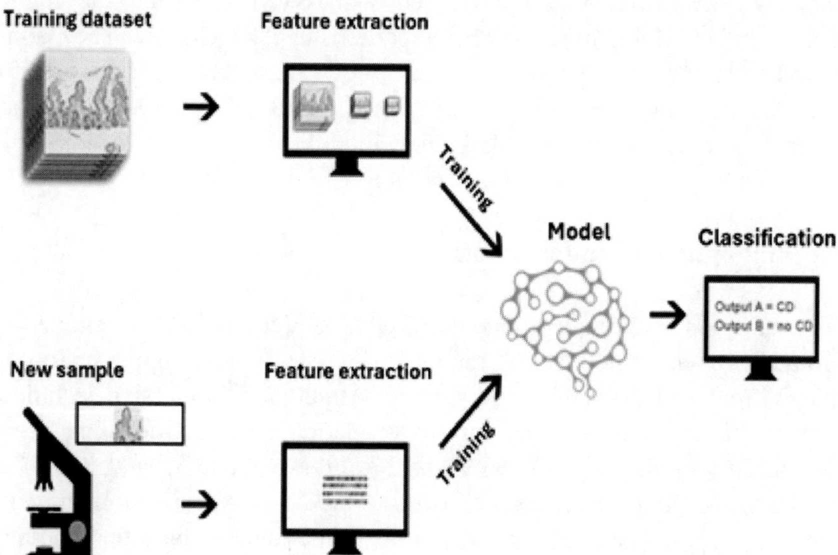

Figure 11. Schematics of a classification model. A training dataset is usually text, video recordings or images. Certain features of data are important and are weighed more than others. Feature extraction techniques are available to achieve that. Once the model is trained, a new sample is fed to the model which then gives out the classification in binary or continuously varying values between 0 and 1 depending on the model.

Zhou et al., (T. Zhou et al., 2017). employed wireless capsule endoscopy (WCE) pictures to train a convolutional neural network (CNN) known as GoogLeNet, attaining a sensitivity (SN) and specificity (SP) of 100%. The research presented a quantitative metric for assessing the severity of CD, referred to as evaluation confidence (EC). The study determined that their methodology effectively identifies CD and assesses its severity level. The primary constraint of this research was the limited sample size. Wang et al., (X. Wang et al., 2020). utilized WCE photos to create a customized module grounded on human visual perception to extract the most significant elements for diagnosing CD and compared these with traditional modules. The specifics on these modules exceed the parameters of this study and are available in other sources (J. Hu, Shen, & Sun, 2018). The components were included into ResNet50 and Inception-v3, two distinct CNN architectures. The output from these modules used as input for three distinct classifiers: Support Vector Machine (SVM), k-Nearest Neighbor (kNN), and Linear Discriminant Analysis (LDA). ResNet50 combined with SVM exhibited the highest efficacy in identifying minor villous alterations in celiac disease. The claimed overall accuracy is 95.9, with a sensitivity of 97.2 and a specificity of 95.6. The primary drawbacks were a small sample size (12 cases/13 controls) and increased computation time with the new module.

Esophagogastroduodenoscopy

Hegenbart and colleagues (Hegenbart, Uhl, & Vécsei, 2011) examined the limitations of machine learning models using conventional upper endoscopy images from CD cases obtained through a modified immersion technique. They evaluated the efficacy of various validation methods, including Leave-one-out cross-validation (LOOCV), k-fold cross-validation, and leave-one-patient-out (LOPO) validation protocols. Three feature extraction strategies were employed: Local Binary Patterns (LBP) and its modified variants, Extended Local Binary Patterns (ELBP), and Extended Local Ternary Patterns (ELTP). An ineffective kNN classifier was used for classification. The study concluded that the LOPO method is optimal when exclusive datasets for training and testing are not available. This technique is particularly useful in research with limited sample sizes. In a subsequent investigation, Hegenbart et al., (Hegenbart, Uhl, Vécsei, & Wimmer, 2013) concluded that scale-variant texture approaches are more effective than invariant methods for detecting CD, using the same input data.

The quantity and quality of data are two limits of AI-based models. In the healthcare sector, the majority of data is unlabeled and necessitates extensive expert annotation for effective model training. Kwitt et al., (Kwitt, Hegenbart, Rasiwasia, Vécsei, & Uhl, 2014). tackled the significant constraint of insufficient specialists to annotate the input data. This pilot study sought to determine whether the label noise from data annotated by non-experts may be mitigated by augmenting the dataset size. Eight non-expert volunteers were selected and provided with a concise 10-minute explanation to the condition, during which they were shown 10 representative endoscopic images of CD and control cases. The study concluded that non-experts can be useful for labeling; however, a substantial training set is necessary to mitigate the heightened label noise. A cited issue was that an expert assisted in selecting the optimal photos for the model, which may have introduced bias into the results.

Gadermayr et al., (2016) utilized upper endoscopy images and implemented a hybrid model combining expert analysis with machine learning (ML) methods to achieve accurate diagnoses. Out of 27 distinct combinations (comprising 3 databases, 3 endoscopists, and 3 classification methodologies), 24 demonstrated superior performance in the hybrid model compared to expert diagnosis. Of these 24 models, 17 showed statistically significant improvement ($P < 0.05$). The study concluded that the effectiveness of medical professionals, particularly those with limited experience, can be enhanced through the integration of computer-aided models into the diagnostic process. The study's limitations included a population limited to children and a small number of endoscopists participating in the dataset chapter.

Electronic Medical Records

Clinical decision support systems (CDSS) are considered essential rather than optional in the foreseeable future (Lisboa, 2002). Tenorio et al., (Tenório et al., 2011).created a web-based Clinical Decision Support System utilizing clinical data from EMR as input parameters. The model executed 270 classifiers employing five distinct ML approaches in Weka 3.6.1. The study indicated that Clinical Decision Support Systems could assist in diagnosing CD, achieving an optimal accuracy of 80%, a SN of 0.78, a SP of 0.80, and an area under the receiver operating characteristic curve (AUROC) of 0.84. It was additionally proposed that a recommendation of CD from CDSS in a patient with a negative confirmatory test should not be considered an error; rather, it should be viewed as a prompt for the clinician to conduct further investigation.

Chen et al., (W. Chen, Huang, Boyle, & Lin, 2016) introduced an automated categorization technique for identifying patients with celiac disease (CD) using data collected from electronic medical records (EMR). The goal was to evaluate clinical data, serology reports, and pathology reports against the International Classification of Diseases (ICD-9) for identifying instances of CD. The input data was derived from preselected CD cases classified using ICD-9 codes in the EMR. This study employed 96 tests with 12 classifications from four distinct techniques, using the three most representative classifiers from each technique, in contrast to Tenorio et al., (Tenório et al., 2011), who analyzed all 270 categories using five machine learning (ML) techniques. The study found that their model outperformed ICD-9, achieving an area under the receiver operating characteristic curve (AUROC) of 0.94 in detecting CD.

Significant limitations identified included the fact that the input data came from prescreened CD cases categorized with ICD-9 codes rather than the general population. As a result, the model's accuracy may fluctuate when applied to the general population or when incorrect ICD-9 labels are used. Furthermore, the model employed a limited number of classes with the default configuration. Employing residual classifications and altering the arrangement may yield different statistical results.

Ludvigsson et al., (Ludvigsson, Pathak, et al., 2013). evaluated the feasibility of developing a model to identify persons at elevated risk of CD who may benefit from screening. Despite the United States Preventive Services Task Force (USPSTF) currently advising against CD screening in the general population due to insufficient evidence (Kivelä & Kurppa, 2017), an effective model may address this issue. The research employed electronic medical records to extract 16 unstructured text elements and utilized ICD-9 codes to identify instances of high-risk CD. The NLP system utilizing free text significantly outperformed the ICD-9 search algorithm, achieving sensitivity scores of 72.9 and 89.9 compared to 17.1, and SP of 88.5, respectively. This study utilized a retrospective EMR-based approach, in contrast to Tenorio et al., (Tenório et al., 2011), which employed a web-based CDSS, hence enhancing its scalability for implementation. The identified limitations include instances from a single tertiary care center, which may not represent the broader population, along with a sample characterized by uneven demographic distribution. Future multicenter studies with appropriate matching can mitigate these limitations.

Hujoel et al., (2018) built ten machine learning (ML) models using electronic medical records (EMR) and serology results to identify previously undetected cases of celiac disease (CD). Various machine learning techniques were employed, and the study reported an area under the receiver operating characteristic (AUROC) range of 0.49 to 0.53. Only two of the ten models were able to exceed random chance. The study concluded that case-finding is largely ineffective, primarily due to the prevalence of asymptomatic and atypical cases among undiagnosed CD patients. The limitations of the study included the lack of family history data, the exclusion of other diseases associated with CD, such as type 1 diabetes mellitus, and the omission of physical examination findings.

Serology

Caetano Dos Santos et al., (Caetano dos Santos et al., 2019). employed serology as the foundation for implementing ML in facilitating the diagnosis of CD. Model 1 utilized all 2579 sample pictures of IgA-class endomysium antibody (EMA) in an AdaBoost framework with SVM. AdaBoost is a meta-algorithm that enhances the efficacy of a weak classifier when integrated (S. Chen, Shen, Wang, & Yoo, 2019). Model 2 utilized random under-sampling, a validation method referred to as Monte Carlo cross-validation, to mitigate multiclass classification mistakes. The two SVM models were developed and evaluated using MATLAB® and exhibited comparable performance metrics. Model 1 exhibited an accuracy of 96.8, sensitivity of 82.84, and specificity (SP) of 99.4, vs Model 2 demonstrated an accuracy of 98.5, sensitivity of 98.91, and specificity of 98.81. A net decrease of 2.05% in classification error was seen in Model 2. This pilot study determined that the classification process of EMA may be automated using ML.

Choung and colleagues (Venuta & Rendina, 2008) focused on the development of novel biomarkers for the diagnosis and monitoring of celiac disease (CD). Serum samples from both cases and controls were used as input data for the machine learning system. Synthetic biomarkers were created and analyzed using the RAPMAD (Robust Analysis of Microarray Data) R program (Renard et al., 2011) to remove unreliable peptides. After eliminating background noise, the training set was executed in the SVM model using the Python package. The study indicated an accuracy of 99%, a sensitivity of 99%, and a specificity of 100%, suggesting that the novel biomarker can effectively identify new cases of CD, facilitating diagnosis and monitoring mucosal healing in established cases. Significant limitations noted were the use of synthetic rather than biological indicators and elevated false-positive rates in treated cases with unresolved mucosal healing.

Genome

Goudey and colleagues (Goudey et al., 2017) investigated celiac disease (CD) to identify SNP-SNP pairwise interactions among unassociated human leukocyte antigen (HLA) haplotype variants. Five datasets from the Genome-Wide Interaction Search (GWIS) database were utilized. Support vector machines (SVM) were executed in SparSNP, a multivariable linear model where sparsity is balanced with penalization, details of which are available elsewhere (Goudey et al., 2017). The study analyzed 500 billion SNP pairs and achieved an AUROC of 0.88, identifying 14 distinct interactions within the HLA class III region, independent of the HLA class II regions that are strongly associated with CD. This finding may influence the application of genetics in therapeutic approaches.

Biopsy

Syed and colleagues (2019) examined the fundamental question of whether machine learning can distinguish between healthy and diseased tissue. The dataset consisted of 3,118 biopsy images of the duodenum from healthy individuals, celiac disease (CD) cases, and instances of environmental enteropathy. A modified CNN version based on AlexNet was developed, achieving an accuracy of 93.4% and a false-negative rate of 2.4%. The integration of CNN with a deconvolutional network enables the model to autonomously learn the microscopic characteristics in the input data images, such as epithelial secretory cells, which are indicative of the diagnosis.

Ion Mobility Spectrometry

Diagnosis and monitoring of celiac disease (CD) require repeated serological testing and multiple biopsy specimens (Rubio-Tapia et al., 2013). Two significant challenges in CD clinics are false-negative serology and reluctance to perform multiple biopsies. Arasaradnam et al., (2014) suggested that the measurement of volatile organic compounds in urine samples could detect alterations in the gut microbiota associated with CD and distinguish it from inflammatory bowel disease. This proposition was based on promising results from research using field asymmetry ion mobility spectrometry (FAIMS) technology to differentiate ulcerative colitis from Crohn's disease (Arasaradnam et al., 2014). The FAIMS data from urine samples were pre-processed using the R package, and statistical analysis was performed with three different machine learning techniques. The algorithms showed strong predictive ability, with an AUROC of 0.91, sensitivity of 0.85, and specificity of 0.85. This pilot study concluded that FAIMS could serve as a viable non-invasive alternative for investigating CD, pending validation through extensive randomized controlled trials.

Limitations

Machine learning, like other technologies, possesses inherent limits. Threats such as data breaches and ransomware attacks that impact technology broadly also encompass ML. However, ML possesses certain inherent limits. Although the data may be extensive and readily accessible, it is crucial to evaluate its quality prior to utilization. Introducing novel data to the ML model may lead to overfitting, an error that arises when a model is excessively tailored to the training dataset, hence undermining the accuracy of subsequent predictions. The majority of accessible ML models are black-box, hence constraining the interpretability of the outcomes. This is especially troubling in the healthcare system, because clinicians must carefully examine systematic bias and confounders to report outcomes accurately. Despite recent advancements in processing power, the expense of such advanced systems remains prohibitive for many healthcare facilities. The healthcare sector is significantly focused on the ethical and legal ramifications of the ML model in application. Machines cannot be accountable for human life. Ultimately, physicians will bear responsibility for the activities undertaken. Physicians may get complacent, relying on machinery more than their clinical sense.

Future Directions

Healthcare has embraced ML in nearly all facets. Given the boundless possible applications, we must concentrate on those that will produce greater returns. The subsequent critical elements require more decisive measures prior to widespread implementation. The integration of ML into electronic medical record systems could be transformative; however, agreement on patient data security and ethical concerns is essential prior to its deployment. Legal culpability must be addressed, as robots cannot be held accountable for their decisions. Doctors will remain accountable for considering machine recommendations for their patients. There is a necessity for the standardization of quality measurements, as many metrics utilized in research, such as accuracy, sensitivity, specificity, precision, F1 score, and the area under the receiver operating characteristic curve, are challenging to compare. High-quality datasets are essential for superior ML models. Enhancements in data mining will yield superior quality ML models. Elimination of black-box labeling can assist the physician in comprehending potential biases and confounders. Research deficiencies must be addressed through enhanced collaboration among major healthcare institutions to finance additional studies in this domain. The integration of cellphones and ML models can be a progressive concept for monitoring health and treatment efficacy. These models can propose new treatment drugs based on clinical and genetic data.

Conclusion

Gluten consumption causes the complex immune-mediated disease known as celiac disease (CD). While our understanding of the disorder is still evolving, we are improving in identifying the distinctive traits of patient subgroups, understanding its connection to other immune-related diseases, developing diagnostic tests, and screening appropriate individuals. Additionally, CD presents a variety of clinical symptoms that differ between children and adults, often leading to challenges in accurate diagnosis. Therefore, a comprehensive approach to CD diagnosis is essential, incorporating clinical signs, gut biopsy, genetic predisposition based on HLA type, and prediction based on response to a gluten-free diet (GFD).

CD involves both the innate and adaptive arms of the immune system, each playing a unique functional role. While CD is primarily an immunological condition triggered by partially digested gluten in the gastrointestinal tract, it can also have a wide range of extraintestinal effects, including cancer and other chronic diseases, in genetically predisposed individuals. In light of this, the GFD remains the most effective treatment; however, for it to be successful globally, the challenges of GFD safety, quality, and cost must be addressed. Therefore, additional clinical trials and research are needed to advance therapeutic interventions for CD. Positive outcomes in therapeutic intervention, particularly the combined use of probiotics, may provide CD patients with simpler treatment options.

Through various mechanisms, *Lactobacillus* and *Bifidobacterium* strains can help prevent CD patients from becoming further debilitated by gliadin intake. These mechanisms include gliadin hydrolysis via enzymatic pathways, modulation of immune system responses, expression of CD-related genes (such as Cox and ZO-1), reinforcement of the mucosal layer, and prevention of toxic peptide entry into intestinal cells. It is recommended to use a combination of the aforementioned probiotics at an adequate functional dose for them to be effective in food products. This is because only a small number of strains typically possess one or more efficient inhibition mechanisms.

Overall, incorporating appropriate and effective probiotics into wheat-based products (particularly in combination form) could offer a potential therapeutic strategy for celiac disease, at least in reducing CD symptoms. The mechanisms of probiotics should be further investigated in clinical trials. It is also crucial to determine whether probiotics can reduce all celiac symptoms and continue to function effectively in cereal-based probiotic products over extended periods, even at high storage temperatures. Lastly, celiac disease support groups and educational initiatives should inform patients about the health benefits of probiotic-enriched cereal products.

A significant number of people have adopted a gluten-free diet (GFD) without seeking expert advice due to the growing media focus on the potential dangers of gluten and the supposed benefits of a GFD. A gluten-free diet has been observed to alleviate symptoms in non-celiac disease (CD) patients, although this is not indicative of any recognized clinical condition. The low levels of fermentable oligosaccharides, disaccharides, monosaccharides, and polyols (FODMAPs) in a GFD may contribute to both the placebo effect and symptom relief. A GFD may also be beneficial for individuals who are allergic to wheat. For now, we recommend that patients who are concerned about undiagnosed CD, gluten sensitivity, or related disorders such as dermatitis herpetiformis (DH) consult with a healthcare professional for proper evaluation. Assessment of concomitant diseases and any nutritional deficiencies should be part of the CD treatment plan.

References

Abadie, V., Sollid, L. M., Barreiro, L. B., & Jabri, B. (2011). Integration of genetic and immunological insights into a model of celiac disease pathogenesis. *Annual review of immunology, 29*(1), 493-525.

Abbasi, A., Aghebati-Maleki, A., Yousefi, M., & Aghebati-Maleki, L. (2021). Probiotic intervention as a potential therapeutic for managing gestational disorders and improving pregnancy outcomes. *Journal of reproductive immunology, 143*, 103244.

Abbasi, A., Rad, A. H., Maleki, L. A., Kafil, H. S., & Baghbanzadeh, A. (2023). Antigenotoxicity and Cytotoxic Potentials of Cell-Free Supernatants Derived from Saccharomyces cerevisiae var. boulardii on HT-29 Human Colon Cancer Cell Lines. *Probiotics and Antimicrobial Proteins*, 1-13.

Abbasi, A., Saadat, T. R., & Saadat, Y. R. (2022). Microbial exopolysaccharides–β-glucans–as promising postbiotic candidates in vaccine adjuvants. *International Journal of Biological Macromolecules*.

Abdalla, A., Saifullah, S. M., Osman, M., Baniya, R., Sidahmed, S., LaChance, J., & Bachuwa, G. (2017). Prevalence of occult celiac disease in females with iron deficiency in the United States: An NHANES analysis. *Journal of Community Hospital Internal Medicine Perspectives, 7*(6), 347-350.

Abdelghany, M., Gonzalez III, L., Slater, J., & Begley, C. (2014). Olmesartan associated sprue -like enteropathy and colon perforation. *Case Reports in Gastrointestinal Medicine, 2014*(1), 494098.

Abedi, A. S., Rismanchi, M., Shahdoostkhany, M., Mohammadi, A., & Hosseini, H. (2016). Microencapsulation of Nigella sativa seeds oil containing thymoquinone by spray-drying for functional yogurt production. *International journal of food science & technology, 51*(10), 2280-2289.

Addolorato, G., Capristo, E., Ghittoni, G., Valeri, C., Mascianà, R., Scarfone, A., ... Gasbarrini, G. (2000). Anxiety but not depression decreases in celiac patients after one-year gluten -free diet. *Digestive and Liver Disease* (32), A113.

Addolorato, G., Mirijello, A., D'Angelo, C., Leggio, L., Ferrulli, A., Vonghia, L., ... Gasbarrini, G. (2008). Social phobia in coeliac disease. *Scandinavian journal of gastroenterology, 43*(4), 410-415.

Adebola, O. O., Corcoran, O., & Morgan, W. A. (2014). Synbiotics: the impact of potential prebiotics inulin, lactulose and lactobionic acid on the survival and growth of lactobacilli probiotics. *Journal of functional foods, 10*, 75-84.

Adedeji, A. A., Alakali, J., Adewale, P. O., & Ngadi, M. O. (2012). Thermophysical properties of Detarium microcarpum seed flour. *LWT, 47*(2), 233-237.

Adriaanse, M., & Leffler, D. A. (2015). Serum markers in the clinical management of celiac disease. *Digestive Diseases, 33*(2), 236-243.

Afik, S., Raulet, G., & Yosef, N. (2019). Reconstructing B-cell receptor sequences from short-read single-cell RNA sequencing with BRAPeS. *Life science alliance, 2*(4).

Afik, S., Yates, K. B., Bi, K., Darko, S., Godec, J., Gerdemann, U., ... Barnes, E. J. (2017). Targeted reconstruction of T cell receptor sequence from single cell RNA-seq links CDR3 length to T cell differentiation state. *Nucleic acids research, 45*(16), e148-e148.

Aguiar, E. V., Santos, F. G., Centeno, A. C. L. S., & Capriles, V. D. (2022). Defining amaranth, buckwheat and quinoa flour levels in gluten -free bread: A simultaneous improvement on physical properties, acceptability and nutrient composition through mixture design. *Foods, 11*(6), 848.

Ahlborn, G. J., Pike, O. A., Hendrix, S. B., Hess, W. M., & Huber, C. S. (2005). Sensory, mechanical, and microscopic evaluation of staling in low-protein and gluten -free breads. *Cereal Chemistry, 82*(3), 328-335.

Akobeng, A. K., Singh, P., Kumar, M., & Al Khodor, S. (2020). Role of the gut microbiota in the pathogenesis of coeliac disease and potential therapeutic implications. *European Journal of Nutrition, 59*(8), 3369-3390.

Aksoy, E., Tıraş-Teber, S., Kansu, A., Deda, G., & Kartal, A. (2016). Neurological findings spectrum in Celiac disease. *The Turkish Journal of Pediatrics, 58*(3), 233-240.

Aleanzi, M., Demonte, A. M., Esper, C., Garcilazo, S., & Waggener, M. (2001). Celiac disease: antibody recognition against native and selectively deamidated gliadin peptides. *Clinical Chemistry, 47*(11), 2023-2028.

Allis, C. D., & Jenuwein, T. (2016). The molecular hallmarks of epigenetic control. *Nature Reviews Genetics, 17*(8), 487-500.

Almallouhi, E., King, K. S., Patel, B., Wi, C., Juhn, Y. J., Murray, J. A., & Absah, I. (2017). Increasing incidence and altered presentation in a population-based study of pediatric celiac disease in North America. *Journal of pediatric gastroenterology and nutrition, 65*(4), 432-437.

Alwitry, A. (2000). Vitamin A deficiency in coeliac disease. *The British Journal of Ophthalmology, 84*(9), 1075.

Amasheh, M., Fromm, A., Krug, S. M., Amasheh, S., Andres, S., Zeitz, M., ... Schulzke, J. D. (2010). TNFα-induced and berberine-antagonized tight junction barrier impairment via tyrosine kinase, Akt and NFκB signaling. *Journal of cell science, 123*(23), 4145-4155.

Amasheh, M., Schlichter, S., Amasheh, S., Mankertz, J., Zeitz, M., Fromm, M., & Schulzke, J. D. (2008). Quercetin Enhances Epithelial Barrier Function and Increases Claudin-4 Expression in Caco-2 Cells3. *The Journal of nutrition, 138*(6), 1067-1073.

AMENT, M. E., OCHS, H. D., & DAVIS, S. D. (1973). Structure and function of the gastrointestinal tract in primary immunodeficiency syndromes a study of 39 patients. *Medicine, 52*(3), 227-248.

Anderson, R. P. (2011). Coeliac disease is on the rise. *The Medical journal of Australia, 194*(6), 278-279.

Anderson, R. P., Degano, P., Godkin, A. J., Jewell, D. P., & Hill, A. V. (2000). *In vivo* antigen challenge in celiac disease identifies a single transglutaminase-modified peptide as the dominant A-gliadin T-cell epitope. *Nature medicine, 6*(3), 337-342.

Anderson, R. P., van Heel, D. A., Tye-Din, J. A., Jewell, D. P., & Hill, A. V. (2006). Antagonists and non-toxic variants of the dominant wheat gliadin T cell epitope in coeliac disease. *Gut, 55*(4), 485-491.

Andrade, F., Albuquerque, P. B., Moraes, G., Farias, M., Teixeira-Sá, D., Vicente, A., & Carneiro-da-Cunha, M. (2018). Influence of hydrocolloids (galactomannan and xanthan gum) on the physicochemical and sensory characteristics of gluten -free cakes based on fava beans (Phaseolus lunatus). *Food & function, 9*(12), 6369-6379.

Antonini, M., Lo Conte, M., Sorini, C., & Falcone, M. (2019). How the interplay between the commensal microbiota, gut barrier integrity, and mucosal immunity regulates brain autoimmunity. *Frontiers in immunology, 10*, 1937.

Arasaradnam, R. P., Westenbrink, E., McFarlane, M. J., Harbord, R., Chambers, S., O'Connell, N., ... Savage, R. (2014). Differentiating coeliac disease from irritable bowel syndrome by urinary volatile organic compound analysis–a pilot study. *PloS one, 9*(10), e107312.

Arendt, E. K., & Moore, M. M. (2006). Gluten-free cereal-based products. *Bakery products: Science and technology, 2006*, 471-496.

Arentz-Hansen, H., Fleckenstein, B., Molberg, Ø., Scott, H., Koning, F., Jung, G., ... Sollid, L. M. (2004). The molecular basis for oat intolerance in patients with celiac disease. *PLoS medicine, 1*(1), e1.

Arentz-Hansen, H., Körner, R., Molberg, Ø., Quarsten, H., Vader, W., Kooy, Y. M., ... Sollid, L. M. (2000). The intestinal T cell response to α-gliadin in adult celiac disease is focused on a single deamidated glutamine targeted by tissue transglutaminase. *The Journal of experimental medicine, 191*(4), 603-612.

Arentz–Hansen, H., Mcadam, S. N., Molberg, Ø., Fleckenstein, B., Lundin, K. E., Jørgensen, T. J., ... Sollid, L. M. (2002). Celiac lesion T cells recognize epitopes that cluster in regions of gliadins rich in proline residues. *Gastroenterology, 123*(3), 803-809.

Arguelles-Grande, C., Tennyson, C. A., Lewis, S. K., Green, P. H., & Bhagat, G. (2012). Variability in small bowel histopathology reporting between different pathology practice settings: impact on the diagnosis of coeliac disease. *Journal of clinical pathology, 65*(3), 242-247.

Ari, A., Morgenstern, S., Chodick, G., Matar, M., Silbermintz, A., Assa, A., ... Shamir, R. (2017). Oesophageal eosinophilia in children with coeliac disease. *Archives of Disease in Childhood, 102*(9), 825-829.

Aronsson, C. A., Lee, H. S., af Segerstad, E. M. H., Uusitalo, U., Yang, J., Koletzko, S., ... Toppari, J. (2019). Association of gluten intake during the first 5 years of life with incidence of celiac disease autoimmunity and celiac disease among children at increased risk. *Jama, 322*(6), 514-523.

Arregui, M. V., Urmeneta, J. M. Z., Brito, H. L., De Esteban, J. P. M., Martínez, C. P., Llenas, L. F., ... Gutierrez, M. R. M. (2016). The role of flow cytometry in celiac disease screening using human leukocyte antigen in adult patients with type 1 diabetes mellitus. *Annals of Gastroenterology: Quarterly Publication of the Hellenic Society of Gastroenterology, 30*(2), 179.

Arroyo, H. A., De Rosa, S., Ruggieri, V., de Dávila, M. T., & Fejerman, N. (2002). Epilepsy, occipital calcifications, and oligosymptomatic celiac disease in childhood. *Journal of child neurology, 17*(11), 800-806.

Ashorn, S., Raukola, H., Välineva, T., Ashorn, M., Wei, B., Braun, J., ... Collin, P. (2008). Elevated serum anti-Saccharomyces cerevisiae, anti-I2 and anti-OmpW antibody levels in patients with suspicion of celiac disease. *Journal of clinical immunology, 28*, 486-494.

Ashraf, R., & Shah, N. P. (2014). Immune system stimulation by probiotic microorganisms. *Critical reviews in food science and nutrition, 54*(7), 938-956.

Assa, A., Frenkel-Nir, Y., Tzur, D., Katz, L. H., & Shamir, R. (2017). Large population study shows that adolescents with celiac disease have an increased risk of multiple autoimmune and nonautoimmune comorbidities. *Acta paediatrica, 106*(6), 967-972.

Atlasy, N., Bujko, A., Brazda, P. B., Janssen-Megens, E., Bækkevold, E. S., Jahnsen, J., ... Stunnenberg, H. G. (2019). Single cell transcriptome atlas of immune cells in human small intestine and in celiac disease. *bioRxiv*, 721258.

Auricchio, R., Galatola, M., Cielo, D., Amoresano, A., Caterino, M., De Vita, E., ... Ruoppolo, M. (2019). A phospholipid profile at 4 months predicts the onset of celiac disease in at-risk infants. *Scientific Reports, 9*(1), 14303.

Aziz, I. (2018). The global phenomenon of self-reported wheat sensitivity. In (Vol. 113, pp. 945-948): LWW.

Aziz, I., Evans, K. E., Hopper, A. D., Smillie, D. M., & Sanders, D. S. (2010). A prospective study into the aetiology of lymphocytic duodenosis. *Alimentary pharmacology & therapeutics, 32*(11-12), 1392-1397.

Babio, N., Alcázar, M., Castillejo, G., Recasens, M., Martínez-Cerezo, F., Gutiérrez-Pensado, V., ... Torres-Moreno, M. (2017). Patients with celiac disease reported higher consumption of added sugar and total fat than healthy individuals. *Journal of pediatric gastroenterology and nutrition, 64*(1), 63-69.

Bach, J. F. (2002). The effect of infections on susceptibility to autoimmune and allergic diseases. *New England Journal of Medicine, 347*(12), 911-920.

Bach, J. F. (2018). The hygiene hypothesis in autoimmunity: the role of pathogens and commensals. *Nature Reviews Immunology, 18*(2), 105-120.

Bagolin do Nascimento, A., Medeiros Rataichesck Fiates, G., dos Anjos, A., & Teixeira, E. (2014). Availability, cost and nutritional composition of gluten -free products. *British Food Journal, 116*(12), 1842-1852.

Bai, J., Gonzalez, D., Mautalen, C., Mazure, R., Pedreira, S., Vazquez, H., ... Niveloni, S. (1997). Long-term effect of gluten restriction on bone mineral density of patients with coeliac disease. *Alimentary pharmacology & therapeutics, 11*(1), 157-164.

Baldino, N., Laitano, F., Lupi, F. R., Curcio, S., & Gabriele, D. (2018). Effect of HPMC and CMC on rheological behavior at different temperatures of gluten -free bread formulations based on rice and buckwheat flours. *European food research and technology, 244*, 1829-1842.

Ballew, J. T., Murray, J. A., Collin, P., Mäki, M., Kagnoff, M. F., Kaukinen, K., & Daugherty, P. S. (2013). Antibody biomarker discovery through *in vitro* directed evolution of consensus recognition epitopes. *Proceedings of the National Academy of Sciences, 110*(48), 19330-19335.

Bamford, R. N., DeFilippis, A. P., Azimi, N., Kurys, G., & Waldmann, T. A. (1998). The 5′ untranslated region, signal peptide, and the coding sequence of the carboxyl terminus of IL-15 participate in its multifaceted translational control. *The Journal of Immunology, 160*(9), 4418-4426.

Barak, S., Mudgil, D., & Taneja, S. (2020). Exudate gums: chemistry, properties and food applications–a review. *Journal of the Science of Food and Agriculture, 100*(7), 2828-2835.

Bárcenas, M. E., & Rosell, C. M. (2006). Different approaches for improving the quality and extending the shelf life of the partially baked bread: low temperatures and HPMC addition. *Journal of food engineering, 72*(1), 92-99.

Bardella, M., Velio, P., Cesana, B. M., Prampolini, L., Casella, G., Di Bella, C., ... Villanacci, V. (2007). Coeliac disease: a histological follow-up study. *Histopathology, 50*(4), 465-471.

Bartolomé-Casado, R., Landsverk, O. J., Chauhan, S. K., Richter, L., Phung, D., Greiff, V., ... Yaqub, S. (2019). Resident memory CD8 T cells persist for years in human small intestine. *Journal of Experimental Medicine, 216*(10), 2412-2426.

Bartolomé-Casado, R., Landsverk, O. J., Chauhan, S. K., Sætre, F., Hagen, K. T., Yaqub, S., ... Aabakken, L. (2021). CD4+ T cells persist for years in the human small intestine and display a TH1 cytokine profile. *Mucosal immunology, 14*(2), 402-410.

Bascuñán, K. A., Pérez-Bravo, F., Gaudioso, G., Vaira, V., Roncoroni, L., Elli, L., ... Araya, M. (2020). A miRNA-based blood and mucosal approach for detecting and monitoring celiac disease. *Digestive diseases and sciences, 65*, 1982-1991.

Bauer, S., Groh, V., Wu, J., Steinle, A., Phillips, J. H., Lanier, L. L., & Spies, T. (1999). Activation of NK cells and T cells by NKG2D, a receptor for stress-inducible MICA. *Science, 285*(5428), 727-729.

Bauman, E. (2008). Gluten Sensitivity : A Rising Concern.

Baunwall, S. M. D., Lee, M. M., Eriksen, M. K., Mullish, B. H., Marchesi, J. R., Dahlerup, J. F., & Hvas, C. L. (2020). Faecal microbiota transplantation for recurrent Clostridioides difficile infection: An updated systematic review and meta-analysis. *EClinicalMedicine, 29*, 100642.

Belei, O., Iacob, E. R., Iacob, D., Amaricai, E., & Marginean, O. (2020). Chemiluminescent Immunoassay versus Enzyme Linked Immunosorbent Assays for IgA Anti-Tissue Transglutaminase Antibodies Assessment in Celiac Disease Children. *Rev. Chim, 71*, 45.

Bellinghausen, I., Weigmann, B., Zevallos, V., Maxeiner, J., Reißig, S., Waisman, A., ... Saloga, J. (2019). Wheat amylase-trypsin inhibitors exacerbate intestinal and airway allergic immune responses in humanized mice. *Journal of Allergy and Clinical Immunology, 143*(1), 201-212. e204.

Belorio, M., & Gómez, M. (2020). Effect of hydration on gluten -free breads made with hydroxypropyl methylcellulose in comparison with psyllium and xanthan gum. *Foods, 9*(11), 1548.

BeMiller, J. N. (2018). *Carbohydrate chemistry for food scientists*: Elsevier.

Beniwal, N., Ameta, G., & Chahar, C. K. (2017). Celiac disease in children with severe acute malnutrition (SAM): a hospital based study. *The Indian Journal of Pediatrics, 84*(5), 339-343.

Benkadri, S., Salvador, A., Sanz, T., & Nasreddine Zidoune, M. (2020). Optimization of xanthan and locust bean gum in a gluten -free infant biscuit based on rice-chickpea flour using response surface methodology. *Foods, 10*(1), 12.

Benkadri, S., Salvador, A., Zidoune, M. N., & Sanz, T. (2018). Gluten-free biscuits based on composite rice–chickpea flour and xanthan gum. *Food Science and Technology International, 24*(7), 607-616.

Bergamo, P., Maurano, F., Mazzarella, G., Iaquinto, G., Vocca, I., Rivelli, A. R., ... Rossi, M. (2011). Immunological evaluation of the alcohol-soluble protein fraction from gluten -free grains in relation to celiac disease. *Molecular nutrition & food research, 55*(8), 1266-1270.

Bernardi, S., Del Bo', C., Marino, M., Gargari, G., Cherubini, A., Andrés-Lacueva, C., ... Kroon, P. (2019). Polyphenols and intestinal permeability: rationale and future perspectives. *Journal of agricultural and food chemistry, 68*(7), 1816-1829.

Bernardo, D. (2013). Human intestinal dendritic cells as controllers of mucosal immunity. *Rev Esp Enferm Dig, 105*(5), 279-290.

Bernstein, C. N., Leslie, W. D., & Leboff, M. S. (2003). AGA technical review on osteoporosis in gastrointestinal diseases. *Gastroenterology, 124*(3), 795-841.

Bethune, M. T., Ribka, E., Khosla, C., & Sestak, K. (2008). Transepithelial transport and enzymatic detoxification of gluten in gluten-sensitive rhesus macaques. *PloS one, 3*(3), e1857.

Bethune, M. T., Strop, P., Tang, Y., Sollid, L. M., & Khosla, C. (2006). Heterologous expression, purification, refolding, and structural-functional characterization of EP-B2, a self-activating barley cysteine endoprotease. *Chemistry & biology, 13*(6), 637-647.

Bhagat, G., Naiyer, A. J., Shah, J. G., Harper, J., Jabri, B., Wang, T. C., ... Manavalan, J. S. (2008). Small intestinal CD8+ TCRγδ+ NKG2A+ intraepithelial lymphocytes have attributes of regulatory cells in patients with celiac disease. *The Journal of clinical investigation, 118*(1), 281-293.

Bhaskar, M. M., Sistla, S., & Kumaravel, S. (2017). A case of pyometrocolpos with Bifidobacterium species. *Anaerobe, 44*, 48-50.

Biagi, F., Luinetti, O., Campanella, J., Klersy, C., Zambelli, C., Villanacci, V., ... Corazza, G. (2004). Intraepithelial lymphocytes in the villous tip: do they indicate potential coeliac disease? *Journal of clinical pathology, 57*(8), 835-839.

Billadeau, D. D., Upshaw, J. L., Schoon, R. A., Dick, C. J., & Leibson, P. J. (2003). NKG2D-DAP10 triggers human NK cell–mediated killing via a Syk-independent regulatory pathway. *Nature immunology, 4*(6), 557-564.

Biswas, S. K. (2016). Does the interdependence between oxidative stress and inflammation explain the antioxidant paradox? *Oxidative medicine and cellular longevity, 2016*(1), 5698931.

Black, K. E., Murray, J. A., & David, C. S. (2002). HLA-DQ determines the response to exogenous wheat proteins: a model of gluten sensitivity in transgenic knockout mice. *The Journal of Immunology, 169*(10), 5595-5600.

Blázquez, A. B., & Berin, M. C. (2017). Microbiome and food allergy. *Translational Research, 179*, 199-203.

Bodd, M., Kim, C. Y., Lundin, K. E., & Sollid, L. M. (2012). T-cell response to gluten in patients with HLA-DQ2. 2 reveals requirement of peptide-MHC stability in celiac disease. *Gastroenterology, 142*(3), 552-561.

Bodd, M., Ráki, M., Bergseng, E., Jahnsen, J., Lundin, K. E., & Sollid, L. M. (2013). Direct cloning and tetramer staining to measure the frequency of intestinal gluten -reactive T cells in celiac disease. *European journal of immunology, 43*(10), 2605-2612.

Bonilla, D. L., Reinin, G., & Chua, E. (2021). Full spectrum flow cytometry as a powerful technology for cancer immunotherapy research. *Frontiers in Molecular Biosciences, 7*, 612801.

Boonen, S., Reginster, J. Y., Kaufman, J. M., Lippuner, K., Zanchetta, J., Langdahl, B., ... Witvrouw, R. (2012). Fracture risk and zoledronic acid therapy in men with osteoporosis. *New England Journal of Medicine, 367*(18), 1714-1723.

Bosscher, D., Van Loo, J., & Franck, A. (2006). Inulin and oligofructose as functional ingredients to improve bone mineralization. *International Dairy Journal, 16*(9), 1092-1097.

Boukid, F., Prandi, B., Sforza, S., Sayar, R., Seo, Y. W., Mejri, M., & Yacoubi, I. (2017). Understanding the effects of genotype, growing year, and breeding on Tunisian durum wheat allergenicity. 2. The celiac disease case. *Journal of agricultural and food chemistry, 65*(28), 5837-5846.

Bouziat, R., Hinterleitner, R., Brown, J. J., Stencel-Baerenwald, J. E., Ikizler, M., Mayassi, T., ... Jabri, B. (2017). Reovirus infection triggers inflammatory responses to dietary antigens and development of celiac disease. *Science, 356*(6333), 44-50. doi:10.1126/science.aah5298

Brandtzaeg, P. (2006). The changing immunological paradigm in coeliac disease. *Immunology letters, 105*(2), 127-139.

Bray, M. S., Loos, R. J., McCaffery, J. M., Ling, C., Franks, P. W., Weinstock, G. M., ... Group, C. W. (2016). NIH working group report—using genomic information to guide weight management: From universal to precision treatment. *Obesity, 24*(1), 14-22.

Brottveit, M., Ráki, M., Bergseng, E., Fallang, L. E., Simonsen, B., Løvik, A., ... Sollid, L. M. (2011). Assessing possible celiac disease by an HLA-DQ2 -gliadin tetramer test. *Official journal of the American College of Gastroenterology| ACG, 106*(7), 1318-1324.

Broughton, S. E., Petersen, J., Theodossis, A., Scally, S. W., Loh, K. L., Thompson, A., ... Beddoe, T. (2012). Biased T cell receptor usage directed against human leukocyte antigen DQ8 -restricted gliadin peptides is associated with celiac disease. *Immunity, 37*(4), 611-621.

Brown, I. S., Bettington, A., Bettington, M., & Rosty, C. (2014). Tropical sprue : revisiting an underrecognized disease. *The American journal of surgical pathology, 38*(5), 666-672.

Brown, I. S., Smith, J., & Rosty, C. (2012). Gastrointestinal pathology in celiac disease: a case series of 150 consecutive newly diagnosed patients. *American journal of clinical pathology, 138*(1), 42-49.

Brown, N. K., Guandalini, S., Semrad, C., & Kupfer, S. S. (2019). A clinician's guide to celiac disease HLA genetics. *Official journal of the American College of Gastroenterology| ACG, 114*(10), 1587-1592.

Brück, J., Holstein, J., Glocova, I., Seidel, U., Geisel, J., Kanno, T., ... Widmaier, K. (2017). Nutritional control of IL-23/Th17-mediated autoimmune disease through HO-1/STAT3 activation. *Scientific reports, 7*(1), 44482.

Brzozowski, B. (2016). Immunoreactivity of wheat proteins modified by hydrolysis and polymerisation. *European Food Research and Technology, 242*(7), 1025-1040.

Büchold, C., Hils, M., Gerlach, U., Weber, J., Pelzer, C., Heil, A., ... Pasternack, R. (2022). Features of ZED1227 : The first-in-class tissue transglutaminase inhibitor undergoing clinical evaluation for the treatment of celiac disease. *Cells, 11*(10), 1667.

Burbure, N., Lebwohl, B., Arguelles-Grande, C., Green, P. H., Bhagat, G., & Lagana, S. (2016). Olmesartan-associated sprue -like enteropathy: a systematic review with emphasis on histopathology. *Human pathology, 50*, 127-134.

Buriánek, F., Gege, C., & Marinković, P. (2024). New developments in celiac disease treatments. *Drug Discovery Today*, 104113.

Burkhardt, J., Chapa-Rodriguez, A., & Bahna, S. (2018). Gluten sensitivities and the allergist: Threshing the grain from the husks. *Allergy, 73*(7), 1359-1368.

Butwicka, A., Lichtenstein, P., Frisén, L., Almqvist, C., Larsson, H., & Ludvigsson, J. F. (2017). Celiac disease is associated with childhood psychiatric disorders: a population-based study. *The Journal of pediatrics, 184*, 87-93. e81.

Bye, A. M., Andermann, F., Robitaille, Y., Oliver, M., Bohane, T., & Andermann, E. (1993). Cortical vascular abnormalities in the syndrome of celiac disease, epilepsy, bilateral occipital calcifications, and folate deficiency. *Annals of Neurology: Official Journal of the American Neurological Association and the Child Neurology Society, 34*(3), 399-403.

Caetano dos Santos, F. L., Michalek, I. M., Laurila, K., Kaukinen, K., Hyttinen, J., & Lindfors, K. (2019). Automatic classification of IgA endomysial antibody test for celiac disease: a new method deploying machine learning. *Scientific reports, 9*(1), 9217.

Caio, G., Volta, U., Sapone, A., Leffler, D. A., De Giorgio, R., Catassi, C., & Fasano, A. (2019). Celiac disease: a comprehensive current review. *BMC medicine, 17*, 1-20.

Cakir, D., Tosun, A., Polat, M., Celebisoy, N., Gokben, S., Aydogdu, S., ... Tekgul, H. (2007). Subclinical neurological abnormalities in children with celiac disease receiving a gluten -free diet. *Journal of pediatric gastroenterology and nutrition, 45*(3), 366-369.

Calleja, S., Vivas, S., Santiuste, M., Arias, L., Hernando, M., Nistal, E., ... Ruiz de Morales, J. G. (2011). Dynamics of non-conventional Intraepithelial lymphocytes—NK, NKT, and γδ T—in celiac disease: relationship with age, diet, and histopathology. *Digestive diseases and sciences, 56*, 2042-2049.

Calvani Jr, M., Parisi, P., Guaitolini, C., Parisi, G., & Paolone, G. (2001). Latent coeliac disease in a child with epilepsy, cerebral calcifications, drug-induced systemic lupus erythematosus and intestinal folic acid malabsorption associated with impairment of folic acid transport across the blood-brain barrier. *European journal of pediatrics, 160*, 288-292.

Camarca, A., Anderson, R. P., Mamone, G., Fierro, O., Facchiano, A., Costantini, S., ... Sette, A. (2009). Intestinal T cell responses to gluten peptides are largely heterogeneous: implications for a peptide-based therapy in celiac disease. *The Journal of Immunology, 182*(7), 4158-4166.

Caminero, A., Galipeau, H. J., McCarville, J. L., Johnston, C. W., Bernier, S. P., Russell, A. K., ... Tye-Din, J. A. (2016). Duodenal bacteria from patients with celiac disease and healthy subjects distinctly affect gluten breakdown and immunogenicity. *Gastroenterology, 151*(4), 670-683.

Caminero, A., McCarville, J. L., Galipeau, H. J., Deraison, C., Bernier, S. P., Constante, M., ... Yu, X. B. (2019). Duodenal bacterial proteolytic activity determines sensitivity to dietary antigen through protease-activated receptor-2. *Nature communications, 10*(1), 1-14.

Campagna, G., Pesce, M., Tatangelo, R., Rizzuto, A., La Fratta, I., & Grilli, A. (2017). The progression of coeliac disease: its neurological and psychiatric implications. *Nutrition Research Reviews, 30*(1), 25-35.

Canova, C., Zabeo, V., Pitter, G., Romor, P., Baldovin, T., Zanotti, R., & Simonato, L. (2014). Association of maternal education, early infections, and antibiotic use with celiac disease: a population-based birth cohort study in northeastern Italy. *American journal of epidemiology, 180*(1), 76-85.

Canzar, S., Neu, K. E., Tang, Q., Wilson, P. C., & Khan, A. A. (2017). BASIC: BCR assembly from single cells. *Bioinformatics, 33*(3), 425-427.

Cao, Z., Sugimura, N., Burgermeister, E., Ebert, M. P., Zuo, T., & Lan, P. (2022). The gut virome: A new microbiome component in health and disease. *EBioMedicine, 81*, 104113.

Cappelli, A., Oliva, N., & Cini, E. (2020). A systematic review of gluten -free dough and bread: Dough rheology, bread characteristics, and improvement strategies. *Applied Sciences, 10*(18), 6559.

Capriles, V. D., & Arêas, J. A. G. (2014). Novel approaches in gluten -free breadmaking: interface between food science, nutrition, and health. *Comprehensive Reviews in Food Science and Food Safety, 13*(5), 871-890.

Cardoso-Silva, D., Delbue, D., Itzlinger, A., Moerkens, R., Withoff, S., Branchi, F., & Schumann, M. (2019). Intestinal barrier function in gluten -related disorders. *Nutrients, 11*(10), 2325.

Carrasco-Pozo, C., Morales, P., & Gotteland, M. (2013). Polyphenols protect the epithelial barrier function of Caco-2 cells exposed to indomethacin through the modulation of occludin and zonula occludens-1 expression. *Journal of agricultural and food chemistry, 61*(22), 5291-5297.

Carta, M. G., Hardoy, M. C., Boi, M. F., Mariotti, S., Carpiniello, B., & Usai, P. (2002). Association between panic disorder, major depressive disorder and celiac disease: a possible role of thyroid autoimmunity. *Journal of psychosomatic research, 53*(3), 789-793.

Caruso, R., Marafini, I., Sedda, S., Del Vecchio Blanco, G., Giuffrida, P., MacDonald, T. T., ... Monteleone, G. (2014). Analysis of the cytokine profile in the duodenal mucosa of refractory coeliac disease patients. *Clinical Science, 126*(6), 451-458.

Castillo, L., & Rivas, C. (2008). Costs of a basic food basket for celiac patients in Chile. *Revista Medica de Chile, 136*(5), 613-619.

Castillo, N. E., Theethira, T. G., & Leffler, D. A. (2015). The present and the future in the diagnosis and management of celiac disease. *Gastroenterology report, 3*(1), 3-11.

Catassi, C., Alaedini, A., Bojarski, C., Bonaz, B., Bouma, G., Carroccio, A., ... Di Liberto, D. (2017). The overlapping area of non-celiac gluten sensitivity (NCGS) and wheat-sensitive irritable bowel syndrome (IBS): an update. *Nutrients, 9*(11), 1268.

Catassi, C., Fabiani, E., Iacono, G., D'Agate, C., Francavilla, R., Biagi, F., ... De Vitis, I. (2007). A prospective, double-blind, placebo-controlled trial to establish a safe gluten threshold for patients with celiac disease. *The American journal of clinical nutrition, 85*(1), 160-166.

Cavaletti, L., Taravella, A., Carrano, L., Carenzi, G., Sigurtà, A., Solinas, N., ... Laezza, M. (2019). E40, a novel microbial protease efficiently detoxifying gluten proteins, for the dietary management of gluten intolerance. *Scientific reports, 9*(1), 1-11.

Cellier, C., Delabesse, E., Helmer, C., Patey, N., Matuchansky, C., Jabri, B., ... Brousse, N. (2000). Refractory sprue, coeliac disease, and enteropathy-associated T-cell lymphoma. *The Lancet, 356*(9225), 203-208.

Cenit, M. C., Olivares, M., Codoñer-Franch, P., & Sanz, Y. (2015). Intestinal microbiota and celiac disease: cause, consequence or co-evolution? *Nutrients, 7*(8), 6900-6923.

Cerf-Bensussan, N., Matysiak-Budnik, T., Cellier, C., & Heyman, M. (2007). Oral proteases: a new approach to managing coeliac disease. *Gut, 56*(2), 157-160.

Cernibori, A., & Gobbi, G. (1995). Partial seizures, cerebral calcifications and celiac disease. *The Italian Journal of Neurological Sciences, 16*, 187-191.

Chakravarthi, S. D., Jain, K., Kochhar, R., Bhadada, S. K., Khandelwal, N., Bhansali, A., ... Singh, K. (2012). Prevalence and predictors of abnormal bone mineral metabolism in recently diagnosed adult celiac patients. *Indian Journal of Gastroenterology, 31*, 165-170.

Chander, U., Leeman-Neill, R. J., & Bhagat, G. (2018). Pathogenesis of enteropathy-associated T cell lymphoma. *Current hematologic malignancy reports, 13*, 308-317.

Chapman, R., Laidlow, J., Colin-Jones, D., Eade, O., & Smith, C. (1978). Increased prevalence of epilepsy in coeliac disease. *British medical journal, 2*(6132), 250.

Charlesworth, R. P. (2020). Diagnosing coeliac disease: out with the old and in with the new? *World Journal of Gastroenterology, 26*(1), 1.

Chen, S., Shen, B., Wang, X., & Yoo, S. J. (2019). A strong machine learning classifier and decision stumps based hybrid adaboost classification algorithm for cognitive radios. *Sensors, 19*(23), 5077.

Chen, W., Huang, Y., Boyle, B., & Lin, S. (2016). The utility of including pathology reports in improving the computational identification of patients. *Journal of Pathology Informatics, 7*(1), 46.

Chen, X., Hnida, K., Graewert, M. A., Andersen, J. T., Iversen, R., Tuukkanen, A., ... Sollid, L. M. (2015). Structural basis for antigen recognition by transglutaminase 2-specific autoantibodies in celiac disease. *Journal of Biological Chemistry, 290*(35), 21365-21375.

Cheng, Y., Wu, T., Tang, S., Liang, F., Fang, Y., Cao, W., ... Xu, X. (2020). Fermented blueberry pomace ameliorates intestinal barrier function through the NF-κB-MLCK signaling pathway in high-fat diet mice. *Food & function, 11*(4), 3167-3179.

Chiba, M., Ohta, H., Yagisawa, H., & Masamune, O. (1987). IgA1 & IgA2 distribution in the intestine. *Gastroenterologia Japonica, 22*, 18-23.

Chin, R. L., Latov, N., Green, P. H., Brannagan III, T. H., Alaedini, A., & Sander, H. W. (2004). Neurologic complications of celiac disease. *Journal of clinical neuromuscular disease, 5*(3), 129-137.

Chin, R., Sander, H., Brannagan, T., Green, P., Hays, A., Alaedini, A., & Latov, N. (2003). Celiac neuropathy. *Neurology, 60*(10), 1581-1585.

Choi, K., Siegel, M., Piper, J. L., Yuan, L., Cho, E., Strnad, P., ... Khosla, C. (2005). Chemistry and biology of dihydroisoxazole derivatives: selective inhibitors of human transglutaminase 2. *Chemistry & biology, 12*(4), 469-475.

Christophersen, A. (2014). Tetramer-visualized gluten -specific CD4+ T cells in blood as a potential diagnostic marker for coeliac disease without oral gluten challenge by Christophersen et al.(vol 2, pg 268, 2014). *United European gastroenterology journal, 2*(4), 550-550.

Christophersen, A., Lund, E. G., Snir, O., Solà, E., Kanduri, C., Dahal-Koirala, S., ... Rohani-Pichavant, M. (2019). Distinct phenotype of CD4+ T cells driving celiac disease identified in multiple autoimmune conditions. *Nature medicine, 25*(5), 734-737.

Christophersen, A., Ráki, M., Bergseng, E., Lundin, K. E., Jahnsen, J., Sollid, L. M., & Qiao, S. W. (2014). Tetramer-visualized gluten -specific CD4+ T cells in blood as a potential diagnostic marker for coeliac disease without oral gluten challenge. *United European gastroenterology journal, 2*(4), 268-278.

Christophersen, A., Risnes, L. F., Bergseng, E., Lundin, K. E., Sollid, L. M., & Qiao, S. W. (2016). Healthy HLA-DQ2. 5+ subjects lack regulatory and memory T cells specific for immunodominant gluten epitopes of celiac disease. *The Journal of Immunology, 196*(6), 2819-2826.

Chung HyunJung, C. H., Liu Qiang, L. Q., & Lim SeungTaik, L. S. (2007). Texture and *in vitro* digestibility of white rice cooked with hydrocolloids.

Chung, S., Yao, H., Caito, S., Hwang, J. w., Arunachalam, G., & Rahman, I. (2010). Regulation of SIRT1 in cellular functions: role of polyphenols. *Archives of biochemistry and biophysics, 501*(1), 79-90.

Ciacci, C., Cavallaro, R., Iovino, P., Sabbatini, F., Palumbo, A., Amoruso, D., ... Mazzacca, G. (2004). Allergy prevalence in adult celiac disease. *Journal of Allergy and Clinical Immunology, 113*(6), 1199-1203.

Ciacci, C., Cirillo, M., Cavallaro, R., & Mazzacca, G. (2002). Long-term follow-up of celiac adults on gluten -free diet : prevalence and correlates of intestinal damage. *Digestion, 66*(3), 178-185.

Ciaccio, E. J., Tennyson, C. A., Bhagat, G., Lewis, S. K., & Green, P. H. (2010). Classification of videocapsule endoscopy image patterns: comparative analysis between patients with celiac disease and normal individuals. *BioMedical Engineering Online, 9*, 1-12.

Cianci, R., Cammarota, G., Frisullo, G., Pagliari, D., Ianiro, G., Martini, M., ... Casciano, F. (2012). Tissue-infiltrating lymphocytes analysis reveals large modifications of the duodenal "immunological niche" in coeliac disease after gluten -free diet. *Clinical and translational gastroenterology, 3*(12), e28.

Cicarelli, G., Della Rocca, G., Amboni, M., Ciacci, C., Mazzacca, G., Filla, A., & Barone, P. (2003). Clinical and neurological abnormalities in adult celiac disease. *Neurological Sciences, 24*, 311-317.

Ciccocioppo, R., Finamore, A., Ara, C., Di Sabatino, A., Mengheri, E., & Corazza, G. R. (2006). Altered expression, localization, and phosphorylation of epithelial junctional proteins in celiac disease. *American Journal of Clinical Pathology, 125*(4), 502-511.

Cirkovic Velickovic, T. D., & Stanic-Vucinic, D. J. (2018). The role of dietary phenolic compounds in protein digestion and processing technologies to improve their antinutritive properties. *Comprehensive Reviews in Food Science and Food Safety, 17*(1), 82-103.

Cohen, A., Stein, E. M., Recker, R. R., Lappe, J. M., Dempster, D. W., Zhou, H., ... Müller, R. (2013). Teriparatide for idiopathic osteoporosis in premenopausal women: a pilot study. *The Journal of Clinical Endocrinology & Metabolism, 98*(5), 1971-1981.

Cohen, I. S., Day, A. S., & Shaoul, R. (2019). To be oats or not to be? An update on the ongoing debate on oats for patients with celiac disease. *Frontiers in Pediatrics, 7*.

Colgrave, M. L., Byrne, K., & Howitt, C. A. (2017). Food for thought: Selecting the right enzyme for the digestion of gluten. *Food Chemistry, 234*, 389-397.

Comino, I., de Lourdes Moreno, M., & Sousa, C. (2015). Role of oats in celiac disease. *World journal of gastroenterology, 21*(41), 11825.

Commission, C. A. (2008). Codex standard for foods for special dietary use for persons intolerant to gluten. *http://www.codexalimentarius.net/download/standards/291/cxs_118e. pdf.*

Compston, J. (2003). Is fracture risk increased in patients with coeliac disease? *Gut, 52*(4), 459-460.

Compston, J., McClung, M., & Leslie, W. Osteoporosis Lancet, 393 (10169)(2019). *View PDF View article View in Scopus*, 364-376.

Consortium, I. W. G. S., Appels, R., Eversole, K., Stein, N., Feuillet, C., Keller, B., ... Distelfeld, A. (2018). Shifting the limits in wheat research and breeding using a fully annotated reference genome. *Science, 361*(6403), eaar7191.

Conte, M., Porpora, M., Nigro, F., Nigro, R., Budelli, A. L., Barone, M. V., & Nanayakkara, M. (2021). Pro-pre and postbiotic in celiac disease. *Applied Sciences, 11*(17), 8185.

Cook, L., Munier, C. M. L., Seddiki, N., van Bockel, D., Ontiveros, N., Hardy, M. Y., ... Petersen, J. (2017). Circulating gluten -specific FOXP3+ CD39+ regulatory T cells have impaired suppressive function in patients with celiac disease. *Journal of Allergy and Clinical Immunology, 140*(6), 1592-1603. e1598.

Cooke, W., & Smith, W. T. (1966). Neurological disorders associated with adult celiac disease. *Brain, 89*(4), 683-722.

Corazza, G. R., Biagi, F., Volta, U., Andreani, M. L., De Franceschi, L., & Gasbarrini, G. (1997). Autoimmune enteropathy and villous atrophy in adults. *The Lancet, 350*(9071), 106-109.

Corazza, G. R., Di Stefano, M., Jorizzo, R. A., Cecchetti, L., Minguzzi, L., & Gasbarrini, G. (1997). Propeptide of type I procollagen is predictive of posttreatment bone mass gain in adult celiac disease. *Gastroenterology, 113*(1), 67-71.

Corazza, G., Di Sario, A., Cecchetti, L., Jorizzo, R., Di Stefano, M., Minguzzi, L., ... Gasbarrini, G. (1996). Influence of pattern of clinical presentation and of gluten -free diet on bone mass and metabolism in adult coeliac disease. *Bone, 18*(6), 525-530.

Correa, M. J., Añon, M. C., Perez, G. T., & Ferrero, C. (2010). Effect of modified celluloses on dough rheology and microstructure. *Food Research International, 43*(3), 780-787.

Crawford, F., Kozono, H., White, J., Marrack, P., & Kappler, J. (1998). Detection of antigen-specific T cells with multivalent soluble class II MHC covalent peptide complexes. *Immunity, 8*(6), 675-682.

Cremonini, E., Mastaloudis, A., Hester, S. N., Verstraeten, S. V., Anderson, M., Wood, S. M., ... Oteiza, P. I. (2017). Anthocyanins inhibit tumor necrosis alpha-induced loss of Caco-2 cell barrier integrity. *Food & function, 8*(8), 2915-2923.

Cremonini, E., Wang, Z., Bettaieb, A., Adamo, A. M., Daveri, E., Mills, D. A., ... Oteiza, P. I. (2018). (-)-Epicatechin protects the intestinal barrier from high fat diet-induced permeabilization: Implications for steatosis and insulin resistance. *Redox biology, 14*, 588-599.

Croese, J., Giacomin, P., Navarro, S., Clouston, A., McCann, L., Dougall, A., ... Howlett, M. (2015). Experimental hookworm infection and gluten microchallenge promote tolerance in celiac disease. *Journal of Allergy and Clinical Immunology, 135*(2), 508-516. e505.

Cronin, C., Jackson, L., Feighery, C., Shanahan, F., Abuzakouk, M., Ryder, D., ... Callaghan, N. (1998). Coeliac disease and epilepsy. *QJM: monthly journal of the Association of Physicians, 91*(4), 303-308.

Crosato, F., & Senter, S. (1992). Cerebral occipital calcifications in celiac disease. *Neuropediatrics, 23*(04), 214-217.

Cross, A. H., & Golumbek, P. T. (2003). Neurologic manifestations of celiac disease: proven, or just a gut feeling? In (Vol. 60, pp. 1566-1568): AAN Enterprises.

Crotty, S. (2011). Follicular helper CD4 T cells (Tfh). *Annual review of immunology, 29*(1), 621-663.

Cruikshank, W. W., Center, D. M., Nisar, N., Wu, M., Natke, B., Theodore, A. C., & Kornfeld, H. (1994). Molecular and functional analysis of a lymphocyte chemoattractant factor: association of biologic function with CD4 expression. *Proceedings of the National Academy of Sciences, 91*(11), 5109-5113.

Cuevas, A., Saavedra, N., Salazar, L. A., & Abdalla, D. S. (2013). Modulation of immune function by polyphenols: possible contribution of epigenetic factors. *Nutrients, 5*(7), 2314-2332.

Cui, S., Luo, Y., Tseng, H. H., Ten Haken, R. K., & El Naqa, I. (2019). Combining handcrafted features with latent variables in machine learning for prediction of radiation-induced lung damage. *Medical physics, 46*(5), 2497-2511.

Culetu, A., Duta, D. E., Papageorgiou, M., & Varzakas, T. (2021). The role of hydrocolloids in gluten -free bread and pasta; rheology, characteristics, staling and glycemic index. *Foods, 10*(12), 3121.

Currie, S., Hadjivassiliou, M., Clark, M. J., Sanders, D. S., Wilkinson, I. D., Griffiths, P. D., & Hoggard, N. (2012). Should we be 'nervous' about coeliac disease? Brain abnormalities in patients with coeliac disease referred for neurological opinion. *Journal of Neurology, Neurosurgery & Psychiatry, 83*(12), 1216-1221.

D'argenio, V., Casaburi, G., Precone, V., Pagliuca, C., Colicchio, R., Sarnataro, D., ... Blanco, G. D. V. (2016). Metagenomics reveals dysbiosis and a potentially pathogenic N. flavescens strain in duodenum of adult celiac patients. *Official journal of the American College of Gastroenterology| ACG, 111*(6), 879-890.

D'Arienzo, R., Maurano, F., Lavermicocca, P., Ricca, E., & Rossi, M. (2009). Modulation of the immune response by probiotic strains in a mouse model of gluten sensitivity. *Cytokine, 48*(3), 254-259.

D'Arienzo, R., Maurano, F., Luongo, D., Mazzarella, G., Stefanile, R., Troncone, R., ... Rossi, M. (2008). Adjuvant effect of Lactobacillus casei in a mouse model of gluten sensitivity. *Immunology letters, 119*(1-2), 78-83.

D'Arienzo, R., Stefanile, R., Maurano, F., Luongo, D., Bergamo, P., Mazzarella, G., ... Rossi, M. (2009). A deregulated immune response to gliadin causes a decreased villus height in DQ8 transgenic mice. *European journal of immunology, 39*(12), 3552-3561.

D'arienzo, R., Stefanile, R., Maurano, F., Mazzarella, G., Ricca, E., Troncone, R., ... Rossi, M. (2011). Immunomodulatory effects of Lactobacillus casei administration in a mouse model of gliadin-sensitive enteropathy. *Scandinavian journal of immunology, 74*(4), 335-341.

Dafik, L., Albertelli, M., Stamnaes, J., Sollid, L. M., & Khosla, C. (2012). Activation and inhibition of transglutaminase 2 in mice. *PloS one, 7*(2), e30642.

Dahal-Koirala, S., Ciacchi, L., Petersen, J., Risnes, L. F., Neumann, R. S., Christophersen, A., ... Rossjohn, J. (2019). Discriminative T-cell receptor recognition of highly homologous HLA-DQ2 –bound gluten epitopes. *Journal of Biological Chemistry, 294*(3), 941-952.

Dahal-Koirala, S., Neumann, R. S., Jahnsen, J., Lundin, K. E., & Sollid, L. M. (2020). On the immune response to barley in celiac disease: Biased and public T-cell receptor usage to a barley unique and immunodominant gluten epitope. *European journal of immunology, 50*(2), 256-269.

Dahal-Koirala, S., Risnes, L. F., Christophersen, A., Sarna, V. K., Lundin, K. E., Sollid, L. M., & Qiao, S. (2016). TCR sequencing of single cells reactive to DQ2. 5-glia-α2 and DQ2. 5-glia-ω2 reveals clonal expansion and epitope-specific V-gene usage. *Mucosal immunology, 9*(3), 587-596.

Dahal-Koirala, S., Risnes, L. F., Neumann, R. S., Christophersen, A., Lundin, K. E., Sandve, G. K., ... Sollid, L. M. (2021). Comprehensive analysis of CDR3 sequences in gluten -specific T-cell receptors reveals a dominant R-motif and several new minor motifs. *Frontiers in Immunology, 12*, 639672.

Dai, A. I., Akcali, A., Varan, C., & Demiryürek, A. T. (2014). Prevalence of resistant occipital lobe epilepsy associated with celiac disease in children. *Child's Nervous System, 30*, 1091-1098.

Dale, H. F., Biesiekierski, J. R., & Lied, G. A. (2019). Non-coeliac gluten sensitivity and the spectrum of gluten-related disorders: An updated overview. *Nutrition Research Reviews, 32*(1), 28-37.

Darwish, G., Helmerhorst, E. J., Schuppan, D., Oppenheim, F. G., & Wei, G. (2019). Pharmaceutically modified subtilisins withstand acidic conditions and effectively degrade gluten *in vivo*. *Scientific reports, 9*(1), 1-10.

Daveson, A. J., Jones, D. M., Gaze, S., McSorley, H., Clouston, A., Pascoe, A., ... Anderson, R. (2011). Effect of hookworm infection on wheat challenge in celiac disease–a randomised double-blinded placebo controlled trial. *PloS one, 6*(3), e17366.

De Angelis, M., Coda, R., Silano, M., Minervini, F., Rizzello, C. G., Di Cagno, R., ... Gobbetti, M. (2006). Fermentation by selected sourdough lactic acid bacteria to decrease coeliac intolerance to rye flour. *Journal of cereal Science, 43*(3), 301-314.

De Angelis, M., Rizzello, C. G., Fasano, A., Clemente, M. G., De Simone, C., Silano, M., ... Gobbetti, M. (2006). VSL# 3 probiotic preparation has the capacity to hydrolyze gliadin polypeptides responsible for celiac sprue probiotics and gluten intolerance. *Biochimica et Biophysica Acta (BBA)-Molecular Basis of Disease, 1762*(1), 80-93.

de Freitas, V., & Mateus, N. (2012). Protein/polyphenol interactions: past and present contributions. Mechanisms of astringency perception. *Current Organic Chemistry, 16*(6), 724-746.

de Kauwe, A. L., Chen, Z., Anderson, R. P., Keech, C. L., Price, J. D., Wijburg, O., ... McCluskey, J. (2009). Resistance to celiac disease in humanized HLA-DR3-DQ2 - transgenic mice expressing specific anti-gliadin CD4+ T cells. *The Journal of Immunology, 182*(12), 7440-7450.

de Lourdes Moreno, M., Segura, V., Ruiz-Carnicer, Á., Nájar, A. M., Comino, I., & Sousa, C. (2021). Oral enzyme strategy in celiac disease. In *Biotechnological Strategies for the Treatment of Gluten Intolerance* (pp. 201-220): Elsevier.

De Palma, G., Kamanova, J., Cinova, J., Olivares, M., Drasarova, H., Tuckova, L., & Sanz, Y. (2012). Modulation of phenotypic and functional maturation of dendritic cells by intestinal bacteria and gliadin: relevance for celiac disease. *Journal of leukocyte biology, 92*(5), 1043-1054.

De Stefano, D., Maiuri, M. C., Simeon, V., Grassia, G., Soscia, A., Cinelli, M. P., & Carnuccio, R. (2007). Lycopene, quercetin and tyrosol prevent macrophage activation induced by gliadin and IFN-γ. *European journal of pharmacology, 566*(1-3), 192-199.

Deconinck, N., Scaillon, M., Segers, V., Groswasser, J. J., & Dan, B. (2006). Opsoclonus-myoclonus associated with celiac disease. *Pediatric neurology, 34*(4), 312-314.

deFonseka, A., Tuskey, A., & Moskaluk, C. (2012). P-10 A Case of Olmesartan Induced Enteropathy. *Inflammatory Bowel Diseases, 18*(suppl_1), S17-S18.

DeGaetani, M., Tennyson, C. A., Lebwohl, B., Lewis, S. K., Daya, H. A., Arguelles-Grande, C., ... Green, P. H. (2013). Villous atrophy and negative celiac serology: a diagnostic and therapeutic dilemma. *Official journal of the American College of Gastroenterology| ACG, 108*(5), 647-653.

Del Pozzo, G., Farina, F., Picascia, S., Laezza, M., Vitale, S., & Gianfrani, C. (2021). HLA class II genes in precision-based care of childhood diseases: what we can learn from celiac disease. *Pediatric Research, 89*(2), 307-312.

Denham, J. M., & Hill, I. D. (2013). Celiac disease and autoimmunity: review and controversies. *Current allergy and asthma reports, 13*(4), 347-353.

Deora, V., Aylward, N., Sokoro, A., & El-Matary, W. (2017). Serum vitamins and minerals at diagnosis and follow-up in children with celiac disease. *Journal of pediatric gastroenterology and nutrition. 65*(2), 185-189.

DePaolo, R., Abadie, V., Tang, F., Fehlner-Peach, H., Hall, J., Wang, W., ... Murray, J. (2011). Co-adjuvant effects of retinoic acid and IL-15 induce inflammatory immunity to dietary antigens. *Nature, 471*(7337), 220-224.

Devisetti, R., Ravi, R., & Bhattacharya, S. (2015). Effect of hydrocolloids on quality of proso millet cookie. *Food and Bioprocess Technology, 8*, 2298-2308.

Dhalwani, N. N., West, J., Sultan, A. A., Ban, L., & Tata, L. J. (2014). Women with celiac disease present with fertility problems no more often than women in the general population. *Gastroenterology, 147*(6), 1267-1274. e1261.

Dhankhar, P., & Tech, M. (2013). A study on development of coconut based gluten free cookies. *International Journal of Engineering Science Invention, 2*(12), 10-19.

Di Cagno, L., & Ravetto, F. (1966). Acute ataxia in the course of the celiac syndrome. Illustration of a case. *Minerva Pediatrica, 18*(15), 753-754.

Di Cagno, R., De Angelis, M., Auricchio, S., Greco, L., Clarke, C., De Vincenzi, M., ... Parrilli, G. (2004). Sourdough bread made from wheat and nontoxic flours and started with selected lactobacilli is tolerated in celiac sprue patients. *Applied and environmental microbiology, 70*(2), 1088-1096.

Di Cagno, R., De Angelis, M., Lavermicocca, P., De Vincenzi, M., Giovannini, C., Faccia, M., & Gobbetti, M. (2002). Proteolysis by sourdough lactic acid bacteria : effects on wheat flour protein fractions and gliadin peptides involved in human cereal intolerance. *Applied and environmental microbiology, 68*(2), 623-633.

Di Niro, R., Mesin, L., Raki, M., Zheng, N. Y., Lund-Johansen, F., Lundin, K. E., ... Sollid, L. M. (2010). Rapid generation of rotavirus-specific human monoclonal antibodies from small-intestinal mucosa. *The Journal of Immunology, 185*(9), 5377-5383.

Di Niro, R., Mesin, L., Zheng, N. Y., Stamnaes, J., Morrissey, M., Lee, J. H., ... Qiao, S. W. (2012). High abundance of plasma cells secreting transglutaminase 2–specific IgA autoantibodies with limited somatic hypermutation in celiac disease intestinal lesions. *Nature medicine, 18*(3), 441-445.

Di Niro, R., Snir, O., Kaukinen, K., Yaari, G., Lundin, K. E., Gupta, N., ... Mäki, M. (2016). Responsive population dynamics and wide seeding into the duodenal lamina propria of transglutaminase-2-specific plasma cells in celiac disease. *Mucosal immunology, 9*(1), 254-264.

Di Sabatino, A., Biagi, F., Lenzi, M., Frulloni, L., Lenti, M. V., Giuffrida, P., & Corazza, G. R. (2017). Clinical usefulness of serum antibodies as biomarkers of gastrointestinal and liver diseases. *Digestive and Liver Disease, 49*(9), 947-956.

Di Sabatino, A., Pickard, K. M., Gordon, J. N., Salvati, V., Mazzarella, G., Beattie, R. M., ... Croft, N. M. (2007). Evidence for the role of interferon-alfa production by dendritic cells in the Th1 response in celiac disease. *Gastroenterology, 133*(4), 1175-1187.

Di Sabatino, A., Vanoli, A., Giuffrida, P., Luinetti, O., Solcia, E., & Corazza, G. R. (2012). The function of tissue transglutaminase in celiac disease. *Autoimmunity reviews, 11*(10), 746-753.

Dias, R., Bras, N. F., Fernandes, I., Perez-Gregorio, M., Mateus, N., & Freitas, V. (2018). Molecular insights on the interaction and preventive potential of epigallocatechin-3-

gallate in Celiac Disease. *International Journal of Biological Macromolecules, 112*, 1029-1037.

Dias, R., Bras, N. F., Perez-Gregorio, M., Fernandes, I., Mateus, N., & Freitas, V. (2019). A multi-spectroscopic study on the interaction of food polyphenols with a bioactive gluten peptide: From chemistry to biological implications. *Food chemistry, 299*, 125051.

Dias, R., Oliveira, H., Fernandes, I., Simal-Gandara, J., & Perez-Gregorio, R. (2021). Recent advances in extracting phenolic compounds from food and their use in disease prevention and as cosmetics. *Critical Reviews in food science and nutrition, 61*(7), 1130-1151.

Dias, R., Perez-Gregorio, M. R., Mateus, N., & De Freitas, V. (2016). Interaction study between wheat-derived peptides and procyanidin B3 by mass spectrometry. *Food chemistry, 194*, 1304-1312.

Dias, R., Perez-Gregorio, R., Mateus, N., & De Freitas, V. (2015). The interaction between tannins and gliadin derived peptides in a celiac disease perspective. *Rsc Advances, 5*(41), 32151-32158.

Dicke, W. K., Weijers, H., & KAMER, J. v. D. (1953). Coeliac disease the presence in wheat of a factor having a deleterious effect in cases of coeliac disease. *Acta paediatrica, 42*(1), 34-42.

Dickinson, E. (2010). Food emulsions and foams: Stabilization by particles. *Current Opinion in Colloid & Interface Science, 15*(1-2), 40-49.

Dickson, B., Streutker, C., & Chetty, R. (2006). Coeliac disease: an update for pathologists. *Journal of clinical pathology, 59*(10), 1008-1016.

Dieterich, W., Schuppan, D., Schink, M., Schwappacher, R., Wirtz, S., Agaimy, A., ... Zopf, Y. (2019). Influence of low FODMAP and gluten -free diets on disease activity and intestinal microbiota in patients with non-celiac gluten sensitivity. *Clinical Nutrition, 38*(2), 697-707.

Ding, S., Jiang, H., & Fang, J. (2018). Regulation of immune function by polyphenols. *Journal of immunology research, 2018*(1), 1264074.

Ditah, I. C., Nadeau, A. M., Rubio-Tapia, A., Marietta, E. V., Brantner, T. L., Camilleri, M. J., ... Murray, J. A. (2015). Trends and racial/ethnic disparities in gluten -sensitive problems in the United States: findings from the National Health and Nutrition Examination Surveys from 1988 to 2012. *Official journal of the American College of Gastroenterology| ACG, 110*(3), 455-461.

Dongyu, Q. (2022). New scenarios on global food security based on Russia-Ukraine conflict. *Food and Agriculture Organization of the United Nations. Brief.*

Dørum, S., Bodd, M., Fallang, L. E., Bergseng, E., Christophersen, A., Johannesen, M. K., ... Sollid, L. M. (2014). HLA-DQ molecules as affinity matrix for identification of gluten T cell epitopes. *The Journal of Immunology, 193*(9), 4497-4506.

Dørum, S., Steinsbø, Ø., Bergseng, E., Arntzen, M. Ø., de Souza, G. A., & Sollid, L. M. (2016). Gluten-specific antibodies of celiac disease gut plasma cells recognize long proteolytic fragments that typically harbor T-cell epitopes. *Scientific Reports, 6*(1), 25565.

dos Santos, F. S., de Figueirędo, R., Queiroz, A., de Lima, T., & Moreira, I. S. (2019). Effect of dehydration methods on okra chemical and physical composition. *Journal of Agricultural Science, 11*(5), 236-249.

Dowd, B., & Walker-Smith, J. (1974). Samuel Gee, Aretaeus, and the coeliac affection. *British medical journal, 2*(5909), 45.

Drabińska, N., Jarocka-Cyrta, E., Markiewicz, L. H., & Krupa-Kozak, U. (2018). The effect of oligofructose-enriched inulin on faecal bacterial counts and microbiota-associated characteristics in celiac disease children following a gluten -free diet : Results of a randomized, placebo-controlled trial. *Nutrients, 10*(2), 201.

Drabińska, N., Jarocka-Cyrta, E., Ratcliffe, N. M., & Krupa-Kozak, U. (2019). The profile of urinary headspace volatile organic compounds after 12-week intake of oligofructose-enriched inulin by children and adolescents with celiac disease on a gluten -free diet : Results of a pilot, randomized, placebo-controlled clinical trial. *Molecules, 24*(7), 1341.

Dreifuss, S. E., Tomizawa, Y., Farber, N. J., Davison, J. M., & Sohnen, A. E. (2013). Spruelike enteropathy associated with olmesartan: an unusual case of severe diarrhea. *Case Reports in Gastrointestinal Medicine, 2013*(1), 618071.

Dryden, G. W., Bunch, A. N., Connors, M. A., Mehta, M. J., & Qazzaz, H. M. (2017). Tu1786–EGCG Reverses LPS-Mediated Changes in Claudin Physiology and Improves Trans-Epithelial Resistance in an Intestinal Epithelium Model. *Gastroenterology, 152.*

Du Pré, M. F., Kozijn, A. E., van Berkel, L. A., Ter Borg, M. N., Lindenbergh–Kortleve, D., Jensen, L. T., ... Nieuwenhuis, E. E. (2011). Tolerance to ingested deamidated gliadin in mice is maintained by splenic, type 1 regulatory T cells. *Gastroenterology, 141*(2), 610-620. e612.

Dubé, C., Rostom, A., Sy, R., Cranney, A., Saloojee, N., Garritty, C., ... Mamaladze, V. (2005). The prevalence of celiac disease in average-risk and at-risk Western European populations: a systematic review. *Gastroenterology, 128*(4), S57-S67.

Dumur, J., Jahier, J., Bancel, E., Laurière, M., Bernard, M., & Branlard, G. (2004). Proteomic analysis of aneuploid lines in the homeologous group 1 of the hexaploid wheat cultivar Courtot. *Proteomics, 4*(9), 2685-2695.

Eaton, W., Mortensen, P. B., Agerbo, E., Byrne, M., Mors, O., & Ewald, H. (2004). Coeliac disease and schizophrenia: population based case control study with linkage of Danish national registers. *Bmj, 328*(7437), 438-439.

Eggesbø, L. M., Risnes, L. F., Neumann, R. S., Lundin, K. E., Christophersen, A., & Sollid, L. M. (2020). Single-cell TCR sequencing of gut intraepithelial γδ T cells reveals a vast and diverse repertoire in celiac disease. *Mucosal immunology, 13*(2), 313-321.

Eggesbø, L. M., Risnes, L. F., Neumann, R. S., Lundin, K. E., Christophersen, A., & Sollid, L. M. (2021). Single-cell TCR repertoire analysis reveals highly polyclonal composition of human intraepithelial CD8+ αβ T lymphocytes in untreated celiac disease. *European journal of immunology, 51*(6).

Ehren, J., Morón, B., Martin, E., Bethune, M. T., Gray, G. M., & Khosla, C. (2009). A food-grade enzyme preparation with modest gluten detoxification properties. *PloS one, 4*(7), e6313.

El Khoury, D., Balfour-Ducharme, S., & Joye, I. J. (2018). A review on the gluten -free diet : Technological and nutritional challenges. *Nutrients, 10*(10), 1410.

El Mouzan, M., Assiri, A., Al Sarkhy, A., Alasmi, M., Saeed, A., Al-Hussaini, A., ... Al Mofarreh, M. (2022). Viral dysbiosis in children with new-onset celiac disease. *PloS one, 17*(1), e0262108.

Eltahla, A. A., Rizzetto, S., Pirozyan, M. R., Betz-Stablein, B. D., Venturi, V., Kedzierska, K., ... Luciani, F. (2016). Linking the T cell receptor to the single cell transcriptome in antigen-specific human T cells. *Immunology and cell biology, 94*(6), 604-611.

Engstrom, N., Saenz-Méndez, P., Scheers, J., & Scheers, N. (2017). Towards Celiac-safe foods: Decreasing the affinity of transglutaminase 2 for gliadin by addition of ascorbyl palmitate and ZnCl2 as detoxifiers. *Scientific reports, 7*(1), 1-8.

Enroth, S., Dahlbom, I., Hansson, T., Johansson, Å., & Gyllensten, U. (2013). Prevalence and sensitization of atopic allergy and coeliac disease in the Northern Sweden Population Health Study. *International journal of circumpolar health, 72*(1), 21403.

Ermarth, A., Bryce, M., Woodward, S., Stoddard, G., Book, L., & Jensen, M. K. (2017). Identification of pediatric patients with celiac disease based on serology and a classification and regression tree analysis. *Clinical gastroenterology and hepatology, 15*(3), 396-402. e392.

Espinosa-Ramirez, J., Garzon, R., Serna-Saldivar, S. O., & Rosell, C. M. (2018). Mimicking gluten functionality with β-conglycinin concentrate: Evaluation in gluten free yeast-leavened breads. *Food Research International, 106*, 64-70.

Fajardo, V., González, M. P., Martínez, M., Samaniego-Vaesken, M. d. L., Achón, M., Úbeda, N., & Alonso-Aperte, E. (2020). Updated food composition database for cereal-based gluten free products in Spain: is reformulation moving on? *Nutrients, 12*(8), 2369.

Fasano, A., Berti, I., Gerarduzzi, T., Not, T., Colletti, R. B., Drago, S., ... Hill, I. D. (2003). Prevalence of celiac disease in at-risk and not-at-risk groups in the United States: a large multicenter study. *Archives of internal medicine, 163*(3), 286-292.

Febvre, H. P., Rao, S., Gindin, M., Goodwin, N. D., Finer, E., Vivanco, J. S., ... Weir, T. L. (2019). PHAGE study: effects of supplemental bacteriophage intake on inflammation and gut microbiota in healthy adults. *Nutrients, 11*(3), 666.

Fehniger, T. A., Suzuki, K., Ponnappan, A., VanDeusen, J. B., Cooper, M. A., Florea, S. M., ... Caligiuri, M. A. (2001). Fatal leukemia in interleukin 15 transgenic mice follows early expansions in natural killer and memory phenotype CD8+ T cells. *The Journal of experimental medicine, 193*(2), 219-232.

Fernández, S., Molina, I. J., Romero, P., González, R., Peña, J., Sánchez, F., ... Ortega, C. (2011). Characterization of gliadin-specific Th17 cells from the mucosa of celiac disease patients. *Official journal of the American College of Gastroenterology| ACG, 106*(3), 528-538.

Ferretti, G., Bacchetti, T., Masciangelo, S., & Saturni, L. (2012). Celiac disease, inflammation and oxidative damage: a nutrigenetic approach. *Nutrients, 4*(4), 243-257.

Filipčev, B., Pojić, M., Šimurina, O., Mišan, A., & Mandić, A. (2021). Psyllium as an improver in gluten -free breads: Effect on volume, crumb texture, moisture binding and staling kinetics. *LWT, 151*, 112156.

Fillatreau, S. (2019). Regulatory functions of B cells and regulatory plasma cells. *biomedical journal, 42*(4), 233-242.

Finamore, A., Roselli, M., Donini, L., Brasili, E., Rami, R., Carnevali, P., ... Mengheri, E. (2019). Supplementation with Bifidobacterium longum Bar33 and Lactobacillus helveticus Bar13 mixture improves immunity in elderly humans (over 75 years) and aged mice. *Nutrition, 63*, 184-192.

Fiorucci, G., Puxeddu, E., Colella, R., Paolo Reboldi, G., Villanacci, V., & Bassotti, G. (2014). Severe spruelike enteropathy due to olmesartan. *Rev Esp Enferm Dig, 106*(2), 142-144.

Fois, A., Vascotto, M., Di Bartolo, R. M., & Di Marco, V. (1994). Celiac disease and epilepsy in pediatric patients. *Child's Nervous System, 10*, 450-454.

Ford, N. D., Patel, S. A., & Narayan, K. V. (2017). Obesity in low-and middle-income countries: burden, drivers, and emerging challenges. *Annual review of public health, 38*(1), 145-164.

Francisco, V., Costa, G., Neves, B., Cruz, M., & Batista, M. (2018). Antiinflammatory activity of polyphenols on dendritic cells. In *Polyphenols : Prevention and treatment of human disease* (pp. 395-415): Elsevier.

Franco, V. A., Garcia, L. G. C., & SILVA, F. A. d. (2020). Addition of hydrocolidics in gluten -free bread and replacement of rice flour for sweet potato flour. *Food Science and Technology, 40*, 88-96.

Franz, B., May Jr, K. F., Dranoff, G., & Wucherpfennig, K. (2011). *Ex vivo* characterization and isolation of rare memory B cells with antigen tetramers. *Blood, The Journal of the American Society of Hematology, 118*(2), 348-357.

Fratelli, C., Santos, F. G., Muniz, D. G., Habu, S., Braga, A. R. C., & Capriles, V. D. (2021). Psyllium improves the quality and shelf life of gluten -free bread. *Foods, 10*(5), 954.

Freeman, H. J. (2016). Olmesartan enteropathy. *Inter J Celiac Dis, 4*, 24-26.

Freeman, H. J. (2017). Dietary compliance in celiac disease. *World Journal of Gastroenterology, 23*(15), 2635.

Freitag, T. L., Loponen, J., Messing, M., Zevallos, V., Andersson, L. C., Sontag-Strohm, T., ... Meri, S. (2014). Testing safety of germinated rye sourdough in a celiac disease model based on the adoptive transfer of prolamin-primed memory T cells into lymphopenic mice. *American Journal of Physiology-Gastrointestinal and Liver Physiology, 306*(6), G526-G534.

Freitag, T. L., Podojil, J. R., Pearson, R. M., Fokta, F. J., Sahl, C., Messing, M., ... Hoover, L. I. (2020). Gliadin nanoparticles induce immune tolerance to gliadin in mouse models of celiac disease. *Gastroenterology, 158*(6), 1667-1681. e1612.

Freitag, T. L., Rietdijk, S., Junker, Y., Popov, Y., Bhan, A. K., Kelly, C. P., ... Schuppan, D. (2009). Gliadin-primed CD4+ CD45RBlowCD25− T cells drive gluten -dependent small intestinal damage after adoptive transfer into lymphopenic mice. *Gut, 58*(12), 1597-1605.

Frick, R., Høydahl, L. S., Petersen, J., Du Pré, M. F., Kumari, S., Berntsen, G., ... Frigstad, T. (2021). A high-affinity human TCR-like antibody detects celiac disease gluten peptide–MHC complexes and inhibits T cell activation. *Science immunology, 6*(62), eabg4925.

Furrie, E., Macfarlane, S., Kennedy, A., Cummings, J., Walsh, S., O'neil, D., & Macfarlane, G. (2005). Synbiotic therapy (Bifidobacterium longum/Synergy 1) initiates resolution of inflammation in patients with active ulcerative colitis: a randomised controlled pilot trial. *Gut, 54*(2), 242-249.

Gabrielli, M., Cremonini, F., Fiore, G., Addolorato, G., Padalino, C., Candelli, M., ... Gasbarrini, A. (2003). Association between migraine and celiac disease: results from a preliminary case-control and therapeutic study. *The American journal of gastroenterology, 98*(3), 625-629.

Gadermayr, M., Kogler, H., Karla, M., Merhof, D., Uhl, A., & Vécsei, A. (2016). Computer-aided texture analysis combined with experts' knowledge: Improving endoscopic celiac disease diagnosis. *World journal of gastroenterology, 22*(31), 7124.

Galipeau, H. J., & Verdu, E. F. (2022). The double-edged sword of gut bacteria in celiac disease and implications for therapeutic potential. *Mucosal immunology, 15*(2), 235-243.

Galipeau, H. J., Rulli, N. E., Jury, J., Huang, X., Araya, R., Murray, J. A., ... Verdu, E. F. (2011). Sensitization to gliadin induces moderate enteropathy and insulitis in nonobese diabetic-DQ8 mice. *The Journal of Immunology, 187*(8), 4338-4346.

Galipeau, H. J., Wiepjes, M., Motta, J. P., Schulz, J. D., Jury, J., Natividad, J. M., ... Martin-Rosique, R. (2014). Novel role of the serine protease inhibitor elafin in gluten -related disorders. *Official journal of the American College of Gastroenterology| ACG, 109*(5), 748-756.

Gallagher, E., Gormley, T. R., & Arendt, E. K. (2004). Recent advances in the formulation of gluten -free cereal-based products. *Trends in Food Science & Technology, 15*(3-4), 143-152.

Gao, J., Li, Y., Wan, Y., Hu, T., Liu, L., Yang, S., ... Yang, W. (2019). A novel postbiotic from Lactobacillus rhamnosus GG with a beneficial effect on intestinal barrier function. *Frontiers in microbiology, 10*, 477.

Gao, Z., Fang, Y., Cao, Y., Liao, H., Nishinari, K., & Phillips, G. O. (2017). Hydrocolloid-food component interactions. *Food Hydrocolloids, 68*, 149-156.

Gao, Z., Wu, H., Zhang, K., Hossen, I., Wang, J., Wang, C., ... Cao, Y. (2020). Protective effects of grape seed procyanidin extract on intestinal barrier dysfunction induced by a long-term high-fat diet. *Journal of Functional Foods, 64*, 103663.

Garmaeva, S., Gulyaeva, A., Sinha, T., Shkoporov, A. N., Clooney, A. G., Stockdale, S. R., ... Dutilh, B. E. (2021). Stability of the human gut virome and effect of gluten -free diet. *Cell reports, 35*(7), 109132.

Gass, J., Bethune, M. T., Siegel, M., Spencer, A., & Khosla, C. (2007). Combination enzyme therapy for gastric digestion of dietary gluten in patients with celiac sprue. *Gastroenterology, 133*(2), 472-480.

Gastroenterology, B. S. o., Lewis, N., & Scott, B. B. (2008). *Guidelines for osteoporosis in inflammatory bowel disease and coeliac disease*: British Society of Gastroenterology.

Geisslitz, S., Ludwig, C., Scherf, K. A., & Koehler, P. (2018). Targeted LC–MS/MS reveals similar contents of α-amylase/trypsin -inhibitors as putative triggers of nonceliac gluten sensitivity in all wheat species except einkorn. *Journal of agricultural and food chemistry, 66*(46), 12395-12403.

Gertner, J., Lilburn, M., & Domenech, M. (1977). 25-Hydroxycholecalciferol absorption in steatorrhoea and postgastrectomy osteomalacia. *Br Med J, 1*(6072), 1310-1312.

Ghadami, M. R. (2016). Celiac disease and epilepsy: the effect of gluten -free diet on seizure control. *Pediatrics, 3*, 52-08.

Ghaffari, S., Abbasi, A., Somi, M. H., Moaddab, S. Y., Nikniaz, L., Kafil, H. S., & Ebrahimzadeh Leylabadlo, H. (2022). Akkermansia muciniphila: from its critical role in human health to strategies for promoting its abundance in human gut microbiome. *Critical reviews in food science and nutrition*, 1-21.

Gil-Humanes, J., Pistón, F., Altamirano-Fortoul, R., Real, A., Comino, I., Sousa, C., ... Barro, F. (2014). Reduced-gliadin wheat bread: an alternative to the gluten -free diet for consumers suffering gluten-related pathologies. *PloS one, 9*(3), e90898.

Gil-Humanes, J., Pistón, F., Tollefsen, S., Sollid, L. M., & Barro, F. (2010). Effective shutdown in the expression of celiac disease-related wheat gliadin T-cell epitopes by RNA interference. *Proceedings of the National Academy of Sciences, 107*(39), 17023-17028.

Gobbi, G. (1993). Coeliac disease, epilepsy and cerebral calcifications. *Biomedicine & Pharmacotherapy, 47*(4), 176.

Gobbi, G. (2005). Coeliac disease, epilepsy and cerebral calcifications. *Brain and Development, 27*(3), 189-200.

Gobbi, G., Ambrosetto, P., Zaniboni, M. G., Lambertini, A., Ambrosioni, G., & Tassinari, C. A. (1992). Celiac disease, posterior cerebral calcifications and epilepsy. *Brain and Development, 14*(1), 23-29.

Goel, G., King, T., Daveson, A. J., Andrews, J. M., Krishnarajah, J., Krause, R., ... Epstein, R. (2017). Epitope-specific immunotherapy targeting CD4-positive T cells in coeliac disease: two randomised, double-blind, placebo-controlled phase 1 studies. *The lancet Gastroenterology & hepatology, 2*(7), 479-493.

Goff, H. D., & Guo, Q. (2019). The role of hydrocolloids in the development of food structure.

Golden, J. A. (2017). Deep learning algorithms for detection of lymph node metastases from breast cancer: helping artificial intelligence be seen. *Jama, 318*(22), 2184-2186.

Goldstein, N. S., & Underhill, J. (2001). Morphologic features suggestive of gluten sensitivity in architecturally normal duodenal biopsy specimens. *American journal of clinical pathology, 116*(1), 63-71.

Gonzalez, S., Gupta, A., Cheng, J., Tennyson, C., Lewis, S. K., Bhagat, G., & Green, P. H. (2010). Prospective study of the role of duodenal bulb biopsies in the diagnosis of celiac disease. *Gastrointestinal endoscopy, 72*(4), 758-765.

Goodman, R. E., Ebisawa, M., Ferreira, F., Sampson, H. A., van Ree, R., Vieths, S., ... Wise, J. (2016). AllergenOnline: a peer-reviewed, curated allergen database to assess novel food proteins for potential cross-reactivity. *Molecular nutrition & food research, 60*(5), 1183-1198.

Goodwin, F. C., Beattie, R. M., Millar, J., & Kirkham, F. J. (2004). Celiac disease and childhood stroke. *Pediatric neurology, 31*(2), 139-142.

Gopalakrishnan, S., Durai, M., Kitchens, K., Tamiz, A. P., Somerville, R., Ginski, M., ... Alkan, S. S. (2012). Larazotide acetate regulates epithelial tight junctions *in vitro* and *in vivo*. *Peptides, 35*(1), 86-94.

Gordon, S. R., Stanley, E. J., Wolf, S., Toland, A., Wu, S. J., Hadidi, D., ... Siegel, J. B. (2012). Computational design of an α-gliadin peptidase. *Journal of the American Chemical Society, 134*(50), 20513-20520.

Goudey, B., Abraham, G., Kikianty, E., Wang, Q., Rawlinson, D., Shi, F., ... Inouye, M. (2017). Interactions within the MHC contribute to the genetic architecture of celiac disease. *PloS one, 12*(3), e0172826.

Greco, L., Gobbetti, M., Auricchio, R., Di Mase, R., Landolfo, F., Paparo, F., ... Cassone, A. (2011). Safety for patients with celiac disease of baked goods made of wheat flour hydrolyzed during food processing. *Clinical gastroenterology and hepatology, 9*(1), 24-29.

Green, P. H. (2005). The many faces of celiac disease: clinical presentation of celiac disease in the adult population. *Gastroenterology, 128*(4), S74-S78.

Green, P. H., & Cellier, C. (2007). Celiac disease. *New england journal of medicine, 357*(17), 1731-1743.

Green, P. H., & Jabri, B. (2003). Coeliac disease. *The Lancet, 362*(9381), 383-391.

Green, P. H., Paski, S., Ko, C. W., & Rubio-Tapia, A. (2022). AGA clinical practice update on management of refractory celiac disease : expert review. *Gastroenterology*.

Grehn, S., Fridell, K., Lilliecreutz, M., & Hallert, C. (2001). Dietary habits of Swedish adult coeliac patients treated by a gluten -free diet for 10 years. *Näringsforskning, 45*(1), 178-182.

Grode, L., Bech, B. H., Jensen, T. M., Humaidan, P., Agerholm, I. E., Plana-Ripoll, O., & Ramlau-Hansen, C. H. (2018). Prevalence, incidence, and autoimmune comorbidities of celiac disease: a nation-wide, population-based study in Denmark from 1977 to 2016. *European journal of gastroenterology & hepatology, 30*(1), 83-91.

Gu, L., Li, N., Gong, J., Li, Q., Zhu, W., & Li, J. (2011). Berberine ameliorates intestinal epithelial tight-junction damage and down-regulates myosin light chain kinase pathways in a mouse model of endotoxinemia. *Journal of Infectious Diseases, 203*(11), 1602-1612.

Guerdrum, L. J., & Bamforth, C. W. (2012). Prolamin levels through brewing and the impact of prolyl endoproteinase. *Journal of the American Society of Brewing Chemists, 70*(1), 35-38.

Guikema, J. E., Hovenga, S., Vellenga, E., Conradie, J. J., Abdulahad, W. H., Bekkema, R., ... Bos, N. A. (2003). CD27 is heterogeneously expressed in multiple myeloma: low CD27 expression in patients with high-risk disease. *British journal of haematology, 121*(1), 36-43.

Gül, H., Hayit, F., Acun, S., & Tekeli, S. G. (2018). *Improvement of quality characteristics of gluten -free cookies with the addition of xanthan gum.* Paper presented at the Agriculture for Life, Life for Agriculture" Conference Proceedings.

Gunnarsen, K. S., Høydahl, L. S., Risnes, L. F., Dahal-Koirala, S., Neumann, R. S., Bergseng, E., ... Dalhus, B. (2017). A TCRα framework–centered codon shapes a biased T cell repertoire through direct MHC and CDR3β interactions. *JCI insight, 2*(17).

Gutiérrez, S., Pérez-Andrés, J., Martínez-Blanco, H., Ferrero, M. A., Vaquero, L., Vivas, S., ... Rodríguez-Aparicio, L. B. (2017). The human digestive tract has proteases capable of gluten hydrolysis. *Molecular metabolism, 6*(7), 693-702.

Guz-Mark, A., Zevit, N., Morgenstern, S., & Shamir, R. (2014). Duodenal intraepithelial lymphocytosis is common in children without coeliac disease, and is not meaningfully influenced by Helicobacter pylori infection. *Alimentary pharmacology & therapeutics, 39*(11), 1314-1320.

Haderslev, K., Tjellesen, L., Sorensen, H., & Staun, M. (2000). Alendronate increases lumbar spine bone mineral density in patients with Crohn's disease. *Gastroenterology, 119*(3), 639-646.

Hadjivassiliou, M., Chattopadhyay, A., Davies Jones, G., Gibson, A., Grünewald, R., & Lobo, A. (1997). Neuromuscular disorder as a presenting feature of coeliac disease. *Journal of Neurology, Neurosurgery & Psychiatry, 63*(6), 770-775.

Hadjivassiliou, M., Sanders, D. D., & Aeschlimann, D. P. (2015). Gluten-related disorders: gluten ataxia. *Digestive Diseases, 33*(2), 264-268.

Hager, A. S., & Arendt, E. K. (2013). Influence of hydroxypropylmethylcellulose (HPMC), xanthan gum and their combination on loaf specific volume, crumb hardness and crumb grain characteristics of gluten -free breads based on rice, maize, teff and buckwheat. *Food Hydrocolloids, 32*(1), 195-203.

Haghshenas, M., Hosseini, H., Nayebzadeh, K., Khanghah, A. M., Kakesh, B. S., & Fonood, R. K. (2014). Production of prebiotic functional shrimp nuggets using ß-glucan and reduction of oil absorption by carboxymethyl cellulose: Impacts on sensory and physical properties. *J. Aquacul. Res. Dev, 5*, 245-248.

Hallert, C., Grant, C., Grehn, S., Grännö, C., Hultén, S., Midhagen, G., ... Valdimarsson, T. (2002). Evidence of poor vitamin status in coeliac patients on a gluten -free diet for 10 years. *Alimentary pharmacology & therapeutics, 16*(7), 1333-1339.

Halstensen, T. S., & Brandtzaeg, P. (1993). Activated T lymphocytes in the celiac lesion: non-proliferative activation (CD25) of CD4+ α/β cells in the lamina propria but proliferation (Ki-67) of α/β and γ/δ cells in the epithelium. *European journal of immunology, 23*(2), 505-510.

Hamilton, J. G., Genoff Garzon, M., Westerman, J. S., Shuk, E., Hay, J. L., Walters, C., ... Daly, B. (2019). "A tool, not a crutch": patient perspectives about IBM Watson for oncology trained by Memorial Sloan Kettering. *Journal of Oncology Practice, 15*(4), e277-e288.

Han, A., Newell, E. W., Glanville, J., Fernandez-Becker, N., Khosla, C., Chien, Y. h., & Davis, M. M. (2013). Dietary gluten triggers concomitant activation of CD4+ and CD8+ αβ T cells and γδ T cells in celiac disease. *Proceedings of the National Academy of Sciences, 110*(32), 13073-13078.

Han, X., Shen, T., & Lou, H. (2007). Dietary polyphenols and their biological significance. *International journal of molecular sciences, 8*(9), 950-988.

Hardy, M. Y., Tye-Din, J. A., Stewart, J. A., Schmitz, F., Dudek, N. L., Hanchapola, I., ... Anderson, R. P. (2015). Ingestion of oats and barley in patients with celiac disease mobilizes cross-reactive T cells activated by avenin peptides and immuno-dominant hordein peptides. *Journal of Autoimmunity, 56*, 56-65.

Harpaz, N., Levi, G. S., Yurovitsky, A., & Kini, S. (2007). Intraepithelial lymphocytosis in architecturally normal small intestinal mucosa: association with morbid obesity. *Archives of pathology & laboratory medicine, 131*(3), 344-344.

Harrer, S., Shah, P., Antony, B., & Hu, J. (2019). Artificial intelligence for clinical trial design. *Trends in pharmacological sciences, 40*(8), 577-591.

Harrison, J. E., Hitchman, A., Finlay, J., & McNeill, K. (1969). Calcium kinetic studies in patients with malabsorption syndrome. *Gastroenterology, 56*(4), 751-757.

Hausch, F., Shan, L., Santiago, N. A., Gray, G. M., & Khosla, C. (2002). Intestinal digestive resistance of immunodominant gliadin peptides. *American Journal of Physiology-Gastrointestinal and Liver Physiology.*

Hayat, M., Cairns, A., Dixon, M., & O'Mahony, S. (2002). Quantitation of intraepithelial lymphocytes in human duodenum: what is normal? *Journal of clinical pathology, 55*(5), 393-394.

Haza, A., Zabala, A., Arranz, N., & Morales, P. (2005). Protective effect of a Lactobacillus salivarius strain of human origin. *Food science and technology international, 11*(4), 251-259.

Héder, M. (2017). From NASA to EU: The evolution of the TRL scale in Public Sector Innovation. *The Innovation Journal, 22*(2), 1-23.

Hegenbart, S., Uhl, A., & Vécsei, A. (2011). *Systematic assessment of performance prediction techniques in medical image classification a case study on celiac disease.* Paper presented at the Information Processing in Medical Imaging: 22nd International Conference, IPMI 2011, Kloster Irsee, Germany, July 3-8, 2011. Proceedings 22.

Hegenbart, S., Uhl, A., Vécsei, A., & Wimmer, G. (2013). Scale invariant texture descriptors for classifying celiac disease. *Medical image analysis, 17*(4), 458-474.

Heikkilä, K., Pearce, J., Mäki, M., & Kaukinen, K. (2015). Celiac disease and bone fractures: a systematic review and meta-analysis. *The Journal of Clinical Endocrinology & Metabolism, 100*(1), 25-34.

Henderson, K. N., Tye-Din, J. A., Reid, H. H., Chen, Z., Borg, N. A., Beissbarth, T., ... Dudek, N. L. (2007). A structural and immunological basis for the role of human leukocyte antigen DQ8 in celiac disease. *Immunity, 27*(1), 23-34.

Heredia-Sandoval, N. G., Islas-Rubio, A. R., Cabrera-Chávez, F., & de la Barca, A. M. C. (2014). Transamidation of gluten proteins during the bread-making process of wheat flour to produce breads with less immunoreactive gluten. *Food & function, 5*(8), 1813-1818.

Herman, M. L., Rubio-Tapia, A., Wu, T. T., & Murray, J. A. (2015). A case of severe sprue -like enteropathy associated with valsartan. *ACG Case Reports Journal, 2*(1), 92-94.

Hernandez, M. A., Colina, G., & Ortigosa, L. (1998). Epilepsy, cerebral calcifications and clinical or subclinical coeliac disease. Course and follow up with gluten -free diet. *Seizure, 7*(1), 49-54.

Heyman, M., Abed, J., Lebreton, C., & Cerf-Bensussan, N. (2012). Intestinal permeability in coeliac disease: insight into mechanisms and relevance to pathogenesis. *Gut, 61*(9), 1355-1364.

Hietikko, M., Koskinen, O., Kurppa, K., Laurila, K., Saavalainen, P., Salmi, T., ... Lindfors, K. (2018). Small-intestinal TG2-specific plasma cells at different stages of coeliac disease. *BMC immunology, 19*, 1-7.

Hmida, N. B., Ahmed, M. B., Moussa, A., Rejeb, M. B., Said, Y., Kourda, N., ... Cerf-Bensussan, N. (2012). Impaired control of effector T cells by regulatory T cells: a clue to loss of oral tolerance and autoimmunity in celiac disease? *Official journal of the American College of Gastroenterology| ACG, 107*(4), 604-611.

Hnida, K., Stamnaes, J., du Pré, M. F., Mysling, S., Jørgensen, T. J., Sollid, L. M., & Iversen, R. (2016). Epitope-dependent functional effects of celiac disease autoantibodies on transglutaminase 2. *Journal of Biological Chemistry, 291*(49), 25542-25552.

Hoehn, K. B., Vander Heiden, J. A., Zhou, J. Q., Lunter, G., Pybus, O. G., & Kleinstein, S. H. (2019). Repertoire-wide phylogenetic models of B cell molecular evolution reveal evolutionary signatures of aging and vaccination. *Proceedings of the National Academy of Sciences, 116*(45), 22664-22672.

Holmes, G. (1996). Non-malignant complications of coeliac disease. *Acta paediatrica, 85*, 68-75.

Holmes, J., Sacchi, L., & Bellazzi, R. (2004). Artificial intelligence in medicine. *Ann R Coll Surg Engl, 86*, 334-338.

Homayouni Rad, A., Aghebati Maleki, L., Samadi Kafil, H., & Abbasi, A. (2021). Postbiotics : A novel strategy in food allergy treatment. *Critical Reviews in Food Science and Nutrition, 61*(3), 492-499.

Hommeida, S., Alsawas, M., Murad, M. H., Katzka, D. A., Grothe, R. M., & Absah, I. (2017). The association between celiac disease and eosinophilic esophagitis : Mayo experience and meta-analysis of the literature. *Journal of pediatric gastroenterology and nutrition, 65*(1), 58-63.

Hopper, A., Cross, S., & Sanders, D. (2008). Patchy villous atrophy in adult patients with suspected gluten -sensitive enteropathy: is a multiple duodenal biopsy strategy appropriate? *Endoscopy, 40*(03), 219-224.

Horstmann, S. W., Axel, C., & Arendt, E. K. (2018). Water absorption as a prediction tool for the application of hydrocolloids in potato starch-based bread. *Food Hydrocolloids, 81*, 129-138.

Houben, A., Höchstötter, A., & Becker, T. (2012). Possibilities to increase the quality in gluten -free bread production: an overview. *European food research and technology, 235*, 195-208.

Høydahl, L. S., Richter, L., Frick, R., Snir, O., Gunnarsen, K. S., Landsverk, O. J., ... Bergseng, E. (2019). Plasma cells are the most abundant gluten peptide MHC-expressing cells in inflamed intestinal tissues from patients with celiac disease. *Gastroenterology, 156*(5), 1428-1439. e1410.

Hu, J., Shen, L., & Sun, G. (2018). *Squeeze-and-excitation networks.* Paper presented at the Proceedings of the IEEE conference on computer vision and pattern recognition.

Hu, X. Z., Xing, X. H., Zhang, Z. M., Wu, R. Q., Guo, Q., Cui, S. W., & Wang, Q. (2011). Antioxidant effects of Artemis sphaerocephala Krasch. gum, on streptozotocin-induced type 2 diabetic rats. *Food Hydrocolloids, 25*(2), 207-213.

Hudacko, R., Kathy Zhou, X., & Yantiss, R. K. (2013). Immunohistochemical stains for CD3 and CD8 do not improve detection of gluten -sensitive enteropathy in duodenal biopsies. *Modern Pathology, 26*(9), 1241-1245.

Huibregtse, I. L., Marietta, E. V., Rashtak, S., Koning, F., Rottiers, P., David, C. S., ... Murray, J. A. (2009). Induction of antigen-specific tolerance by oral administration of Lactococcus lactis delivered immunodominant DQ8 -restricted gliadin peptide in sensitized nonobese diabetic Ab Dq8 transgenic mice. *The Journal of Immunology, 183*(4), 2390-2396.

Hujoel, I. A., & Murray, J. A. (2020). Refractory celiac disease. *Current gastroenterology reports, 22*(4), 1-8.

Hujoel, I. A., Murphree, D. H., Van Dyke, C. T., Sharma, A., Murray, J. A., & Rubio-Tapia, A. (2018). Machine learning in detection of undiagnosed celiac disease. *Clinical Gastroenterology and Hepatology, 16*(8), 1354-1355. e1351.

Hurtado-Romero, A., Del Toro-Barbosa, M., Garcia-Amezquita, L. E., & García-Cayuela, T. (2020). Innovative technologies for the production of food ingredients with prebiotic potential: Modifications, applications, and validation methods. *Trends in Food Science & Technology, 104*, 117-131.

Husby, S., Murray, J. A., & Katzka, D. A. (2019). AGA clinical practice update on diagnosis and monitoring of celiac disease—changing utility of serology and histologic measures: expert review. *Gastroenterology, 156*(4), 885-889.

Hussain, T., & Tan, B. (2016). yin y, Blachier F, Tossou MC, Rahu N. *Oxidative stress and inflammation: What polyphenols can do for us.*

Ianiro, G., Bibbò, S., Montalto, M., Ricci, R., Gasbarrini, A., & Cammarota, G. (2014). Systematic review: sprue -like enteropathy associated with olmesartan. *Alimentary pharmacology & therapeutics, 40*(1), 16-23.

Iglesias, D. E., Cremonini, E., Fraga, C. G., & Oteiza, P. I. (2020). Ellagic acid protects Caco-2 cell monolayers against inflammation-induced permeabilization. *Free Radical Biology and Medicine, 152*, 776-786.

Ilus, T., Kaukinen, K., Virta, L. J., Pukkala, E., & Collin, P. (2014). Incidence of malignancies in diagnosed celiac patients: a population-based estimate. *Official journal of the American College of Gastroenterology| ACG, 109*(9), 1471-1477.

Inns, T., Fleming, K. M., Iturriza-Gomara, M., & Hungerford, D. (2021). Paediatric rotavirus vaccination, coeliac disease and type 1 diabetes in children: a population-based cohort study. *BMC medicine, 19*(1), 1-9.

Irondi, E. A., Imam, Y. T., & Ajani, E. O. (2021). Effect of Flour Addition on the Physicochemical Properties of Whole Millet Flour and the Sensory Attributes of its Gluten-Free Bread. *Acta Universitatis Cibiniensis. Series E: Food Technology, 25*(1), 43-52.

Irondi, E. A., Imam, Y. T., & Ajani, E. O. (2022). Physicochemical, antioxidant and starch-digesting enzymes inhibitory properties of pearl millet and sweet detar gluten -free flour blends, and sensory qualities of their breads. *Frontiers in Food Science and Technology, 2*, 974588.

Irondi, E. A., Imam, Y. T., Ajani, E. O., & Alamu, E. O. Grain & Oil Science and Technology. *Food Hydrocolloids, 3*, 10.

Işikay, S., & Kocamaz, H. (2015). The neurological face of celiac disease. *Arquivos de Gastroenterologia, 52*(3), 167-170.

Islam, M. S., Jhily, N. J., Hasan, R., Parvin, N., Islam, M. A., Hossain, I., & Akter, K. (2021). Nutritional Transition in Unindustrialized Countries: Causes and Consequences on Public Health. *Indian Journal of Public Health, 12*(4), 343.

Ivarsson, A., Persson, L., Nyström, L., Ascher, H., Cavell, B., Danielsson, L., ... Stenhammar, L. (2000). Epidemic of coeliac disease in Swedish children. *Acta paediatrica, 89*(2), 165-171.

Iversen, R. (2013). Transglutaminase 2-specific autoantibodies in celiac disease.

Iversen, R., Mysling, S., Hnida, K., Jørgensen, T. J., & Sollid, L. M. (2014). Activity-regulating structural changes and autoantibody epitopes in transglutaminase 2 assessed by hydrogen/deuterium exchange. *Proceedings of the National Academy of Sciences, 111*(48), 17146-17151.

Iversen, R., Roy, B., Stamnaes, J., Høydahl, L. S., Hnida, K., Neumann, R. S., ... Sollid, L. M. (2019). Efficient T cell–B cell collaboration guides autoantibody epitope bias and onset of celiac disease. *Proceedings of the National Academy of Sciences, 116*(30), 15134-15139.

Iversen, R., Snir, O., Stensland, M., Kroll, J. E., Steinsbø, Ø., Korponay-Szabó, I. R., ... Sollid, L. M. (2017). Strong clonal relatedness between serum and gut IgA despite different plasma cell origins. *Cell reports, 20*(10), 2357-2367.

Iyer, A., Rathnasabapathi, D., Elsone, L., Mutch, K., Terlizzo, M., Footitt, D., & Jacob, A. (2014). Transverse myelitis associated with an itchy rash and hyperckemia: neuromyelitis optica associated with dermatitis herpetiformis. *JAMA neurology, 71*(5), 630-633.

Jabri, B. (2021). Transglutaminase 2 Inhibition for Prevention of Mucosal Damage in Celiac Disease. The New England journal of medicine, 385(1), 76.

Jabri, B., & Abadie, V. (2015). IL-15 functions as a danger signal to regulate tissue-resident T cells and tissue destruction. *Nature Reviews Immunology, 15*(12), 771-783.

Jabri, B., & Sollid, L. M. (2009). Tissue-mediated control of immunopathology in coeliac disease. *Nature Reviews Immunology, 9*(12), 858-870.

Jabri, B., & Sollid, L. M. (2017). T cells in celiac disease. *The Journal of Immunology, 198*(8), 3005-3014.

Jafri, M. R., Nordstrom, C. W., Murray, J. A., Van Dyke, C. T., Dierkhising, R. A., Zinsmeister, A. R., & Melton, L. J. (2008). Long-term fracture risk in patients with celiac disease: a population-based study in Olmsted County, Minnesota. *Digestive diseases and sciences, 53*, 964-971.

Jakobek, L. (2015). Interactions of polyphenols with carbohydrates, lipids and proteins. *Food chemistry, 175*, 556-567.

Janssen, G., Christis, C., Kooy-Winkelaar, Y., Edens, L., Smith, D., van Veelen, P., & Koning, F. (2015). Ineffective degradation of immunogenic gluten epitopes by currently available digestive enzyme supplements. *PloS one, 10*(6), e0128065.

Jansson-Knodell, C. L., Hujoel, I. A., West, C. P., Taneja, V., Prokop, L. J., Rubio-Tapia, A., & Murray, J. A. (2019). Sex difference in celiac disease in undiagnosed populations: a systematic review and meta-analysis. *Clinical gastroenterology and hepatology, 17*(10), 1954-1968. e1913.

Jd, A. (1996). Phenotypic analysis of antigen-specific T lymphocytes. *Science, 274*, 94.

Jenks, S. A., Cashman, K. S., Woodruff, M. C., Lee, F. E. H., & Sanz, I. (2019). Extrafollicular responses in humans and SLE. *Immunological reviews, 288*(1), 136-148.

Jensen, E. T., Eluri, S., Lebwohl, B., Genta, R. M., & Dellon, E. S. (2015). Increased risk of esophageal eosinophilia and eosinophilic esophagitis in patients with active celiac disease on biopsy. *Clinical gastroenterology and hepatology, 13*(8), 1426-1431.

Johnson, J., Boynton, K., & Peterson, K. (2016). Co-occurrence of eosinophilic esophagitis and potential/probable celiac disease in an adult cohort: a possible association with implications for clinical practice. *Diseases of the Esophagus, 29*(8), 977-982.

Juhász, A., Belova, T., Florides, C. G., Maulis, C., Fischer, I., Gell, G., ... Maharajan, A. (2018). Genome mapping of seed-borne allergens and immunoresponsive proteins in wheat. *Science advances, 4*(8), eaar8602.

Jüse, U., van de Wal, Y., Koning, F., Sollid, L. M., & Fleckenstein, B. (2010). Design of new high-affinity peptide ligands for human leukocyte antigen -DQ2 using a positional scanning peptide library. *Human immunology, 71*(5), 475-481.

Kakar, S., Nehra, V., Murray, J. A., Dayharsh, G. A., & Burgart, L. J. (2003). Significance of intraepithelial lymphocytosis in small bowel biopsy samples with normal mucosal architecture. *Official journal of the American College of Gastroenterology| ACG, 98*(9), 2027-2033.

Kalayci, A. G., Kansu, A., Girgin, N., Kucuk, O., & Aras, G. (2001). Bone mineral density and importance of a gluten -free diet in patients with celiac disease in childhood. *Pediatrics, 108*(5), e89-e89.

KAMER, J. V. D., Weijers, H. A., & Dicke, W. K. (1953). Coeliac disease: an investigation into the injurious constituents of wheat in connection with their action on patients with coeliac disease. *Acta paediatrica, 42*(3), 223-231.

Kamycheva, E., Goto, T., & Camargo, C. (2017). Celiac disease is associated with reduced bone mineral density and increased FRAX scores in the US National Health and Nutrition Examination Survey. *Osteoporosis International, 28*, 781-790.

Kan, S., Cen, Y., He, Z., Zhang, Z., Zhang, L., & Wang, Y. (2019). Supervised deep feature embedding with handcrafted feature. *IEEE Transactions on Image Processing, 28*(12), 5809-5823.

Kang, H. K., Ecklund, D., Liu, M., & Datta, S. K. (2009). Apigenin, a non-mutagenic dietary flavonoid, suppresses lupus by inhibiting autoantigen presentation for expansion of autoreactive Th1 and Th17 cells. *Arthritis research & therapy, 11*, 1-13.

Kaplan, J., Pack, D., Horoupian, D., DeSouza, T., Brin, M., & Schaumburg, H. (1988). Distal axonopathy associated with chronic gluten enteropathy: a treatable disorder. *Neurology, 38*(4), 642-642.

Karell, K., Louka, A. S., Moodie, S. J., Ascher, H., Clot, F., Greco, L., ... Disease, E. G. C. o. C. (2003). HLA types in celiac disease patients not carrying the DQA1* 05-DQB1* 02 (DQ2) heterodimer: results from the European Genetics Cluster on Celiac Disease. Human immunology, 64(4), 469-477.

Karimi, N., Jabbari, V., Nazemi, A., Ganbarov, K., Karimi, N., Tanomand, A., ... Khodadadi, E. (2020). Thymol, cardamom and Lactobacillus plantarum nanoparticles as a functional candy with high protection against Streptococcus mutans and tooth decay. *Microbial pathogenesis, 148*, 104481.

Karwautz, A., Wagner, G., Berger, G., Sinnreich, U., Grylli, V., & Huber, W. D. (2008). Eating pathology in adolescents with celiac disease. *Psychosomatics, 49*(5), 399-406.

Katz, K. D., Rashtak, S., Lahr, B. D., Melton III, L. J., Krause, P. K., Maggi, K., ... Murray, J. A. (2011). Screening for celiac disease in a North American population: sequential serology and gastrointestinal symptoms. *The American journal of gastroenterology, 106*(7), 1333.

Kaukinen, K., Peräaho, M., Lindfors, K., Partanen, J., Woolley, N., Pikkarainen, P., ... Mäki, M. (2007). Persistent small bowel mucosal villous atrophy without symptoms in coeliac disease. *Alimentary pharmacology & therapeutics, 25*(10), 1237-1245.

Kaur, M., Sandhu, K. S., Arora, A., & Sharma, A. (2015). Gluten free biscuits prepared from buckwheat flour by incorporation of various gums: Physicochemical and sensory properties. *LWT-Food Science and Technology, 62*(1), 628-632.

Kavuncu, V., Dundar, U., Ciftci, I., Evcik, D., & Yigit, I. (2009). Is there any requirement for celiac disease screening routinely in postmenapausal women with osteoporosis ? *Rheumatology international, 29*, 841-845.

Kawabata, K., Yoshioka, Y., & Terao, J. (2019). Role of intestinal microbiota in the bioavailability and physiological functions of dietary polyphenols. *Molecules, 24*(2), 370.

Keijzer, C., Zee, R. v. d., Eden, W. v., & Broere, F. (2013). Treg inducing adjuvants for therapeutic vaccination against chronic inflammatory diseases. *Frontiers in immunology, 4*, 245.

Kelly, C., Green, P., Murray, J., Dimarino, A., Colatrella, A., Leffler, D., ... Jiang, J. (2013). Larazotide acetate in patients with coeliac disease undergoing a gluten challenge: a randomised placebo-controlled study. *Alimentary pharmacology & therapeutics, 37*(2), 252-262.

Kemppainen, K. M., Lynch, K. F., Liu, E., Lönnrot, M., Simell, V., Briese, T., ... She, J. X. (2017). Factors that increase risk of celiac disease autoimmunity after a gastrointestinal infection in early life. *Clinical gastroenterology and hepatology, 15*(5), 694-702. e695.

Kemppainen, T., Heikkinen, M., Ristikankare, M., Kosma, V., & Julkunen, R. (2010). Nutrient intakes during diets including unkilned and large amounts of oats in celiac disease. *European journal of clinical nutrition, 64*(1), 62-67.

Kemppainen, T., Kröger, H., Janatuinen, E., Arnala, I., Kosma, V. M., Pikkarainen, P., ... Uusitupa, M. (1999). Osteoporosis in adult patients with celiac disease. *Bone, 24*(3), 249-255.

Kemppainen, T., Kröger, H., Janatuinen, E., Arnala, I., Lamberg-Allardt, C., Kärkkäinen, M., ... Alhava, E. (1999). Bone recovery after a gluten -free diet : a 5-year follow-up study. *Bone, 25*(3), 355-360.

Kerkman, P. F., Dernstedt, A., Tadala, L., Mittler, E., Dannborg, M., Sundling, C., ... Wigren Byström, J. (2021). Generation of plasma cells and CD27− IgD− B cells during hantavirus infection is associated with distinct pathological findings. *Clinical & Translational Immunology, 10*(7), e1313.

Kerr, M., & Cherney, K. (2015). Gluten allergies food list: what to avoid & what to eat. *Health Line*, 1-6.

Khairuddin, M. A. N., & Lasekan, O. (2021). Gluten-free cereal products and beverages: A review of their health benefits in the last five years. *Foods, 10*(11), 2523.

Khan, A. S., Peter, S., & Wilcox, C. M. (2014). Olmesartan-induced enteropathy resembling celiac disease. *Endoscopy, 46*(S 01), E97-E98.

Khan, H., Sureda, A., Belwal, T., Çetinkaya, S., Süntar, İ., Tejada, S., ... Aschner, M. (2019). Polyphenols in the treatment of autoimmune diseases. *Autoimmunity reviews, 18*(7), 647-657.

Kieslich, M., Errázuriz, G., Posselt, H. G., Moeller-Hartmann, W., Zanella, F., & Boehles, H. (2001). Brain white-matter lesions in celiac disease: a prospective study of 75 diet-treated patients. *Pediatrics, 108*(2), e21-e21.

Kim, C. Y., Quarsten, H., Bergseng, E., Khosla, C., & Sollid, L. M. (2004). Structural basis for HLA-DQ2 -mediated presentation of gluten epitopes in celiac disease. *Proceedings of the National Academy of Sciences, 101*(12), 4175-4179.

Kim, H. J., Kim, S. H., & Yun, J. M. (2012). Fisetin inhibits hyperglycemia-induced proinflammatory cytokine production by epigenetic mechanisms. *Evidence-Based Complementary and Alternative Medicine, 2012*(1), 639469.

Kim, H. S., Quon, M. J., & Kim, J. a. (2014). New insights into the mechanisms of polyphenols beyond antioxidant properties; lessons from the green tea polyphenol, epigallocatechin 3-gallate. *Redox biology, 2*, 187-195.

Kim, H. s., Unalp-Arida, A., Ruhl, C. E., & Murray, J. A. (2019). Autoimmune and allergic disorders are more common in people with celiac disease or on a gluten -free diet in the United States. *Journal of clinical gastroenterology, 53*(10), e416-e423.

King, A., Moodie, S., Fraser, J., Curtis, D., Reid, E., Dearlove, A., ... Ciclitira, P. (2002). CTLA-4/CD28 gene region is associated with genetic susceptibility to coeliac disease in UK families. *Journal of medical genetics, 39*(1), 51-54.

King, J. A., Jeong, J., Underwood, F. E., Quan, J., Panaccione, N., Windsor, J. W., ... Shaheen, A. A. (2020). Incidence of celiac disease is increasing over time: a systematic review and meta-analysis. *Official journal of the American College of Gastroenterology| ACG, 115*(4), 507-525.

Kivelä, L., & Kurppa, K. (2017). USPSTF celiac disease screening recommendations. *The Journal of Pediatrics, 188*, 308-311.

Kivelä, L., Caminero, A., Leffler, D. A., Pinto-Sanchez, M. I., Tye-Din, J. A., & Lindfors, K. (2021). Current and emerging therapies for coeliac disease. *Nature Reviews Gastroenterology & Hepatology, 18*(3), 181-195.

Kmieciak, M., Gowda, M., Graham, L., Godder, K., Bear, H. D., Marincola, F. M., & Manjili, M. H. (2009). Human T cells express CD25 and Foxp3 upon activation and exhibit effector/memory phenotypes without any regulatory/suppressor function. *Journal of translational medicine, 7*, 1-7.

Kockova, M., & Valík, Ľ. (2014). Development of new cereal-, pseudocereal-, and cereal-leguminous-based probiotic foods. *Czech Journal of Food Sciences, 32*(4), 391-397.

Koletzko, S., Lee, H. S., Beyerlein, A., Aronsson, C. A., Hummel, M., Liu, E., ... Hagopian, W. (2018). Caesarean section on the risk of celiac disease in the offspring: The Teddy Study. *Journal of pediatric gastroenterology and nutrition, 66*(3), 417.

Komeroski, M. R., Homem, R. V., Schmidt, H. d. O., Rockett, F. C., de Lira, L., da Farias, D. V., ... de Oliveira, V. R. (2021). Effect of whey protein and mixed flours on the quality parameters of gluten -free breads. *International Journal of Gastronomy and Food Science, 24*, 100361.

Kondrashova, A., Mustalahti, K., Kaukinen, K., Viskari, H., Volodicheva, V., Haapala, A. M., ... Hyöty, H. (2008). Lower economic status and inferior hygienic environment may protect against celiac disease. *Annals of medicine, 40*(3), 223-231.

Koning, F. (2005). Celiac disease: caught between a rock and a hard place. *Gastroenterology, 129*(4), 1294-1301.

Kooy-Winkelaar, Y. M., Bouwer, D., Janssen, G. M., Thompson, A., Brugman, M. H., Schmitz, F., ... van Rood, J. J. (2017). CD4 T-cell cytokines synergize to induce proliferation of malignant and nonmalignant innate intraepithelial lymphocytes. *Proceedings of the National Academy of Sciences, 114*(6), E980-E989.

Kooy-Winkelaar, Y., van Lummel, M., Moustakas, A. K., Schweizer, J., Mearin, M. L., Mulder, C. J., ... van Bergen, J. (2011). Gluten-specific T cells cross-react between HLA-DQ8 and the HLA-DQ2α/DQ8β transdimer. *The Journal of Immunology, 187*(10), 5123-5129.

Korneychuk, N., Ramiro-Puig, E., Ettersperger, J., Schulthess, J., Montcuquet, N., Kiyono, H., ... Cerf-Bensussan, N. (2014). Interleukin 15 and CD4+ T cells cooperate to promote small intestinal enteropathy in response to dietary antigen. *Gastroenterology, 146*(4), 1017-1027.

Korponay-Szabo, I., Tumpek, J., Gyimesi, J., Laurila, K., Papp, M., Maki, M., & Khosla, C. (2010). *Food-grade gluten degrading enzymes to treat dietary transgressions in coeliac adolescents.* Paper presented at the Journal of pediatric gastroenterology and nutrition .

Krigel, A., Turner, K. O., Makharia, G. K., Green, P. H., Genta, R. M., & Lebwohl, B. (2016). Ethnic variations in duodenal villous atrophy consistent with celiac disease in the United States. *Clinical gastroenterology and hepatology, 14*(8), 1105-1111.

Krishnareddy, S., Stier, K., Recanati, M., Lebwohl, B., & Green, P. H. (2017). Commercially available glutenases: a potential hazard in coeliac disease. *Therapeutic advances in gastroenterology, 10*(6), 473-481.

Krom, H., Sprangers, F., van den Berg, R., Benninga, M. A., & Kindermann, A. (2017). Transverse myelitis as manifestation of celiac disease in a toddler. *Pediatrics, 139*(3).

Krupa-Kozak, U., Bączek, N., Capriles, V. D., & Łopusiewicz, Ł. (2022). Novel gluten - free bread with an extract from flaxseed by-product: the relationship between water replacement level and nutritional value, antioxidant properties, and sensory quality. *Molecules, 27*(9), 2690.

Kuja-Halkola, R., Lebwohl, B., Halfvarson, J., Emilsson, L., Magnusson, P. K., & Ludvigsson, J. F. (2017). Birth weight, sex, and celiac disease: a nationwide twin study. *Clinical Epidemiology, 9*, 567.

Kumar Singh, A., Cabral, C., Kumar, R., Ganguly, R., Kumar Rana, H., Gupta, A., ... Pandey, A. K. (2019). Beneficial effects of dietary polyphenols on gut microbiota and strategies to improve delivery efficiency. *Nutrients, 11*(9), 2216.

Kumar, J., Kumar, M., Pandey, R., & Chauhan, N. S. (2017). Physiopathology and management of gluten -induced celiac disease. *Journal of Food Science, 82*(2), 270-277.

Kumar, M., Rastogi, A., Bhadada, S. K., Bhansali, A., Vaiphei, K., & Kochhar, R. (2013). Effect of zoledronic acid on bone mineral density in patients of celiac disease: a prospective, randomized, pilot study. *Indian Journal of Medical Research, 138*(6), 882-887.

Kwitt, R., Hegenbart, S., Rasiwasia, N., Vécsei, A., & Uhl, A. (2014). *Do we need annotation experts? A case study in celiac disease classification.* Paper presented at the Medical Image Computing and Computer-Assisted Intervention–MICCAI 2014: 17th International Conference, Boston, MA, USA, September 14-18, 2014, Proceedings, Part II 17.

Labate, A., Gambardella, A., Messina, D., Tammaro, S., Le Piane, E., Pirritano, D., ... Oliveri, R. (2001). Silent celiac disease in patients with childhood localization-related epilepsies. *Epilepsia, 42*(9), 1153-1155.

Lähdeaho, M. L., Kaukinen, K., Laurila, K., Vuotikka, P., Koivurova, O. P., Kärjä-Lahdensuu, T., ... Mäki, M. (2014). Glutenase ALV003 attenuates gluten -induced mucosal injury in patients with celiac disease. *Gastroenterology, 146*(7), 1649-1658.

Laignier, F., Akutsu, R. d. C. d. A., Lima, B. R. d., Zandonadi, R. P., Raposo, A., Saraiva, A., & Botelho, R. B. A. (2022). Amorphophallus konjac: Sensory profile of this novel alternative flour on gluten -free bread. *Foods, 11*(10), 1379.

Lamacchia, C., Camarca, A., Picascia, S., Di Luccia, A., & Gianfrani, C. (2014). Cereal-based gluten -free food: How to reconcile nutritional and technological properties of wheat proteins with safety for celiac disease patients. *Nutrients, 6*(2), 575-590.

Lambert, K., & Ficken, C. (2016). Cost and affordability of a nutritionally balanced gluten -free diet: Is following a gluten-free diet affordable? *Nutrition & Dietetics, 73*(1), 36-42.

Lammers, K. M., Lu, R., Brownley, J., Lu, B., Gerard, C., Thomas, K., ... Alkan, S. (2008). Gliadin induces an increase in intestinal permeability and zonulin release by binding to the chemokine receptor CXCR3. *Gastroenterology, 135*(1), 194-204. e193.

Landsverk, O. J., Snir, O., Casado, R. B., Richter, L., Mold, J. E., Réu, P., ... Aandahl, E. M. (2017). Antibody-secreting plasma cells persist for decades in human intestine. *Journal of Experimental Medicine, 214*(2), 309-317.

Lang, A., Salomon, N., Wu, J. C., Kopylov, U., Lahat, A., Har-Noy, O., ... Gamus, D. (2015). Curcumin in combination with mesalamine induces remission in patients with mild-to-moderate ulcerative colitis in a randomized controlled trial. *Clinical Gastroenterology and Hepatology, 13*(8), 1444-1449. e1441.

Lang, T., & McKee, M. (2022). The reinvasion of Ukraine threatens global food supplies. In (Vol. 376): British Medical Journal Publishing Group.

Laparra, J. M., & Sanz, Y. (2010). Bifidobacteria inhibit the inflammatory response induced by gliadins in intestinal epithelial cells via modifications of toxic peptide generation during digestion. *Journal of cellular biochemistry, 109*(4), 801-807.

Laparra, J. M., Olivares, M., Gallina, O., & Sanz, Y. (2012). Bifidobacterium longum CECT 7347 modulates immune responses in a gliadin-induced enteropathy animal model. *PloS one, 7*(2), e30744.

Latorre, M., Lagana, S. M., Freedberg, D. E., Lewis, S. K., Lebwohl, B., Bhagat, G., & Green, P. H. (2015). Endoscopic biopsy technique in the diagnosis of celiac disease: one bite or two? *Gastrointestinal endoscopy, 81*(5), 1228-1233.

Laursen, L. (2016). Erratum: Will Europe toast GM wheat for gluten sufferers? *Nature Biotechnology, 34*(10), 1072-1072.

Lauwers, G. Y., Fasano, A., & Brown, I. S. (2015). Duodenal lymphocytosis with no or minimal enteropathy: much ado about nothing? *Modern Pathology, 28*, S22-S29.

Le Bras, S., & Geha, R. S. (2006). IPEX and the role of Foxp3 in the development and function of human Tregs. *The Journal of clinical investigation, 116*(6), 1473-1475.

Lebreton, C., Ménard, S., Abed, J., Moura, I. C., Coppo, R., Dugave, C., ... Griffin, M. (2012). Interactions among secretory immunoglobulin A, CD71, and transglutaminase-2 affect permeability of intestinal epithelial cells to gliadin peptides. *Gastroenterology, 143*(3), 698-707. e694.

Lebwohl, B., Granath, F., Ekbom, A., Smedby, K. E., Murray, J. A., Neugut, A. I., ... Ludvigsson, J. F. (2013). Mucosal healing and risk for lymphoproliferative malignancy in celiac disease: a population-based cohort study. *Annals of internal medicine, 159*(3), 169-175.

Lebwohl, B., Kapel, R. C., Neugut, A. I., Green, P. H., & Genta, R. M. (2011). Adherence to biopsy guidelines increases celiac disease diagnosis. *Gastrointestinal endoscopy, 74*(1), 103-109.

Lebwohl, B., Michaëlsson, K., Green, P. H., & Ludvigsson, J. F. (2014). Persistent mucosal damage and risk of fracture in celiac disease. *The Journal of Clinical Endocrinology & Metabolism, 99*(2), 609-616.

Lebwohl, B., Spechler, S. J., Wang, T. C., Green, P. H., & Ludvigsson, J. F. (2014). Use of proton pump inhibitors and subsequent risk of celiac disease. *Digestive and liver disease, 46*(1), 36-40.

Lebwohl, B., Tennyson, C. A., Holub, J. L., Lieberman, D. A., Neugut, A. I., & Green, P. H. (2012). Sex and racial disparities in duodenal biopsy to evaluate for celiac disease. *Gastrointestinal endoscopy, 76*(4), 779-785.

Lee, A. R., Ng, D., Zivin, J., & Green, P. (2007). Economic burden of a gluten -free diet. *Journal of human Nutrition and Dietetics, 20*(5), 423-430.

Leffler, D. A., Dennis, M., Hyett, B., Kelly, E., Schuppan, D., & Kelly, C. P. (2007). Etiologies and predictors of diagnosis in nonresponsive celiac disease. *Clinical gastroenterology and hepatology, 5*(4), 445-450.

Leffler, D. A., Kelly, C. P., Abdallah, H., Colatrella, A., Harris, L., Leon, F., ... Murray, J. (2012). A randomized, double-blind study of larazotide acetate to prevent the activation of celiac disease during gluten challenge. *Official journal of the American College of Gastroenterology| ACG, 107*(10), 1554-1562.

Leffler, D. A., Kelly, C. P., Green, P. H., Fedorak, R. N., DiMarino, A., Perrow, W., ... Bachir, N. M. (2015). Larazotide acetate for persistent symptoms of celiac disease despite a gluten -free diet : a randomized controlled trial. *Gastroenterology, 148*(7), 1311-1319. e1316.

Lefranc, M. P. (2011). IMGT, the international ImMunoGeneTics information system. *Cold Spring Harbor Protocols, 2011*(6), pdb. top115.

Leišová-Svobodová, L., Sovová, T., & Dvořáček, V. (2022). Analysis of oat seed transcriptome with regards to proteins involved in celiac disease. *Scientific reports, 12*(1), 1-11.

Leonard, M. M., Bai, Y., Serena, G., Nickerson, K. P., Camhi, S., Sturgeon, C., ... Nath, B. (2019). RNA sequencing of intestinal mucosa reveals novel pathways functionally linked to celiac disease pathogenesis. *PloS one, 14*(4), e0215132.

Leonard, M. M., Camhi, S., Huedo-Medina, T. B., & Fasano, A. (2015). Celiac disease genomic, environmental, microbiome, and metabolomic (CDGEMM) study design: approach to the future of personalized prevention of celiac disease. *Nutrients, 7*(11), 9325-9336.

Leonard, M. M., Sapone, A., Catassi, C., & Fasano, A. (2017). Celiac disease and nonceliac gluten sensitivity: a review. *Jama, 318*(7), 647-656.

Leonard, M. M., Silvester, J. A., Leffler, D., Fasano, A., Kelly, C. P., Lewis, S. K., ... McAuliffe, W. J. (2021). Evaluating responses to gluten challenge: a randomized, double-blind, 2-dose gluten challenge trial. *Gastroenterology, 160*(3), 720-733. e728.

Leonard, M. M., Weir, D. C., DeGroote, M., Mitchell, P. D., Singh, P., Silvester, J. A., ... Fasano, A. (2017). Value of IgA tTG in predicting mucosal recovery in children with celiac disease on a gluten -free diet. *Journal of pediatric gastroenterology and nutrition, 64*(2), 286-291.

Lerner, A., Ramesh, A., & Matthias, T. (2019). The revival of the battle between David and Goliath in the enteric viruses and microbiota struggle: potential implication for celiac disease. *Microorganisms, 7*(6), 173.

Lexhaller, B., Tompos, C., & Scherf, K. A. (2017). Fundamental study on reactivities of gluten protein types from wheat, rye and barley with five sandwich ELISA test kits. *Food Chemistry, 237*, 320-330.

Li, H., Song, W., Liu, T., Xu, S., Zhang, S., Zhang, Y., ... Yu, J. (2022). Developing novel synbiotic yoghurt with Lacticaseibacillus paracasei and lactitol: Investigation of the microbiology, textural and rheological properties. *International Dairy Journal, 135*, 105475.

Li, J. M., & Nie, S. P. (2016). The functional and nutritional aspects of hydrocolloids in foods. *Food Hydrocolloids, 53*, 46-61.

Li, J., Wu, T., Li, N., Wang, X., Chen, G., & Lyu, X. (2019). Bilberry anthocyanin extract promotes intestinal barrier function and inhibits digestive enzyme activity by regulating the gut microbiota in aging rats. *Food & function, 10*(1), 333-343.

Li, L., Wang, L., Wu, Z., Yao, L., Wu, Y., Huang, L., ... Gou, D. (2014). Anthocyanin-rich fractions from red raspberries attenuate inflammation in both RAW264. 7 macrophages and a mouse model of colitis. *Scientific reports, 4*(1), 6234.

Li, W., Yang, H., Zhao, Q., Wang, X., Zhang, J., & Zhao, X. (2019). Polyphenol-rich loquat fruit extract prevents fructose-induced nonalcoholic fatty liver disease by modulating glycometabolism, lipometabolism, oxidative stress, inflammation, intestinal barrier, and gut microbiota in mice. *Journal of agricultural and food chemistry, 67*(27), 7726-7737.

Li, Y., Rahman, S. U., Huang, Y., Zhang, Y., Ming, P., Zhu, L., ... Wang, X. (2020). Green tea polyphenols decrease weight gain, ameliorate alteration of gut microbiota, and mitigate intestinal inflammation in canines with high-fat-diet-induced obesity. *The Journal of Nutritional Biochemistry, 78*, 108324.

Liang, L., Pinier, M., Leroux, J. C., & Subirade, M. (2009). Interaction of α-gliadin with poly (HEMA-co-SS): Structural characterization and biological implication. *Biopolymers: Original Research on Biomolecules, 91*(2), 169-178.

Lim, J. J., Jones, C. M., Loh, T. J., Ting, Y. T., Zareie, P., Loh, K. L., ... Stevenaert, F. (2021). The shared susceptibility epitope of HLA-DR4 binds citrullinated self-antigens and the TCR. *Science immunology, 6*(58), eabe0896.

Lindeman, I., Emerton, G., Mamanova, L., Snir, O., Polanski, K., Qiao, S. W., ... Stubbington, M. J. (2018). BraCeR: B-cell-receptor reconstruction and clonality inference from single-cell RNA-seq. *Nature methods, 15*(8), 563-565.

Lindeman, I., Zhou, C., Eggesbø, L. M., Miao, Z., Polak, J., Lundin, K. E., ... Sollid, L. M. (2020). Longevity, clonal relationship, and transcriptional program of celiac disease–specific plasma cells. *Journal of Experimental Medicine, 218*(2), e20200852.

Lindfors, K., Blomqvist, T., Juuti-Uusitalo, K., Stenman, S., Venäläinen, J., Mäki, M., & Kaukinen, K. (2008). Live probiotic Bifidobacterium lactis bacteria inhibit the toxic effects induced by wheat gliadin in epithelial cell culture. *Clinical & Experimental Immunology, 152*(3), 552-558.

Lindfors, K., Kaukinen, K., & Mäki, M. (2009). A role for anti-transglutaminase 2 autoantibodies in the pathogenesis of coeliac disease? *Amino acids, 36*, 685-691.

Lionetti, E., Castellaneta, S., Francavilla, R., Pulvirenti, A., Tonutti, E., Amarri, S., ... Bellantoni, A. (2014). Introduction of gluten, HLA status, and the risk of celiac disease in children. *New England Journal of Medicine, 371*(14), 1295-1303.

Lionetti, E., Francavilla, R., Pavone, P., Pavone, L., Francavilla, T., Pulvirenti, A., ... Ruggieri, M. (2010). The neurology of coeliac disease in childhood: what is the evidence? A systematic review and meta-analysis. *Developmental Medicine & Child Neurology, 52*(8), 700-707.

Lisboa, P. J. (2002). A review of evidence of health benefit from artificial neural networks in medical intervention. *Neural networks, 15*(1), 11-39.

Littmann, E. R., Lee, J. J., Denny, J. E., Alam, Z., Maslanka, J. R., Zarin, I., ... Saffern, M. S. (2021). Host immunity modulates the efficacy of microbiota transplantation for treatment of Clostridioides difficile infection. *Nature communications, 12*(1), 1-15.

Liu, E., Dong, F., Barón, A. E., Taki, I., Norris, J. M., Frohnert, B. I., ... Rewers, M. (2017). High incidence of celiac disease in a long-term study of adolescents with susceptibility genotypes. *Gastroenterology, 152*(6), 1329-1336. e1321.

Liu, E., Lee, H. S., Aronsson, C. A., Hagopian, W. A., Koletzko, S., Rewers, M. J., ... Simell, V. (2014). Risk of pediatric celiac disease according to HLA haplotype and country. *New England Journal of Medicine, 371*(1), 42-49.

Liu, X., Mu, T., Sun, H., Zhang, M., Chen, J., & Fauconnier, M. L. (2018). Influence of different hydrocolloids on dough thermo-mechanical properties and *in vitro* starch digestibility of gluten -free steamed bread based on potato flour. *Food chemistry, 239*, 1064-1074.

Liu, X., Mu, T., Sun, H., Zhang, M., Chen, J., & Fauconnier, M. L. (2019). Effect of ingredients on the quality of gluten -free steamed bread based on potato flour. *Journal of food science and technology, 56*, 2863-2873.

Liu, Y., Wang, X., Chen, Q., Luo, L., Ma, M., Xiao, B., & Zeng, L. (2020). Camellia sinensis and Litsea coreana ameliorate intestinal inflammation and modulate gut microbiota in dextran sulfate sodium -induced colitis mice. *Molecular nutrition & food research, 64*(6), 1900943.

Lobo de Sá, F. D., Butkevych, E., Nattramilarasu, P. K., Fromm, A., Mousavi, S., Moos, V., ... Seinige, D. (2019). Curcumin mitigates immune-induced epithelial barrier dysfunction by Campylobacter jejuni. *International journal of molecular sciences, 20*(19), 4830.

Lohi, S., Mustalahti, K., Kaukinen, K., Laurila, K., Collin, P., Rissanen, H., ... Reunanen, A. (2007). Increasing prevalence of coeliac disease over time. *Alimentary pharmacology & therapeutics, 26*(9), 1217-1225.

Lohiniemi, S., Mäki, M., Kaukinen, K., Laippala, P., & Collin, P. (2000). Gastrointestinal symptoms rating scale in coeliac disease patients on wheat starch-based gluten -free diets. *Scandinavian journal of gastroenterology, 35*(9), 947-949.

López-Palacios, N., Pascual, V., Castaño, M., Bodas, A., Fernández-Prieto, M., Espino-Paisán, L., ... Rey, E. (2018). Evaluation of T cells in blood after a short gluten challenge for coeliac disease diagnosis. *Digestive and Liver Disease, 50*(11), 1183-1188.

Lu, W., Nishinari, K., Matsukawa, S., & Fang, Y. (2020). The future trends of food hydrocolloids. *Food Hydrocolloids, 103*, 105713.

Ludvigsson, J. F., & Lebwohl, B. (2019). Three papers indicate that amount of gluten play a role for celiac disease-But only a minor role. *Acta Paediatrica (Oslo, Norway: 1992), 109*(1), 8-10.

Ludvigsson, J. F., Bai, J. C., Biagi, F., Card, T. R., Ciacci, C., Ciclitira, P. J., ... Van Heel, D. A. (2014). Diagnosis and management of adult coeliac disease: guidelines from the British Society of Gastroenterology. *Gut, 63*(8), 1210-1228.

Ludvigsson, J. F., Hemminki, K., Wahlström, J., & Almqvist, C. (2011). Celiac disease confers a 1.6-fold increased risk of asthma: a nationwide population-based cohort study. *Journal of Allergy and Clinical Immunology, 127*(4), 1071-1073. e1074.

Ludvigsson, J. F., Leffler, D. A., Bai, J. C., Biagi, F., Fasano, A., Green, P. H., ... Leonard, J. N. (2013). The Oslo definitions for coeliac disease and related terms. *Gut, 62*(1), 43-52.

Ludvigsson, J. F., Pathak, J., Murphy, S., Durski, M., Kirsch, P. S., Chute, C. G., ... Murray, J. A. (2013). Use of computerized algorithm to identify individuals in need of testing for celiac disease. *Journal of the American Medical Informatics Association, 20*(e2), e306-e310.

Ludvigsson, J. F., Rubio-Tapia, A., Van Dyke, C. T., Melton III, L. J., Zinsmeister, A. R., Lahr, B. D., & Murray, J. A. (2013). Increasing incidence of celiac disease in a North American population. *The American journal of gastroenterology, 108*(5), 818.

Ludvigsson, J. F., Zingone, F., Tomson, T., Ekbom, A., & Ciacci, C. (2012). Increased risk of epilepsy in biopsy -verified celiac disease: a population-based cohort study. *Neurology, 78*(18), 1401-1407.

Lund-Blix, N. A., Mårild, K., Tapia, G., Norris, J. M., Stene, L. C., & Størdal, K. (2019). Gluten intake in early childhood and risk of celiac disease in childhood: a nationwide cohort study. *Official journal of the American College of Gastroenterology| ACG, 114*(8), 1299-1306.

Lundin, K. E. (2014). Non-celiac gluten sensitivity-why worry? *BMC medicine, 12*(1), 1-3.

Lundin, K. E., & Sollid, L. M. (2014). Advances in coeliac disease. *Current opinion in gastroenterology, 30*(2), 154-162.

Lundin, K. E., & Wijmenga, C. (2015). Coeliac disease and autoimmune disease—genetic overlap and screening. *Nature reviews Gastroenterology & hepatology, 12*(9), 507-515.

Lundin, K. E., Brottveit, M., & Skodje, G. (2022). Noncoeliac gluten sensitivity. *Coeliac Disease and Gluten-Related Disorders*, 177-195.

Lundin, K. E., Qiao, S. W., Snir, O., & Sollid, L. M. (2015). Coeliac disease–from genetic and immunological studies to clinical applications. *Scandinavian journal of gastroenterology, 50*(6), 708-717.

Lundin, K., Scott, H., Hansen, T., Paulsen, G., Halstensen, T., Fausa, O., ... Sollid, L. (1993). Gliadin-specific, HLA-DQ (alpha 1* 0501, beta 1* 0201) restricted T cells isolated from the small intestinal mucosa of celiac disease patients. *The Journal of experimental medicine, 178*(1), 187-196.

Luostarinen, L., Himanen, S., Luostarinen, M., Collin, P., & Pirttilä, T. (2003). Neuromuscular and sensory disturbances in patients with well treated coeliac disease. *Journal of Neurology, Neurosurgery & Psychiatry, 74*(4), 490-494.

Macaulay, I. C., Haerty, W., Kumar, P., Li, Y. I., Hu, T. X., Teng, M. J., ... Shirley, L. M. (2015). G&T-seq: parallel sequencing of single-cell genomes and transcriptomes. *Nature methods, 12*(6), 519-522.

Magaudda, A., Dalla Bernardina, B., De Marco, P., Sfaello, Z., Longo, M., Colamaria, V., ... Di Perri, R. (1993). Bilateral occipital calcification, epilepsy and coeliac disease: clinical and neuroimaging features of a new syndrome. *Journal of Neurology, Neurosurgery & Psychiatry, 56*(8), 885-889.

Mahmoud, R., Yousif, E., Gadallah, M., & Alawneh, A. (2013). Formulations and quality characterization of gluten -free Egyptian balady flat bread. *Annals of Agricultural Sciences, 58*(1), 19-25.

Maiuri, L., Ciacci, C., Auricchio, S., Brown, V., Quaratino, S., & Londei, M. (2000). Interleukin 15 mediates epithelial changes in celiac disease. *Gastroenterology, 119*(4), 996-1006.

Maiuri, L., Ciacci, C., Ricciardelli, I., Vacca, L., Raia, V., Auricchio, S., ... Londei, M. (2003). Association between innate response to gliadin and activation of pathogenic T cells in coeliac disease. *The Lancet, 362*(9377), 30-37.

Makharia, G. K. (2014). Current and emerging therapy for celiac disease. *Frontiers in medicine, 1*, 6.

Malamut, G., & Cellier, C. (2019). Refractory celiac disease. *Gastroenterology Clinics of North America, 48*(1), 137-144.

Malamut, G., El Machhour, R., Montcuquet, N., Martin-Lannerée, S., Dusanter-Fourt, I., Verkarre, V., ... Butz, E. A. (2010). IL-15 triggers an antiapoptotic pathway in human intraepithelial lymphocytes that is a potential new target in celiac disease–associated inflammation and lymphomagenesis. *The Journal of clinical investigation, 120*(6), 2131-2143.

Malamut, G., Meresse, B., Cellier, C., & Cerf-Bensussan, N. (2012). *Refractory celiac disease: from bench to bedside.* Paper presented at the Seminars in immunopathology.

Malamut, G., Verkarre, V., Suarez, F., Viallard, J. F., Lascaux, A. S., Cosnes, J., ... Ziol, M. (2010). The enteropathy associated with common variable immunodeficiency: the delineated frontiers with celiac disease. *Official journal of the American College of Gastroenterology| ACG, 105*(10), 2262-2275.

Malcolmson, L., Matsuo, R., & Balshaw, R. (1993). Effects of drying temperature and farina blending on spaghetti quality using response surface methodology. *Cereal Chemistry, 70*, 1-1.

Malfertheiner, P., Ripellino, C., & Cataldo, N. (2018). Severe intestinal malabsorption associated with ACE inhibitor or angiotensin receptor blocker treatment. An observational cohort study in Germany and Italy. *Pharmacoepidemiology and Drug Safety, 27*(6), 581-586.

Manavalan, J. S., Hernandez, L., Shah, J. G., Konikkara, J., Naiyer, A. J., Lee, A. R., ... Bhagat, G. (2010). Serum cytokine elevations in celiac disease: association with disease presentation. *Human immunology, 71*(1), 50-57.

Manzoor, M., Singh, J., Bandral, J. D., Gani, A., & Shams, R. (2020). Food hydrocolloids : Functional, nutraceutical and novel applications for delivery of bioactive compounds. *International Journal of Biological Macromolecules, 165*, 554-567.

Marasco, G., Cirota, G. G., Rossini, B., Lungaro, L., Di Biase, A. R., Colecchia, A., ... Caio, G. (2020). Probiotics, prebiotics and other dietary supplements for gut microbiota modulation in celiac disease patients. *Nutrients, 12*(9), 2674.

Marco, C., & Rosell, C. M. (2008). Breadmaking performance of protein enriched, gluten -free breads. *European food research and technology, 227*, 1205-1213.

Mårild, K., Dong, F., Lund-Blix, N. A., Seifert, J., Barón, A. E., Waugh, K. C., ... Stene, L. C. (2019). Gluten intake and risk of celiac disease: long-term follow-up of an at-risk birth cohort. *The American journal of gastroenterology, 114*(8), 1307.

Mårild, K., Stephansson, O., Montgomery, S., Murray, J. A., & Ludvigsson, J. F. (2012). Pregnancy outcome and risk of celiac disease in offspring: a nationwide case-control study. *Gastroenterology, 142*(1), 39-45. e33.

Mårild, K., Ye, W., Lebwohl, B., Green, P. H., Blaser, M. J., Card, T., & Ludvigsson, J. F. (2013). Antibiotic exposure and the development of coeliac disease: a nationwide case–control study. *BMC gastroenterology, 13*(1), 1-9.

Mariotti, M., Pagani, M. A., & Lucisano, M. (2013). The role of buckwheat and HPMC on the breadmaking properties of some commercial gluten -free bread mixtures. *Food Hydrocolloids, 30*(1), 393-400.

Marsh, M. N. (1992). Gluten, major histocompatibility complex, and the small intestine: a molecular and immunobiologic approach to the spectrum of gluten sensitivity ('celiac sprue '). *Gastroenterology, 102*(1), 330-354.

Marthey, L., Cadiot, G., Seksik, P., Pouderoux, P., Lacroute, J., Skinazi, F., ... Druez, A. (2014). Olmesartan-associated enteropathy: results of a national survey. *Alimentary pharmacology & therapeutics, 40*(9), 1103-1109.

Martinez, M., Gómez-Cabellos, S., Giménez, M. J., Barro, F., Diaz, I., & Diaz-Mendoza, M. (2019). Plant proteases: from key enzymes in germination to allies for fighting human gluten -related disorders. *Frontiers in plant science, 10*, 721.

Martorell, P., Alvarez, B., Llopis, S., Navarro, V., Ortiz, P., Gonzalez, N., ... Ramón, D. (2021). Heat-treated Bifidobacterium longum CECT-7347: a whole-cell postbiotic with antioxidant, anti-inflammatory, and gut-barrier protection properties. *Antioxidants, 10*(4), 536.

Masia, R., Peyton, S., Lauwers, G. Y., & Brown, I. (2014). Gastrointestinal biopsy findings of autoimmune enteropathy : a review of 25 cases. *The American journal of surgical pathology, 38*(10), 1319-1329.

Mather, K. J., Meddings, J. B., Beck, P. L., Scott, B. R., & Hanley, D. A. (2001). Prevalence of IgA-antiendomysial antibody in asymptomatic low bone mineral density. *Official journal of the American College of Gastroenterology| ACG, 96*(1), 120-125.

Matos, M. E., & Rosell, C. M. (2015). Understanding gluten -free dough for reaching breads with physical quality and nutritional balance. *Journal of the Science of Food and Agriculture, 95*(4), 653-661.

Matysiak–Budnik, T., Candalh, C., Cellier, C., Dugave, C., Namane, A., Vidal–Martinez, T., ... Heyman, M. (2005). Limited efficiency of prolyl-endopeptidase in the detoxification of gliadin peptides in celiac disease. *Gastroenterology, 129*(3), 786-796.

Matysiak-Budnik, T., Moura, I. C., Arcos-Fajardo, M., Lebreton, C., Ménard, S., Candalh, C., ... Van Niel, G. (2008). Secretory IgA mediates retrotranscytosis of intact gliadin peptides via the transferrin receptor in celiac disease. *The Journal of experimental medicine, 205*(1), 143-154.

Mauro, A., Orsi, L., Mortara, P., Costa, P., & Schiffer, D. (1991). Cerebellar syndrome in adult celiac disease with vitamin E deficiency. *Acta neurologica scandinavica, 84*(2), 167-170.

Mayangsari, Y., & Suzuki, T. (2018). Resveratrol enhances intestinal barrier function by ameliorating barrier disruption in Caco-2 cell monolayers. *Journal of Functional Foods, 51*, 39-46.

Mayassi, T., & Jabri, B. (2018). Human intraepithelial lymphocytes. *Mucosal immunology, 11*(5), 1281-1289.

Mayassi, T., Ladell, K., Gudjonson, H., McLaren, J. E., Shaw, D. G., Tran, M. T., ... van Unen, V. (2019). Chronic inflammation permanently reshapes tissue-resident immunity in celiac disease. *Cell, 176*(5), 967-981. e919.

Mazzarella, G., Salvati, V. M., Iaquinto, G., Stefanile, R., Capobianco, F., Luongo, D., ... Malamisura, B. (2012). Reintroduction of gluten following flour transamidation in adult celiac patients: a randomized, controlled clinical study. *Clinical and Developmental Immunology, 2012*.

Mazzini, E., Massimiliano, L., Penna, G., & Rescigno, M. (2014). Oral tolerance can be established via gap junction transfer of fed antigens from CX3CR1+ macrophages to CD103+ dendritic cells. *Immunity, 40*(2), 248-261.

McCarville, J. L., Nisemblat, Y., Galipeau, H. J., Jury, J., Tabakman, R., Cohen, A., ... Murray, J. A. (2014). BL-7010 demonstrates specific binding to gliadin and reduces gluten -associated pathology in a chronic mouse model of gliadin sensitivity. *PloS one, 9*(11), e109972.

McFarlane, X., Bhalla, A., Reeves, D., Morgan, L., & Robertson, D. (1995). Osteoporosis in treated adult coeliac disease. *Gut, 36*(5), 710-714.

McKinnon, K. M. (2018). Flow cytometry : an overview. *Current protocols in immunology, 120*(1), 5.1. 1-5.1. 11.

Mei, H. E., Frölich, D., Giesecke, C., Loddenkemper, C., Reiter, K., Schmidt, S., ... Radbruch, A. (2010). Steady-state generation of mucosal IgA+ plasmablasts is not abrogated by B-cell depletion therapy with rituximab. *Blood, The Journal of the American Society of Hematology, 116*(24), 5181-5190.

Memeo, L., Jhang, J., Hibshoosh, H., Green, P. H., Rotterdam, H., & Bhagat, G. (2005). Duodenal intraepithelial lymphocytosis with normal villous architecture: common occurrence in H. pylori gastritis. *Modern Pathology, 18*(8), 1134-1144.

Ménard, S., Lebreton, C., Schumann, M., Matysiak-Budnik, T., Dugave, C., Bouhnik, Y., ... Crenn, P. (2012). Paracellular versus transcellular intestinal permeability to gliadin peptides in active celiac disease. *The American journal of pathology, 180*(2), 608-615.

Mention, J. J., Ahmed, M. B., Bègue, B., Barbe, U., Verkarre, V., Asnafi, V., ... Mcintyre, E. (2003). Interleukin 15: a key to disrupted intraepithelial lymphocyte homeostasis and lymphomagenesis in celiac disease. *Gastroenterology, 125*(3), 730-745.

Meresse, B., Chen, Z., Ciszewski, C., Tretiakova, M., Bhagat, G., Krausz, T. N., ... Spies, T. (2004). Coordinated induction by IL15 of a TCR-independent NKG2D signaling pathway converts CTL into lymphokine-activated killer cells in celiac disease. *Immunity, 21*(3), 357-366.

Meresse, B., Korneychuk, N., Malamut, G., & Cerf-Bensussan, N. (2015). Interleukin-15, a master piece in the immunological jigsaw of celiac disease. *Digestive Diseases, 33*(2), 122-130.

Meresse, B., Ripoche, J., Heyman, M., & Cerf-Bensussan, N. (2009). Celiac disease: from oral tolerance to intestinal inflammation, autoimmunity and lymphomagenesis. *Mucosal immunology, 2*(1), 8-23.

Mesin, L., Sollid, L. M., & Niro, R. D. (2012). The intestinal B-cell response in celiac disease. *Frontiers in Immunology, 3*, 313.

Meyer, D., Stavropolous, S., Diamond, B., Shane, E., & Green, P. H. (2001). Osteoporosis in a North American adult population with celiac disease. *Official journal of the American College of Gastroenterology| ACG, 96*(1), 112-119.

Midhagen, G., Åberg, A. K., Olcén, P., Järnerot, G., Valdimarsson, T., Dahlbom, I., ... Ström, M. (2004). Antibody levels in adult patients with coeliac disease during gluten -free diet: a rapid initial decrease of clinical importance. *Journal of internal medicine, 256*(6), 519-524.

Mika, N., Zorn, H., & Rühl, M. (2015). Prolyl-specific peptidases for applications in food protein hydrolysis. *Applied microbiology and biotechnology, 99*(19), 7837-7846.

Milani, J., & Maleki, G. (2012). Hydrocolloids in food industry. *Food industrial processes–Methods and equipment, 2*, 2-37.

Miles, J. J., Douek, D. C., & Price, D. A. (2011). Bias in the αβ T-cell repertoire: implications for disease pathogenesis and vaccination. *Immunology and cell biology, 89*(3), 375-387.

Mills, S., Shanahan, F., Stanton, C., Hill, C., Coffey, A., & Ross, R. P. (2013). Movers and shakers: influence of bacteriophages in shaping the mammalian gut microbiota. *Gut microbes, 4*(1), 4-16.

Min, S., Lee, B., & Yoon, S. (2017). Deep learning in bioinformatics. *Briefings in bioinformatics, 18*(5), 851-869.

Mino, M., & Lauwers, G. Y. (2003). Role of lymphocytic immunophenotyping in the diagnosis of gluten -sensitive enteropathy with preserved villous architecture. *The American journal of surgical pathology, 27*(9), 1237-1242.

Mir, S. A., Shah, M. A., Naik, H. R., & Zargar, I. A. (2016). Influence of hydrocolloids on dough handling and technological properties of gluten -free breads. *Trends in Food Science & Technology, 51*, 49-57.

Miranda, J., Lasa, A., Bustamante, M., Churruca, I., & Simon, E. (2014). Nutritional differences between a gluten -free diet and a diet containing equivalent products with gluten. *Plant foods for human nutrition, 69*, 182-187.

Mishra, A., Sullivan, L., & Caligiuri, M. A. (2014). Molecular pathways: interleukin-15 signaling in health and in cancer. *Clinical Cancer Research, 20*(8), 2044-2050.

Mishra, S., Sinha, S., Dey, K. P., & Sen, G. (2014). Synthesis, characterization and applications of polymethylmethacrylate grafted psyllium as flocculant. *Carbohydrate polymers, 99*, 462-468.

Missbach, B., Schwingshackl, L., Billmann, A., Mystek, A., Hickelsberger, M., Bauer, G., & König, J. (2015). Gluten-free food database: the nutritional quality and cost of packaged gluten -free foods. *PeerJ, 3*, e1337.

Mitea, C., Salentijn, E. M., van Veelen, P., Goryunova, S. V., van der Meer, I. M., van den Broeck, H. C., ... Drijfhout, J. W. (2010). A universal approach to eliminate antigenic properties of alpha-gliadin peptides in celiac disease. *PloS one, 5*(12), e15637.

Mitoma, H., Adhikari, K., Aeschlimann, D., Chattopadhyay, P., Hadjivassiliou, M., Hampe, C. S., ... Lee, J. (2016). Consensus paper: neuroimmune mechanisms of cerebellar ataxias. *The Cerebellum, 15*, 213-232.

Miyake, M., Sasaki, K., Ide, K., Matsukura, Y., Shijima, K., & Fujiwara, D. (2006). Highly oligomeric procyanidins ameliorate experimental autoimmune encephalomyelitis via suppression of Th1 immunity. *The Journal of Immunology, 176*(10), 5797-5804.

Mohammadi, M., Khorshidian, N., Yousefi, M., & Khaneghah, A. M. (2022). Physicochemical, Rheological, and Sensory Properties of Gluten-Free Cookie Produced by Flour of Chestnut, Date Seed, and Modified Starch. *Journal of Food Quality, 2022*(1), 5159084.

Mohammadi, M., Sadeghnia, N., Azizi, M. H., Neyestani, T. R., & Mortazavian, A. M. (2014). Development of gluten -free flat bread using hydrocolloids: Xanthan and CMC. *Journal of Industrial and Engineering Chemistry, 20*(4), 1812-1818.

Molberg, Ø., Kett, K., Scott, H., Thorsby, E., Sollid, L., & Lundin, K. (1997). Gliadin specific, HLA DQ2 -restricted T cells are commonly found in small intestinal biopsies from coeliac disease patients, but not from controls. *Scandinavian journal of immunology, 46*(3), 103-109.

Molberg, Ø., Uhlen, A. K., Jensen, T., Flæte, N. S., Fleckenstein, B., Arentz–Hansen, H., ... Sollid, L. M. (2005). Mapping of gluten T-cell epitopes in the bread wheat ancestors: implications for celiac disease. *Gastroenterology, 128*(2), 393-401.

Molina-Infante, J., & Carroccio, A. (2017). Suspected nonceliac gluten sensitivity confirmed in few patients after gluten challenge in double-blind, placebo-controlled trials. *Clinical gastroenterology and hepatology, 15*(3), 339-348.

Montalto, M., D'Onofrio, F., Santoro, L., Gallo, A., Gasbarrini, A., & Gasbarrini, G. (2009). Autoimmune enteropathy in children and adults. *Scandinavian journal of gastroenterology, 44*(9), 1029-1036.

Monteagudo-Mera, A., Rodríguez-Aparicio, L., Rúa, J., Martínez-Blanco, H., Navasa, N., García-Armesto, M. R., & Ferrero, M. Á. (2012). *In vitro* evaluation of physiological probiotic properties of different lactic acid bacteria strains of dairy and human origin. *Journal of functional foods, 4*(2), 531-541.

Moreira, R., Chenlo, F., & Torres, M. D. (2013). Rheology of gluten -free doughs from blends of chestnut and rice flours. *Food and Bioprocess Technology, 6*, 1476-1485.

Moreno Amador, M. d. L., Arevalo-Rodriguez, M., Durán, E. M., Martinez Reyes, J. C., & Sousa Martin, C. (2019). A new microbial gluten -degrading prolyl endopeptidase: Potential application in celiac disease to reduce gluten immunogenic peptides. *PloS one, 14*(6), e0218346.

Moreno Amador, M. d. L., Comino Montilla, I. M., & Sousa Martín, C. (2014). Alternative grains as potential raw material for gluten –free food development in the diet of celiac and gluten–sensitive patients. *Austin Journal of Nutrition and Metabolism, 2 (3), 1-9.*

Morreale, F., Garzón, R., & Rosell, C. M. (2018). Understanding the role of hydrocolloids viscosity and hydration in developing gluten -free bread. A study with hydroxypropylmethylcellulose. *Food Hydrocolloids, 77*, 629-635.

Muir, J. G., Varney, J., Ajamian, M., & Gibson, P. (2019). Gluten-free and low-FODMAP sourdoughs for patients with coeliac disease and irritable bowel syndrome: A clinical perspective. *International journal of food microbiology, 290*, 237-246.

Multimers, P. D. (2001). Staining of Celiac Disease -Relevant T Cells by. *J Immunol, 167*, 4861-4868.

Murray, J. A., Van Dyke, C., Plevak, M. F., Dierkhising, R. A., Zinsmeister, A. R., & Melton III, L. J. (2003). Trends in the identification and clinical features of celiac disease in a North American community, 1950–2001. *Clinical gastroenterology and hepatology, 1*(1), 19-27.

Nair, N., Newell, E. W., Vollmers, C., Quake, S. R., Morton, J. M., Davis, M. M., ... Greenberg, H. B. (2016). High-dimensional immune profiling of total and rotavirus VP6-specific intestinal and circulating B cells by mass cytometry. *Mucosal immunology, 9*(1), 68-82.

Naji-Tabasi, S., & Mohebbi, M. (2015). Evaluation of cress seed gum and xanthan gum effect on macrostructure properties of gluten -free bread by image processing. *Journal of Food Measurement and characterization, 9*, 110-119.

Nakai, J. (2018). Food and Agriculture Organization of the United Nations and the sustainable development goals. *Sustainable development, 22*, 1-450.

Nardecchia, S., Auricchio, R., Discepolo, V., & Troncone, R. (2019). Extra-intestinal manifestations of coeliac disease in children: clinical features and mechanisms. *Frontiers in pediatrics, 7*, 56.

Nassiri, M. (2022). Production of Functional Ice Cream Fortified by Immunoglobulin Y against Escherichia coli O157: H7 and Helicobacter Pylori. *Biointerface Research in Applied Chemistry, 13*.

Nautiyal, O. (2011). Hydrocolloids, modified hydrocolloids as food recipes and formulating agents.

Nazareth, S., Lebwohl, B., Tennyson, C. A., Simpson, S., Greenlee, H., & Green, P. H. (2015). Dietary supplement use in patients with celiac disease in the United States. *Journal of clinical gastroenterology, 49*(7), 577-581.

Nenna, R., Petrarca, L., Verdecchia, P., Florio, M., Pietropaoli, N., Mastrogiorgio, G., ... Cucchiara, S. (2016). Celiac disease in a large cohort of children and adolescents with recurrent headache : a retrospective study. *Digestive and Liver Disease, 48*(5), 495-498.

Newberry, R. D., Stenson, W. F., & Lorenz, R. G. (1999). Cyclooxygenase-2 -dependent arachidonic acid metabolites are essential modulators of the intestinal immune response to dietary antigen. *Nature medicine, 5*(8), 900-906.

Nielsen, J. A., Steephen, A., & Lewin, M. (2013). Angiotensin-II inhibitor (olmesartan)-induced collagenous sprue with resolution following discontinuation of drug. *World Journal of Gastroenterology: WJG, 19*(40), 6928.

Nilsen, E. M., Jahnsen, F. L., Lundin, K. E., Johansen, F. E., Fausa, O., Sollid, L. M., ... Brandtzaeg, P. (1998). Gluten induces an intestinal cytokine response strongly dominated by interferon gamma in patients with celiac disease. *Gastroenterology, 115*(3), 551-563.

Nishimura, H., Yajima, T., Naiki, Y., Tsunobuchi, H., Umemura, M., Itano, K., ... Yoshikai, Y. (2000). Differential roles of interleukin 15 mRNA isoforms generated by alternative splicing in immune responses *in vivo*. *The Journal of experimental medicine, 191*(1), 157-170.

Noorlaila, A., Hasanah, H. N., Asmeda, R., & Yusoff, A. (2020). The effects of xanthan gum and hydroxypropylmethylcellulose on physical properties of sponge cakes. *Journal of the Saudi Society of Agricultural Sciences, 19*(2), 128-135.

Norris, J. M., Barriga, K., Hoffenberg, E. J., Taki, I., Miao, D., Haas, J. E., ... Eisenbarth, G. S. (2005). Risk of celiac disease autoimmunity and timing of gluten introduction in the diet of infants at increased risk of disease. *Jama, 293*(19), 2343-2351.

Nunes, C., Freitas, V., Almeida, L., & Laranjinha, J. (2019). Red wine extract preserves tight junctions in intestinal epithelial cells under inflammatory conditions: Implications for intestinal inflammation. *Food & function, 10*(3), 1364-1374.

Núñez, C., & Fernández-Bañares, F. (2021). Some considerations about γδ and CD8+ T-cell responses in blood after gluten challenge in treated celiac disease. *Mucosal immunology, 14*(5), 1214-1215.

Nwaru, B., Hickstein, L., Panesar, S., Roberts, G., Muraro, A., Sheikh, A., ... Group, A. G. (2014). Prevalence of common food allergies in Europe: a systematic review and meta-analysis. *Allergy, 69*(8), 992-1007.

Nwokocha, L. M., & Williams, P. A. (2012). Evaluating the potential of Nigerian plants as a source of industrial hydrocolloids. *Gums and stabilizers for the food industry, 16*, 27-44.

Odenwald, M. A., & Turner, J. R. (2017). The intestinal epithelial barrier: a therapeutic target? *Nature reviews Gastroenterology & hepatology, 14*(1), 9-21.

Ohimain, E. I. (2014). The prospects and challenges of cassava inclusion in wheat bread policy in Nigeria. *International Journal of Science, Technology and Society, 2*(1), 6-17.

Olivares, M., Benítez-Páez, A., de Palma, G., Capilla, A., Nova, E., Castillejo, G., ... Polanco, I. (2018). Increased prevalence of pathogenic bacteria in the gut microbiota of infants at risk of developing celiac disease: The PROFICEL study. *Gut Microbes, 9*(6), 551-558.

Olivares, M., Laparra, M., & Sanz, Y. (2012). Oral administration of Bifidobacterium longum CECT 7347 modulates jejunal proteome in an *in vivo* gliadin-induced enteropathy animal model. *Journal of proteomics, 77*, 310-320.

Olivares, M., Neef, A., Castillejo, G., De Palma, G., Varea, V., Capilla, A., ... Polanco, I. (2015). The HLA-DQ2 genotype selects for early intestinal microbiota composition in infants at high risk of developing coeliac disease. *Gut, 64*(3), 406-417.

Olivera, A., Moore, T. W., Hu, F., Brown, A. P., Sun, A., Liotta, D. C., ... Marcus, A. I. (2012). Inhibition of the NF-κB signaling pathway by the curcumin analog, 3, 5-Bis (2-pyridinylmethylidene)-4-piperidone (EF31): Anti-inflammatory and anti-cancer properties. *International immunopharmacology, 12*(2), 368-377.

Orlando, A., Linsalata, M., Bianco, G., Notarnicola, M., D'Attoma, B., Scavo, M. P., ... Russo, F. (2018). Lactobacillus rhamnosus GG protects the epithelial barrier of wistar rats from the pepsin -trypsin -digested gliadin (PTG)-induced enteropathy. *Nutrients, 10*(11), 1698.

Orlando, A., Linsalata, M., D'Attoma, B., & Russo, F. (2017). Changes in paracellular permeability induced by Pepsin-Trypsin digested Gliadin (PTG): Role of polyamines in the Lactobacillus rhamnosus GG protective action. *Journal of functional foods, 36*, 52-62.

Orlando, A., Linsalata, M., Notarnicola, M., Tutino, V., & Russo, F. (2014). Lactobacillus GG restoration of the gliadin induced epithelial barrier disruption: the role of cellular polyamines. *BMC microbiology, 14*(1), 1-12.

Orwoll, E., Ettinger, M., Weiss, S., Miller, P., Kendler, D., Graham, J., ... Pietschmann, P. (2000). Alendronate for the treatment of osteoporosis in men. *New England Journal of Medicine, 343*(9), 604-610.

Osborne, T. (1907). The Proteins of the Wheat Kernel Washington. *DC: Carnegie Inst.*

Oscarsson, E., Håkansson, Å., Andrén Aronsson, C., Molin, G., & Agardh, D. (2021). Effects of probiotic bacteria Lactobacillaceae on the gut microbiota in children with celiac disease autoimmunity: A placebo-controlled and randomized clinical trial. *Frontiers in Nutrition, 8*, 354.

Osman, A., Günnel, T., Dietl, A., Uhlig, H., Amin, M., Fleckenstein, B., ... Mothes, T. (2000). B cell epitopes of gliadin. *Clinical & Experimental Immunology, 121*(2), 248-254.

Osorio, C. E., Mejías, J. H., & Rustgi, S. (2019). Gluten detection methods and their critical role in assuring safe diets for celiac patients. *Nutrients, 11*(12), 2920.

Osorio, C. E., Wen, N., Mejías, J. H., Mitchell, S., Von Wettstein, D., & Rustgi, S. (2020). Directed-Mutagenesis of Flavobacterium meningosepticum prolyl-oligopeptidase and a glutamine-specific endopeptidase from barley. *Frontiers in Nutrition, 7*, 11.

Osterhoff, G., Morgan, E. F., Shefelbine, S. J., Karim, L., McNamara, L. M., & Augat, P. (2016). Bone mechanical properties and changes with osteoporosis. *Injury, 47*, S11-S20.

Ostermann-Porcel, M. V., Quiroga-Panelo, N., Rinaldoni, A. N., & Campderrós, M. E. (2017). Incorporation of okara into gluten -free cookies with high quality and nutritional value. *Journal of Food Quality, 2017*(1), 4071585.

Ozma, M. A., Abbasi, A., & Sabahi, S. (2022). Characterization of Postbiotics Derived from Lactobacillus paracasei ATCC 55544 and its Application in Malva sylvestris Seed Mucilage Edible Coating to the Improvement of the Microbiological, and Sensory Properties of Lamb Meat During Storage. *Biointerface Res Appl Chem., 13*(3).

Ozma, M. A., Abbasi, A., Ahangarzadeh Rezaee, M., Hosseini, H., Hosseinzadeh, N., Sabahi, S., ... Lahouty, M. (2022). A critical review on the nutritional and medicinal profiles of garlic's (Allium sativum L.) Bioactive Compounds. *Food Reviews International*, 1-38.

Pabst, O., & Mowat, A. (2012). Oral tolerance to food protein. *Mucosal immunology, 5*(3), 232-239.

Palová-Jelínková, L., Dáňová, K., Drašarová, H., Dvořák, M., Funda, D. P., Fundová, P., ... Martin, S. F. (2013). Pepsin digest of wheat gliadin fraction increases production of IL-1β via TLR4/MyD88/TRIF/MAPK/NF-κB signaling pathway and an NLRP3 inflammasome activation. *PloS one, 8*(4), e62426.

Parenti, O., Guerrini, L., & Zanoni, B. (2020). Techniques and technologies for the breadmaking process with unrefined wheat flours. *Trends in Food Science & Technology, 99*, 152-166.

Parisi, P., Pietropaoli, N., Ferretti, A., Nenna, R., Mastrogiorgio, G., Del Pozzo, M., ... Villa, M. (2015). Role of the gluten -free diet on neurological-EEG findings and sleep disordered breathing in children with celiac disease. *Seizure, 25*, 181-183.

Park, H. Y., Kunitake, Y., Hirasaki, N., Tanaka, M., & Matsui, T. (2015). Theaflavins enhance intestinal barrier of Caco-2 Cell monolayers through the expression of AMP-activated protein kinase-mediated Occludin, Claudin-1, and ZO-1. *Bioscience, biotechnology, and biochemistry, 79*(1), 130-137.

Park, K., Tsai, R., Wang, L., Khavari, N., Bachrach, L., & Bass, D. (2013). Cost-effectiveness of universal serologic screening to prevent nontraumatic hip and vertebral fractures in patients with celiac disease. *Clinical gastroenterology and hepatology, 11*(6), 645-653.

Passananti, V., Santonicola, A., Bucci, C., Andreozzi, P., Ranaudo, A., Di Giacomo, D. V., & Ciacci, C. (2012). Bone mass in women with celiac disease: role of exercise and gluten -free diet. *Digestive and Liver Disease, 44*(5), 379-383.

Paterson, B., Lammers, K., Arrieta, M., Fasano, A., & Meddings, J. (2007). The safety, tolerance, pharmacokinetic and pharmacodynamic effects of single doses of AT-1001 in coeliac disease subjects: a proof of concept study. *Alimentary pharmacology & therapeutics, 26*(5), 757-766.

Patterson, E. R., Shmidt, E., Oxentenko, A. S., Enders, F. T., & Smyrk, T. C. (2015). Normal villous architecture with increased intraepithelial lymphocytes : a duodenal manifestation of Crohn disease. *American journal of clinical pathology, 143*(3), 445-450.

Paulley, J. (1954). Observations on the aetiology of idiopathic steatorrhoea. *British medical journal, 2*(4900), 1318.

Pellecchia, M. T., Scala, R., Filla, A., De Michele, G., Ciacci, C., & Barone, P. (1999). Idiopathic cerebellar ataxia associated with celiac disease: lack of distinctive neurological features. *Journal of Neurology, Neurosurgery & Psychiatry, 66*(1), 32-35.

Pennisi, M., Bramanti, A., Cantone, M., Pennisi, G., Bella, R., & Lanza, G. (2017). Neurophysiology of the "celiac brain": Disentangling gut-brain connections. *Frontiers in neuroscience, 11*, 498.

Perera, D. R., Weinstein, W. M., & Rubin, C. E. (1975). Small intestinal biopsy. *Human pathology, 6*(2), 157-217.

Perot, M., Lupi, R., Guyot, S., Delayre-Orthez, C., Gadonna-Widehem, P., Thébaudin, J. Y., ... Larre, C. (2017). Polyphenol interactions mitigate the immunogenicity and allergenicity of gliadins. *Journal of agricultural and food chemistry, 65*(31), 6442-6451.

Pessanha, K. L. F., de Menezes, J. P., dos Anjos Silva, A., da Silva Ferreira, M. V., Takeiti, C. Y., & Carvalho, C. W. P. (2021). Impact of whole millet extruded flour on the physicochemical properties and antihyperglycemic activity of gluten free bread. *LWT, 147*, 111495.

Petersen, J., Ciacchi, L., Tran, M. T., Loh, K. L., Kooy-Winkelaar, Y., Croft, N. P., ... Anderson, R. P. (2020). T cell receptor cross-reactivity between gliadin and bacterial peptides in celiac disease. *Nature Structural & Molecular Biology, 27*(1), 49-61.

Petersen, J., Kooy-Winkelaar, Y., Loh, K. L., Tran, M., Van Bergen, J., Koning, F., ... Reid, H. H. (2016). Diverse T cell receptor gene usage in HLA-DQ8 -associated celiac disease converges into a consensus binding solution. *Structure, 24*(10), 1643-1657.

Petersen, J., Montserrat, V., Mujico, J. R., Loh, K. L., Beringer, D. X., Van Lummel, M., ... Kooy-Winkelaar, Y. (2014). T-cell receptor recognition of HLA-DQ2 –gliadin complexes associated with celiac disease. *Nature Structural & Molecular Biology, 21*(5), 480-488.

Petersen, J., van Bergen, J., Loh, K. L., Kooy-Winkelaar, Y., Beringer, D. X., Thompson, A., ... McLaren, J. E. (2015). Determinants of gliadin-specific T cell selection in celiac disease. *The Journal of Immunology, 194*(12), 6112-6122.

Piga, A., Conte, P., Fois, S., Catzeddu, P., Del Caro, A., Sanguinetti, A. M., & Fadda, C. (2021). Technological, nutritional and sensory properties of an innovative gluten -free double-layered flat bread enriched with amaranth flour. *Foods, 10*(5), 920.

Pillon, R., Ziberna, F., Badina, L., Ventura, A., Longo, G., Quaglia, S., ... Patano, G. (2015). Prevalence of celiac disease in patients with severe food allergy. *Allergy, 70*(10), 1346-1349.

Pinier, M., Fuhrmann, G., Galipeau, H. J., Rivard, N., Murray, J. A., David, C. S., ... Verdu, E. F. (2012). The copolymer P (HEMA-co-SS) binds gluten and reduces immune response in gluten-sensitized mice and human tissues. *Gastroenterology, 142*(2), 316-325. e312.

Pinier, M., Verdu, E. F., Nasser–Eddine, M., David, C. S., Vézina, A., Rivard, N., & Leroux, J. C. (2009). Polymeric binders suppress gliadin-induced toxicity in the intestinal epithelium. *Gastroenterology, 136*(1), 288-298.

Pinto, D., Montani, E., Bolli, M., Garavaglia, G., Sallusto, F., Lanzavecchia, A., & Jarrossay, D. (2013). A functional BCR in human IgA and IgM plasma cells. *Blood, The Journal of the American Society of Hematology, 121*(20), 4110-4114.

Piper, J. L., Gray, G. M., & Khosla, C. (2004). Effect of prolyl endopeptidase on digestive-resistant gliadin peptides *in vivo. Journal of Pharmacology and Experimental Therapeutics, 311*(1), 213-219.

Plant, G. T., James-Galton, M., & Wilkinson, D. (2015). Progressive cortical visual failure associated with occipital calcification and coeliac disease with relative preservation of the dorsal 'action'pathway. *cortex, 71*, 160-170.

Plotkin, G. R., & Isselbacher, K. J. (1964). Secondary disaccharidase deficiency in adult celiac disease (nontropical sprue) and other malabsorption states. *New England Journal of Medicine, 271*(20), 1033-1037.

Polgar, L. (2002). The prolyl oligopeptidase family. *Cellular and Molecular Life Sciences CMLS, 59*(2), 349-362.

Polizzi, A., Finocchiaro, M., Parano, E., Pavone, P., & Musumeci, S. (2000). Recurrent peripheral neuropathy in a girl with celiac disease. *Journal of Neurology, Neurosurgery & Psychiatry, 68*(1), 104-105.

Potter, M. D., Walker, M. M., Jones, M. P., Koloski, N. A., Keely, S., & Talley, N. J. (2018). Wheat intolerance and chronic gastrointestinal symptoms in an Australian population-based study: association between wheat sensitivity, celiac disease and functional gastrointestinal disorders. *Official journal of the American College of Gastroenterology| ACG, 113*(7), 1036-1044.

Powrie, F., Leach, M. W., Mauze, S., Menon, S., Caddle, L. B., & Coffman, R. L. (1994). Inhibition of Thl responses prevents inflammatory bowel disease in scid mice reconstituted with CD45RBhi CD4+ T cells. *Immunity, 1*(7), 553-562.

Prandi, B., Tedeschi, T., Folloni, S., Galaverna, G., & Sforza, S. (2017). Peptides from gluten digestion: A comparison between old and modern wheat varieties. *Food Research International, 91*, 92-102.

Pratesi, R., Gandolfi, L., Martins, R. C., Tauil, P. L., Nobrega, Y. K., & Teixeira, W. A. (2003). Is the prevalence of celiac disease increased among epileptic patients? *Arquivos de neuro-psiquiatria, 61*, 330-334.

Pratesi, R., Modelli, I., Martins, R., Almeida, P., & Gandolfi, L. (2003). Celiac disease and epilepsy: favorable outcome in a child with difficult to control seizures. *Acta neurologica scandinavica, 108*(4), 290-293.

Pronin, D., Börner, A., & Scherf, K. A. (2021). Old and modern wheat (Triticum aestivum L.) cultivars and their potential to elicit celiac disease. *Food Chemistry, 339*, 127952.

Pultz, I. S., Hill, M., Vitanza, J. M., Wolf, C., Saaby, L., Liu, T., ... Leffler, D. A. (2021). Gluten degradation, pharmacokinetics, safety, and tolerability of TAK-062, an engineered enzyme to treat celiac disease. *Gastroenterology, 161*(1), 81-93. e83.

Pyle, G. G., Paaso, B., Anderson, B. E., Allen, D. D., Marti, T., Li, Q., ... Gray, G. M. (2005). Effect of pretreatment of food gluten with prolyl endopeptidase on gluten-induced malabsorption in celiac sprue. *Clinical gastroenterology and hepatology, 3*(7), 687-694.

Qiao, S. W., & Sollid, L. M. (2019). Two novel HLA-DQ2. 5-restricted gluten T cell epitopes in the DQ2. 5-glia-γ4 epitope family. *Immunogenetics, 71*(10), 665-667.

Qiao, S. W., Bergseng, E., Molberg, Ø., Jung, G., Fleckenstein, B., & Sollid, L. M. (2005). Refining the rules of gliadin T cell epitope binding to the disease-associated DQ2 molecule in celiac disease: importance of proline spacing and glutamine deamidation. *The Journal of Immunology, 175*(1), 254-261.

Qiao, S. W., Christophersen, A., Lundin, K. E., & Sollid, L. M. (2014). Biased usage and preferred pairing of α-and β-chains of TCRs specific for an immunodominant gluten epitope in coeliac disease. *International immunology, 26*(1), 13-19.

Qiao, S. W., Piper, J., Haraldsen, G., Øynebråten, I., Fleckenstein, B., Molberg, Ø., ... Sollid, L. M. (2005). Tissue transglutaminase-mediated formation and cleavage of histamine-gliadin complexes: biological effects and implications for celiac disease. *The Journal of Immunology, 174*(3), 1657-1663.

Qiao, S. W., Ráki, M., Gunnarsen, K. S., Løset, G. Å., Lundin, K. E., Sandlie, I., & Sollid, L. M. (2011). Posttranslational modification of gluten shapes TCR usage in celiac disease. *The Journal of Immunology, 187*(6), 3064-3071.

Qin, S., & Hou, D. X. (2016). Multiple regulations of Keap1/Nrf2 system by dietary phytochemicals. *Molecular nutrition & food research, 60*(8), 1731-1755.

Quarsten, H., McAdam, S. N., Jensen, T., Arentz-Hansen, H., Molberg, Ø., Lundin, K. E., & Sollid, L. M. (2001). Staining of celiac disease-relevant T cells by peptide-DQ2 multimers. *The Journal of Immunology, 167*(9), 4861-4868.

Quirce, S., Boyano-Martínez, T., & Díaz-Perales, A. (2016). Clinical presentation, allergens, and management of wheat allergy. *Expert Review of Clinical Immunology, 12*(5), 563-572.

Rachlin, H. (2012). Making IBM's computer, Watson, human. *The Behavior Analyst, 35*(1), 1-16.

Rai, S., Kaur, A., & Chopra, C. (2018). Gluten-free products for celiac susceptible people. *Frontiers in nutrition, 5*, 116.

Raj, S. (2020). Influences of the nutrition transition on chronic disease. *Integrative and Functional Medical Nutrition Therapy: Principles and Practices*, 17-29.

Rajpoot, P., & Makharia, G. K. (2013). Problems and challenges to adaptation of gluten free diet by Indian patients with celiac disease. *Nutrients, 5*(12), 4869-4879.

Ráki, M., Fallang, L. E., Brottveit, M., Bergseng, E., Quarsten, H., Lundin, K. E., & Sollid, L. M. (2007). Tetramer visualization of gut-homing gluten -specific T cells in the peripheral blood of celiac disease patients. *Proceedings of the National Academy of Sciences, 104*(8), 2831-2836.

Ramakrishna, B., Makharia, G. K., Chetri, K., Dutta, S., Mathur, P., Ahuja, V., ... Daniel, D. (2016). Prevalence of adult celiac disease in India: regional variations and associations. *Official journal of the American College of Gastroenterology| ACG, 111*(1), 115-123.

Rani, U., Imdad, A., & Beg, M. (2015). Rare neurological manifestation of celiac disease. *Case reports in gastroenterology, 9*(2), 200-205.

Rashmi, B. S., Gayathri, D., Vasudha, M., Prashantkumar, C. S., Swamy, C. T., Sunil, K. S., ... Prakash, P. (2020). Gluten hydrolyzing activity of Bacillus spp isolated from sourdough. *Microbial cell factories, 19*(1), 1-11.

Rea, D., & Fülöp, V. (2006). Structure-function properties of prolyl oligopeptidase family enzymes. *Cell biochemistry and biophysics, 44*(3), 349-365.

Remely, M., Lovrecic, L., De La Garza, A., Migliore, L., Peterlin, B., Milagro, F., ... Haslberger, A. (2015). Therapeutic perspectives of epigenetically active nutrients. *British journal of pharmacology, 172*(11), 2756-2768.

Renard, B. Y., Löwer, M., Kühne, Y., Reimer, U., Rothermel, A., Türeci, Ö., ... Sahin, U. (2011). rapmad: Robust analysis of peptide microarray data. *BMC bioinformatics, 12*, 1-10.

Ress, K., Annus, T., Putnik, U., Luts, K., Uibo, R., & Uibo, O. (2014). Celiac disease in children with atopic dermatitis. *Pediatric dermatology, 31*(4), 483-488.

Rey, M., Yang, M., Lee, L., Zhang, Y., Sheff, J. G., Sensen, C. W., ... McCarville, J. L. (2016). Addressing proteolytic efficiency in enzymatic degradation therapy for celiac disease. *Scientific reports, 6*(1), 1-13.

Rhein-Knudsen, N., & Meyer, A. S. (2021). Chemistry, gelation, and enzymatic modification of seaweed food hydrocolloids. *Trends in Food Science & Technology, 109*, 608-621.

Ribeiro, M., Nunes, F. M., Guedes, S., Domingues, P., Silva, A. M., Carrillo, J. M., ... Igrejas, G. (2015). Efficient chemo-enzymatic gluten detoxification: reducing toxic epitopes for celiac patients improving functional properties. *Scientific reports, 5*(1), 1-17.

Ribeiro, M., Rodriguez-Quijano, M., Nunes, F. M., Carrillo, J. M., Branlard, G., & Igrejas, G. (2016). New insights into wheat toxicity: Breeding did not seem to contribute to a prevalence of potential celiac disease's immunostimulatory epitopes. *Food Chemistry, 213*, 8-18.

Riddle, M. S., Murray, J. A., & Porter, C. K. (2012). The incidence and risk of celiac disease in a healthy US adult population. *Official journal of the American College of Gastroenterology| ACG, 107*(8), 1248-1255.

Riddle, M. S., Murray, J. A., Cash, B. D., Pimentel, M., & Porter, C. K. (2013a). Pathogen-specific risk of celiac disease following bacterial causes of foodborne illness: a retrospective cohort study. *Digestive diseases and sciences, 58*, 3242-3245.

Riddle, M. S., Murray, J. A., Cash, B. D., Pimentel, M., & Porter, C. K. (2013b). Pathogen-specific risk of celiac disease following bacterial causes of foodborne illness: a retrospective cohort study. *Digestive diseases and sciences, 58*(11), 3242-3245.

Risnes, L. F., Christophersen, A., Dahal-Koirala, S., Neumann, R. S., Sandve, G. K., Sarna, V. K., ... Sollid, L. M. (2018). Disease-driving CD4+ T cell clonotypes persist for decades in celiac disease. *The Journal of clinical investigation, 128*(6), 2642-2650.

Risnes, L. F., Eggesbø, L. M., Christophersen, A., & Sollid, L. M. (2021). Response to:"Some considerations about γδ and CD8+ T-cell responses in blood after gluten challenge in treated celiac disease." *Mucosal immunology, 14*(5), 1216-1217.

Risnes, L. F., Eggesbø, L. M., Zühlke, S., Dahal-Koirala, S., Neumann, R. S., Lundin, K. E., ... Sollid, L. M. (2021). Circulating CD103+ γδ and CD8+ T cells are clonally shared with tissue-resident intraepithelial lymphocytes in celiac disease. *Mucosal immunology, 14*(4), 842-851.

Rizzetto, S., Koppstein, D. N., Samir, J., Singh, M., Reed, J. H., Cai, C. H., ... Luciani, F. (2018). B-cell receptor reconstruction from single-cell RNA-seq with VDJPuzzle. *Bioinformatics, 34*(16), 2846-2847.

Rodríguez-Daza, M. C., Daoust, L., Boutkrabt, L., Pilon, G., Varin, T., Dudonné, S., ... Desjardins, Y. (2020). Wild reberry proanthocyanidins shape distinct gut microbiota profile and influence glucose homeostasis and intestinal phenotypes in high-fat high-sucrose fed mice. *Scientific reports, 10*(1), 2217.

Romanos, J., Rosén, A., Kumar, V., Trynka, G., Franke, L., Szperl, A., ... Jankipersadsing, S. A. (2014). Improving coeliac disease risk prediction by testing non-HLA variants additional to HLA variants. *Gut, 63*(3), 415-422.

Ronie, M. E., Mamat, H., Abdul Aziz, A. H., & Zainol, M. K. (2023). Proximate compositions, texture, and sensory profiles of gluten -free Bario Rice bread supplemented with potato starch. *Foods, 12*(6), 1172.

Rosell, C. M., Barro, F., Sousa, C., & Mena, M. C. (2014). Cereals for developing gluten - free products and analytical tools for gluten detection. *Journal of cereal science, 59*(3), 354-364.

Rosell, C. M., Collar, C., & Haros, M. (2007). Assessment of hydrocolloid effects on the thermo-mechanical properties of wheat using the Mixolab. *Food Hydrocolloids, 21*(3), 452-462.

Rosell, C. M., Rojas, J. A., & De Barber, C. B. (2001). Influence of hydrocolloids on dough rheology and bread quality. *Food Hydrocolloids, 15*(1), 75-81.

Roshan, B., Leffler, D. A., Jamma, S., Dennis, M., Sheth, S., Falchuk, K., ... Schuppan, D. (2011). The incidence and clinical spectrum of refractory celiac disease in a north american referral center. *Official journal of the American College of Gastroenterology| ACG, 106*(5), 923-928.

Rostami, K., Marsh, M. N., Johnson, M. W., Mohaghegh, H., Heal, C., Holmes, G., ... Bassotti, G. (2017). ROC-king onwards: intraepithelial lymphocyte counts, distribution & role in coeliac disease mucosal interpretation. *Gut, 66*(12), 2080-2086.

Rotsch, A. (1954). Chemische und technische Untersuchungen an künstlichen Teigen. *Brot Gebaeck, 8*, 129.

Roy, B., Neumann, R. S., Snir, O., Iversen, R., Sandve, G. K., Lundin, K. E., & Sollid, L. M. (2017). High-throughput single-cell analysis of B cell receptor usage among autoantigen-specific plasma cells in celiac disease. *The Journal of Immunology, 199*(2), 782-791.

Rubio-Tapia, A., & Murray, J. A. (2010). Classification and management of refractory coeliac disease. *Gut, 59*(4), 547-557.

Rubio-Tapia, A., Herman, M. L., Ludvigsson, J. F., Kelly, D. G., Mangan, T. F., Wu, T. T., & Murray, J. A. (2012). *Severe spruelike enteropathy associated with olmesartan.* Paper presented at the Mayo clinic proceedings.

Rubio-Tapia, A., Hill, I. D., Kelly, C. P., Calderwood, A. H., & Murray, J. A. (2013). ACG clinical guidelines: diagnosis and management of celiac disease. *Official journal of the American College of Gastroenterology| ACG, 108*(5), 656-676.

Rubio–Tapia, A., Kyle, R. A., Kaplan, E. L., Johnson, D. R., Page, W., Erdtmann, F., ... Lahr, B. D. (2009). Increased prevalence and mortality in undiagnosed celiac disease. *Gastroenterology, 137*(1), 88-93.

Rubio-Tapia, A., Malamut, G., Verbeek, W. H., van Wanrooij, R. L., Leffler, D. A., Niveloni, S. I., ... Murray, J. A. (2016). Creation of a model to predict survival in patients with refractory coeliac disease using a multinational registry. *Alimentary pharmacology & therapeutics, 44*(7), 704-714.

Rubio-Tapia, A., Rahim, M. W., See, J. A., Lahr, B. D., Wu, T. T., & Murray, J. A. (2010). Mucosal recovery and mortality in adults with celiac disease after treatment with a gluten -free diet. *Official journal of the American College of Gastroenterology| ACG, 105*(6), 1412-1420.

Ruggieri, M., Incorpora, G., Polizzi, A., Parano, E., Spina, M., & Pavone, P. (2008). Low prevalence of neurologic and psychiatric manifestations in children with gluten sensitivity. *The Journal of pediatrics, 152*(2), 244-249. e241.

Russo, P. A., Brochu, P., Seidman, E. G., & Roy, C. C. (1999). Autoimmune enteropathy. *Pediatric and Developmental Pathology, 2*(1), 65-71.

Saag, K. G., Shane, E., Boonen, S., Marín, F., Donley, D. W., Taylor, K. A., ... Marcus, R. (2007). Teriparatide or alendronate in glucocorticoid-induced osteoporosis. *New England Journal of Medicine, 357*(20), 2028-2039.

Sabahi, S., Abbasi, A., & Mortazavi, S. A. (2022). Characterization of cinnamon essential oil and its application in Malva sylvestris seed mucilage edible coating to the enhancement of the microbiological, physicochemical and sensory properties of lamb meat during storage. *Journal of Applied Microbiology*.

Sabahi, S., Homayouni Rad, A., Aghebati-Maleki, L., Sangtarash, N., Ozma, M. A., Karimi, A., ... Abbasi, A. (2022). Postbiotics as the new frontier in food and pharmaceutical research. *Critical reviews in food science and nutrition,* 1-28.

Sabatino, D., Bertrandi, Maldini, C., Pennese, Proietti, & Corazza. (1998). Phenotyping of peripheral blood lymphocytes in adult coeliac disease. *Immunology, 95*(4), 572-576.

Sadegh Nia, N., Azizi, M. H., Seyedin Ardebili, M., & Mohammadi, M. (2016). Effect of xanthan and CMC on rheological properties of Gluten-free bread dough. *Journal of food science and technology (Iran), 13*(51), 137-148.

Saha, D., & Bhattacharya, S. (2010). Hydrocolloids as thickening and gelling agents in food: a critical review. *Journal of food science and technology, 47*, 587-597.

Salden, B., Monserrat, V., Troost, F., Bruins, M., Edens, L., Bartholomé, R., ... Masclee, A. (2015). Randomised clinical study: Aspergillus niger-derived enzyme digests gluten in the stomach of healthy volunteers. *Alimentary pharmacology & therapeutics, 42*(3), 273-285.

Salehi, F. (2019). Improvement of gluten -free bread and cake properties using natural hydrocolloids: A review. *Food science & nutrition, 7*(11), 3391-3402.

Samaroo, D., Dickerson, F., Kasarda, D. D., Green, P. H., Briani, C., Yolken, R. H., & Alaedini, A. (2010). Novel immune response to gluten in individuals with schizophrenia. *Schizophrenia research, 118*(1-3), 248-255.

Sammaritano, M. (1985). The syndrome of epilepsy and bilateral occipital cortical calcifications. *Epilepsia, 26*, 530.

Sánchez, E., Donat, E., Ribes-Koninckx, C., Fernández-Murga, M. L., & Sanz, Y. (2013). Duodenal-mucosal bacteria associated with celiac disease in children. *Applied and environmental microbiology, 79*(18), 5472-5479.

Sanchez, H., Osella, C., & De La Torre, M. (2002). Optimization of gluten -free bread prepared from cornstarch, rice flour, and cassava starch. *Journal of Food Science, 67*(1), 416-419.

Sánchez-León, S., Gil-Humanes, J., Ozuna, C. V., Giménez, M. J., Sousa, C., Voytas, D. F., & Barro, F. (2018). Low-gluten, nontransgenic wheat engineered with CRISPR/Cas9. *Plant biotechnology journal, 16*(4), 902-910.

Sanchez-Muñoz, L. B., Santón, A., Cano, A., Lopez, A., Almeida, J., Orfao, A., ... Roy, G. (2008). Flow cytometric analysis of intestinal intraepithelial lymphocytes in the diagnosis of refractory celiac sprue. *European journal of gastroenterology & hepatology, 20*(5), 478-487.

Sander, G. R., Cummins, A. G., & Powell, B. C. (2005). Rapid disruption of intestinal barrier function by gliadin involves altered expression of apical junctional proteins. *FEBS letters, 579*(21), 4851-4855.

Sanders, D. S., Patel, D., Khan, F. B., Westbrook, R. H., Webber, C. V., Milford-Ward, A., & McCloskey, E. V. (2005). Case-finding for adult celiac disease in patients with reduced bone mineral density. *Digestive diseases and sciences, 50*, 587-592.

Santaguida, M. G., Gatto, I., Mangino, G., Virili, C., Stramazzo, I., Fallahi, P., ... Centanni, M. (2018). Breg cells in celiac disease isolated or associated to Hashimoto's thyroiditis. *International journal of endocrinology, 2018*(1), 5290865.

Santos, F. G., Aguiar, E. V., Centeno, A. C. L., Rosell, C. M., & Capriles, V. D. (2020). Effect of added psyllium and food enzymes on quality attributes and shelf life of chickpea-based gluten -free bread. *LWT, 134*, 110025.

Santos, F. G., Aguiar, E. V., Rosell, C. M., & Capriles, V. D. (2021). Potential of chickpea and psyllium in gluten -free breadmaking: Assessing bread's quality, sensory acceptability, and glycemic and satiety indexes. *Food Hydrocolloids, 113*, 106487.

Sarang, Z., Tóth, B., Balajthy, Z., Köröskényi, K., Garabuczi, E., Fésüs, L., & Szondy, Z. (2009). Some lessons from the tissue transglutaminase knockout mouse. *Amino acids, 36*, 625-631.

Sarna, V. K., Lundin, K. E., Mørkrid, L., Qiao, S. W., Sollid, L. M., & Christophersen, A. (2018). HLA-DQ–gluten tetramer blood test accurately identifies patients with and without celiac disease in absence of gluten consumption. *Gastroenterology, 154*(4), 886-896. e886.

Sarna, V. K., Skodje, G. I., Reims, H. M., Risnes, L. F., Dahal-Koirala, S., Sollid, L. M., & Lundin, K. E. (2018). HLA-DQ: gluten tetramer test in blood gives better detection of coeliac patients than biopsy after 14-day gluten challenge. *Gut, 67*(9), 1606-1613.

Sarno, M., Lania, G., Cuomo, M., Nigro, F., Passannanti, F., Budelli, A., ... Barone, M. V. (2014). Lactobacillus paracasei CBA L74 interferes with gliadin peptides entrance in Caco-2 cells. *International Journal of food sciences and nutrition, 65*(8), 953-959.

Sarra, M., Cupi, M., Monteleone, I., Franzè, E., Ronchetti, G., Di Sabatino, A., ... Sica, G. (2013). IL-15 positively regulates IL-21 production in celiac disease mucosa. *Mucosal immunology, 6*(2), 244-255.

Sarteshnizi, R. A., Hosseini, H., Bondarianzadeh, D., & Colmenero, F. J. (2015). Optimization of prebiotic sausage formulation: Effect of using β-glucan and resistant starch by D-optimal mixture design approach. *LWT-Food Science and Technology, 62*(1), 704-710.

Sarteshnizi, R. A., Hosseini, H., Khosroshahi, N. K., Shahraz, F., Khaneghah, A. M., Kamran, M., ... Chiavaro, E. (2017). Effect of resistant starch and β-glucan combination on oxidative stability, frying performance, microbial count and shelf life of prebiotic sausage during refrigerated storage. *Food Technology and Biotechnology, 55*(4), 475.

Sartor, R. B., & Wu, G. D. (2017). Roles for intestinal bacteria, viruses, and fungi in pathogenesis of inflammatory bowel diseases and therapeutic approaches. *Gastroenterology, 152*(2), 327-339. e324.

Saturni, L., Ferretti, G., & Bacchetti, T. (2010). The gluten -free diet : safety and nutritional quality. *Nutrients, 2*(1), 16-34.

Savvateeva, L. V., Gorokhovets, N. V., Makarov, V. A., Serebryakova, M. V., Solovyev, A. G., Morozov, S. Y., ... Aliev, G. (2015). Glutenase and collagenase activities of wheat cysteine protease Triticain-α: Feasibility for enzymatic therapy assays. *The international journal of biochemistry & cell biology, 62*, 115-124.

Schalk, K., Lang, C., Wieser, H., Koehler, P., & Scherf, K. A. (2017). Quantitation of the immunodominant 33-mer peptide from α-gliadin in wheat flours by liquid chromatography tandem mass spectrometry. *Scientific Reports, 7*(1), 45092.

Schalk, K., Lexhaller, B., Koehler, P., & Scherf, K. A. (2017). Isolation and characterization of gluten protein types from wheat, rye, barley and oats for use as reference materials. *PloS one, 12*(2), e0172819.

Scherf, K. A., Koehler, P., & Wieser, H. (2016). Gluten and wheat sensitivities–an overview. *Journal of cereal science, 67*, 2-11.

Scherf, K. A., Umseher, L., Kieffer, R., & Koehler, P. (2016). Optimization of a micro-scale extension test for rehydrated vital wheat gluten. *Journal of cereal science, 68*, 140-147.

Scherf, K. A., Wieser, H., & Koehler, P. (2018). Novel approaches for enzymatic gluten degradation to create high-quality gluten-free products. *Food Research International, 110*, 62-72.

Scherf, K., Brockow, K., Biedermann, T., Koehler, P., & Wieser, H. (2016). Wheat-dependent exercise-induced anaphylaxis. *Clinical & Experimental Allergy, 46*(1), 10-20.

Schumann, M., Günzel, D., Buergel, N., Richter, J. F., Troeger, H., May, C., ... Bojarski, C. (2012). Cell polarity-determining proteins Par-3 and PP-1 are involved in epithelial tight junction defects in coeliac disease. *Gut, 61*(2), 220-228.

Scialom, S., Malamut, G., Meresse, B., Guegan, N., Brousse, N., Verkarre, V., ... Savoye, G. (2015). Gastrointestinal disorder associated with olmesartan mimics autoimmune enteropathy. *PloS one, 10*(6), e0125024.

Scott, E. M., Gaywood, I., & Scott, B. B. (2000). Guidelines for osteoporosis in coeliac disease and inflammatory bowel disease. *Gut, 46*(suppl 1), I1-I8.

Seeman, E., & Delmas, P. D. (2006). Bone quality—the material and structural basis of bone strength and fragility. *New England Journal of Medicine, 354*(21), 2250-2261.

Seisun, D., & Zalesny, N. (2021). Strides in food texture and hydrocolloids. *Food Hydrocolloids, 117*, 106575.

Sel, Ç. G., Aksoy, E., Aksoy, A., Yüksel, D., & Özbay, F. (2017). Neurological manifestations of atypical celiac disease in childhood. *Acta Neurologica Belgica, 117*(3), 719-727.

Serra, S., & Jani, P. A. (2006). An approach to duodenal biopsies. *Journal of clinical pathology, 59*(11), 1133-1150.

Serratrice, J., Disdier, P., De Roux, C., Christides, C., & Weiller, P. (1998). Migraine and coeliac disease. *Headache: The Journal of Head and Face Pain, 38*(8), 627-628.

Shahzad, S. A., Hussain, S., Mohamed, A. A., Alamri, M. S., Qasem, A. A. A., Ibraheem, M. A., ... El-Din, M. F. S. (2020). Gluten-free cookies from sorghum and Turkish beans; effect of some non-conventional and commercial hydrocolloids on their technological and sensory attributes. *Food Science and Technology, 41*(1), 15-24.

Shalimar, D., Das, P., Sreenivas, V., Gupta, S. D., Panda, S. K., & Makharia, G. K. (2013). Mechanism of villous atrophy in celiac disease: role of apoptosis and epithelial regeneration. *Archives of Pathology and Laboratory Medicine, 137*(9), 1262-1269.

Shams, P., Waldman, A., Dogan, A., MacKenzie, J., & Plant, G. (2002). Ataxia in the setting of complicated enteropathy: double jeopardy. *Journal of Neurology, Neurosurgery & Psychiatry, 72*(4), 527-529.

Shan, L., Marti, T., Sollid, L. M., Gray, G. M., & Khosla, C. (2004). Comparative biochemical analysis of three bacterial prolyl endopeptidases: implications for coeliac sprue. *Biochemical journal, 383*(2), 311-318.

Shewry, P. R. (2018). Do ancient types of wheat have health benefits compared with modern bread wheat? *Journal of cereal science, 79*, 469-476.

Shewry, P. R., & Tatham, A. S. (1990). The prolamin storage proteins of cereal seeds: structure and evolution. *Biochemical journal, 267*(1), 1.

Shewry, P. R., Pellny, T. K., & Lovegrove, A. (2016). Is modern wheat bad for health? *Nature plants, 2*(7), 1-3.

Shewry, P., & Hey, S. (2016). Do we need to worry about eating wheat? *Nutrition bulletin, 41*(1), 6-13.

Shmidt, E., Smyrk, T. C., Boswell, C. L., Enders, F. T., & Oxentenko, A. S. (2014). Increasing duodenal intraepithelial lymphocytosis found at upper endoscopy: time trends and associations. *Gastrointestinal endoscopy, 80*(1), 105-111.

Shrilakshmi, B. (2012). Recommended dietary allowances. *Nutrition Science, New Age International Publishers, New Delhi*, 11-20.

Siegel, M., & Khosla, C. (2007). Transglutaminase 2 inhibitors and their therapeutic role in disease states. *Pharmacology & therapeutics, 115*(2), 232-245.

Siegel, M., Bethune, M. T., Gass, J., Ehren, J., Xia, J., Johannsen, A., ... Khosla, C. (2006). Rational design of combination enzyme therapy for celiac sprue. *Chemistry & biology, 13*(6), 649-658.

Siegel, M., Strnad, P., Watts, R. E., Choi, K., Jabri, B., Omary, M. B., & Khosla, C. (2008). Extracellular transglutaminase 2 is catalytically inactive, but is transiently activated upon tissue injury. *PloS one, 3*(3), e1861.

Silva, R. F., & Pogačnik, L. (2020). Polyphenols from food and natural products: Neuroprotection and safety. *Antioxidants, 9*(1), 61.

Silvester, J. A., Kurada, S., Szwajcer, A., Kelly, C. P., Leffler, D. A., & Duerksen, D. R. (2017). Tests for serum transglutaminase and endomysial antibodies do not detect most patients with celiac disease and persistent villous atrophy on gluten -free diets: a meta-analysis. *Gastroenterology, 153*(3), 689-701. e681.

Sima, H., Hekmatdoost, A., Ghaziani, T., Alavian, S. M., Mashayekh, A., & Zali, M. (2010). The prevalence of celiac autoantibodies in hepatitis patients. *Iranian Journal of Allergy, Asthma and Immunology*, 157-162.

Simonati, A., Battistella, P., Guariso, C., Clementi, M., & Rizzuto, N. (1998). Coeliac disease associated with peripheral neuropathy in a child: a case report. *Neuropediatrics, 29*(03), 155-158.

Simpson, D. J. (2001). Proteolytic degradation of cereal prolamins—the problem with proline. *Plant Science, 161*(5), 825-838.

Singh, J., & Whelan, K. (2011). Limited availability and higher cost of gluten -free foods. *Journal of human Nutrition and Dietetics, 24*(5), 479-486.

Singh, P., Arora, A., Strand, T. A., Leffler, D. A., Catassi, C., Green, P. H., ... Makharia, G. K. (2018). Global prevalence of celiac disease: systematic review and meta-analysis. *Clinical gastroenterology and hepatology, 16*(6), 823-836. e822.

Singh, R., Chandrashekharappa, S., Bodduluri, S. R., Baby, B. V., Hegde, B., Kotla, N. G., ... Vijay-Kumar, M. (2019). Enhancement of the gut barrier integrity by a microbial metabolite through the Nrf2 pathway. *Nature communications, 10*(1), 89.

Sjöström, H., Lundin, K., Molberg, O., Körner, R., McAdam, S., Anthonsen, D., ... Thorsby, E. (1998). Identification of a gliadin T-cell epitope in coeliac disease: general importance of gliadin deamidation for intestinal T-cell recognition. *Scandinavian journal of immunology, 48*, 111-115.

Skendi, A., Papageorgiou, M., & Varzakas, T. (2021). High protein substitutes for gluten in gluten-free bread. *Foods, 10*(9), 1997.

Slim, M., Rico-Villademoros, F., & Calandre, E. P. (2018). Psychiatric comorbidity in children and adults with gluten -related disorders: a narrative review. *Nutrients, 10*(7), 875.

Smedby, K., Åkerman, M., Hildebrand, H., Glimelius, B., Ekbom, A., & Askling, J. (2005). Malignant lymphomas in coeliac disease: evidence of increased risks for lymphoma types other than enteropathy-type T cell lymphoma. *Gut, 54*(1), 54-59.

Smith, D., & Gerdes, L. (2012). Meta-analysis on anxiety and depression in adult celiac disease. *Acta Psychiatrica Scandinavica, 125*(3), 189-193.

Smith, L. B., Lynch, K. F., Kurppa, K., Koletzko, S., Krischer, J., Liu, E., ... Group, T. S. (2017). Psychological manifestations of celiac disease autoimmunity in young children. *Pediatrics, 139*(3).

Snir, O., Chen, X., Gidoni, M., du Pré, M. F., Zhao, Y., Steinsbø, Ø., ... Sollid, L. M. (2017). Stereotyped antibody responses target posttranslationally modified gluten in celiac disease. *JCI insight, 2*(17).

Snir, O., Kanduri, C., Lundin, K. E., Sandve, G. K., & Sollid, L. M. (2019). Transcriptional profiling of human intestinal plasma cells reveals effector functions beyond antibody production. *United European gastroenterology journal, 7*(10), 1399-1407.

Snir, O., Mesin, L., Gidoni, M., Lundin, K. E., Yaari, G., & Sollid, L. M. (2015). Analysis of celiac disease autoreactive gut plasma cells and their corresponding memory compartment in peripheral blood using high-throughput sequencing. *The Journal of Immunology, 194*(12), 5703-5712.

Socha, P., Mickowska, B., Urminská, D., & Kačmárová, K. (2021). The use of different proteases to hydrolyze gliadins. *Journal of Microbiology, Biotechnology and Food Sciences, 2021*, 101-104.

Sollid, L. M. (2002). Coeliac disease: dissecting a complex inflammatory disorder. *Nature Reviews Immunology, 2*(9), 647-655.

Sollid, L. M., & Jabri, B. (2011). Celiac disease and transglutaminase 2: a model for posttranslational modification of antigens and HLA association in the pathogenesis of autoimmune disorders. *Current opinion in immunology, 23*(6), 732-738.

Sollid, L. M., Tye-Din, J. A., Qiao, S. W., Anderson, R. P., Gianfrani, C., & Koning, F. (2020a). Update 2020: nomcnclature and listing of celiac disease–relevant gluten epitopes recognized by CD4+ T cells. *Immunogenetics, 72*(1), 85-88.

Sollid, L. M., Tye-Din, J. A., Qiao, S. W., Anderson, R. P., Gianfrani, C., & Koning, F. (2020b). Update 2020: nomenclature and listing of celiac disease–relevant gluten epitopes recognized by CD4+ T cells. *Immunogenetics, 72*, 85-88.

Sowa, M., Hiemann, R., Schierack, P., Reinhold, D., Conrad, K., & Roggenbuck, D. (2017). Next-Generation Autoantibody Testing by Combination of Screening and Confirmation—the CytoBead® Technology. *Clinical Reviews in Allergy & Immunology, 53*, 87-104.

Sozer, N., Bruins, R., Dietzel, C., Franke, W., & Kokini, J. L. (2011). Improvement of shelf life stability of cakes. *Journal of Food Quality, 34*(3), 151-162.

Spaenij–Dekking, L., Kooy–Winkelaar, Y., van Veelen, P., Drijfhout, J. W., Jonker, H., van Soest, L., ... Koning, F. (2005). Natural variation in toxicity of wheat: potential for selection of nontoxic varieties for celiac disease patients. *Gastroenterology, 129*(3), 797-806.

Stanich, P. P., Yearsley, M., & Meyer, M. M. (2013). Olmesartan-associated sprue -like enteropathy. *Journal of clinical gastroenterology, 47*(10), 894-895.

Steenholt, J. V., Nielsen, C., Baudewijn, L., Staal, A., Rasmussen, K. S., Sabir, H. J., ... Toft-Hansen, H. (2017). The composition of T cell subtypes in duodenal biopsies are altered in coeliac disease patients. *PloS one, 12*(2), e0170270.

Steinsbø, Ø., Dunand, C. J. H., Huang, M., Mesin, L., Salgado-Ferrer, M., Lundin, K. E., ... Sollid, L. M. (2014). Restricted VH/VL usage and limited mutations in gluten -specific IgA of coeliac disease lesion plasma cells. *Nature Communications, 5*(1), 4041.

Stepniak, D., Spaenij-Dekking, L., Mitea, C., Moester, M., de Ru, A., Baak-Pablo, R., ... Koning, F. (2006). Highly efficient gluten degradation with a newly identified prolyl endoprotease: implications for celiac disease. *American Journal of Physiology-Gastrointestinal and Liver Physiology, 291*(4), G621-G629.

Stepniak, D., Vader, L. W., Kooy, Y., van Veelen, P. A., Moustakas, A., Papandreou, N. A., ... Koning, F. (2005). T-cell recognition of HLA-DQ2 -bound gluten peptides can be influenced by an N-terminal proline at p-1. *Immunogenetics, 57*(1), 8-15.

Stepniak, D., Wiesner, M., de Ru, A. H., Moustakas, A. K., Drijfhout, J. W., Papadopoulos, G. K., ... Koning, F. (2008). Large-scale characterization of natural ligands explains the unique gluten -binding properties of HLA-DQ2. *The Journal of Immunology, 180*(5), 3268-3278.

Stern, J. N., Yaari, G., Vander Heiden, J. A., Church, G., Donahue, W. F., Hintzen, R. Q., ... Nylander, A. (2014). B cells populating the multiple sclerosis brain mature in the draining cervical lymph nodes. *Science translational medicine, 6*(248), 248ra107-248ra107.

Stevens, L., & Rashid, M. (2008). Gluten-free and regular foods: a cost comparison. *Canadian journal of dietetic practice and research, 69*(3), 147-150.

Stoeckius, M., Hafemeister, C., Stephenson, W., Houck-Loomis, B., Chattopadhyay, P. K., Swerdlow, H., ... Smibert, P. (2017). Simultaneous epitope and transcriptome measurement in single cells. *Nature methods, 14*(9), 865-868.

Story, M., & Stang, J. (2005). Nutrition needs of adolescents. *Guidelines for adolescent nutrition services, 3*(1), 21-34.

Stubbington, M. J., Lönnberg, T., Proserpio, V., Clare, S., Speak, A. O., Dougan, G., & Teichmann, S. A. (2016). T cell fate and clonality inference from single-cell transcriptomes. *Nature methods, 13*(4), 329-332.

Stubbington, M. J., Rozenblatt-Rosen, O., Regev, A., & Teichmann, S. A. (2017). Single-cell transcriptomics to explore the immune system in health and disease. *Science, 358*(6359), 58-63.

Sturgeon, C., & Fasano, A. (2016). Zonulin, a regulator of epithelial and endothelial barrier functions, and its involvement in chronic inflammatory diseases. *Tissue barriers, 4*(4), e1251384.

Sugai, E., Vázquez, H., Nachman, F., Moreno, M. L., Mazure, R., Smecuol, E., ... Gómez, J. C. (2006). Accuracy of testing for antibodies to synthetic gliadin–related peptides in celiac disease. *Clinical gastroenterology and hepatology, 4*(9), 1112-1117.

Suk, J. S., Xu, Q., Kim, N., Hanes, J., & Ensign, L. M. (2016). PEGylation as a strategy for improving nanoparticle-based drug and gene delivery. *Advanced drug delivery reviews, 99*, 28-51.

Šuligoj, T., Gregorini, A., Colomba, M., Ellis, H. J., & Ciclitira, P. J. (2013). Evaluation of the safety of ancient strains of wheat in coeliac disease reveals heterogeneous small intestinal T cell responses suggestive of coeliac toxicity. *Clinical Nutrition, 32*(6), 1043-1049.

Sulkanen, S., Halttunen, T., Laurila, K., Kolho, K. L., Korponay-Szabó, I. R., Sarnesto, A., ... Mäki, M. (1998). Tissue transglutaminase autoantibody enzyme-linked immunosorbent assay in detecting celiac disease. *Gastroenterology, 115*(6), 1322-1328.

Svensson, V., Natarajan, K. N., Ly, L. H., Miragaia, R. J., Labalette, C., Macaulay, I. C., ... Teichmann, S. A. (2017). Power analysis of single-cell RNA-sequencing experiments. *Nature methods, 14*(4), 381-387.

Syage, J. A., Green, P. H., Khosla, C., Adelman, D. C., Sealey-Voyksner, J. A., & Murray, J. A. (2019). Latiglutenase treatment for celiac disease: symptom and quality of life improvement for seropositive patients on a gluten -free diet. *GastroHep, 1*(6), 293-301.

Syage, J. A., Kelly, C. P., Dickason, M. A., Ramirez, A. C., Leon, F., Dominguez, R., & Sealey-Voyksner, J. A. (2018). Determination of gluten consumption in celiac disease patients on a gluten-free diet. *The American journal of clinical nutrition, 107*(2), 201-207.

Syage, J. A., Murray, J. A., Green, P. H., & Khosla, C. (2017). Latiglutenase improves symptoms in seropositive celiac disease patients while on a gluten -free diet. *Digestive diseases and sciences, 62*(9), 2428-2432.

Syed, S., Al-Boni, M., Khan, M. N., Sadiq, K., Iqbal, N. T., Moskaluk, C. A., ... Moore, S. R. (2019). Assessment of machine learning detection of environmental enteropathy and celiac disease in children. *JAMA network open, 2*(6), e195822-e195822.

Szajewska, H., Shamir, R., Mearin, L., Ribes-Koninckx, C., Catassi, C., Domellöf, M., ... Vandenplas, Y. (2016). Gluten introduction and the risk of coeliac disease: a position paper by the European Society for Pediatric Gastroenterology, Hepatology, and Nutrition. *Journal of pediatric gastroenterology and nutrition, 62*(3), 507-513.

Tack, G. J., Van de Water, J. M., Bruins, M. J., Kooy-Winkelaar, E. M., van Bergen, J., Bonnet, P., ... von Blomberg, B. M. E. (2013). Consumption of gluten with gluten-degrading enzyme by celiac patients: a pilot-study. *World journal of gastroenterology : WJG, 19*(35), 5837.

Taddei, P., Zanna, N., & Tozzi, S. (2013). Raman characterization of the interactions between gliadins and anthocyanins. *Journal of Raman Spectroscopy, 44*(10), 1435-1439.

Tagaya, Y., Kurys, G., Thies, T. A., Losi, J. M., Azimi, N., Hanover, J. A., ... Waldmann, T. A. (1997). Generation of secretable and nonsecretable interleukin 15 isoforms through alternate usage of signal peptides. *Proceedings of the National Academy of Sciences, 94*(26), 14444-14449.

Talbot, G. H. (2012). *Small bowel histopathologic findings suggestive of celiac disease in an asymptomatic patient receiving olmesartan.* Paper presented at the Mayo Clinic Proceedings.

Taranta, A., Fortunati, D., Longo, M., Rucci, N., Iacomino, E., Aliberti, F., ... Dubini, A. (2004). Imbalance of osteoclastogenesis-regulating factors in patients with celiac disease. *Journal of Bone and Mineral Research, 19*(7), 1112-1121.

Tata, L., Card, T., Logan, R., Hubbard, R., Smith, C., & West, J. (2005). Fertility and pregnancy-related events in women with celiac disease: a population-based cohort study. *Gastroenterology, 128*(4), 849-855.

Tatham, A., & Shewry, P. (2008). Allergens to wheat and related cereals. *Clinical & Experimental Allergy, 38*(11), 1712-1726.

Tenório, J. M., Hummel, A. D., Cohrs, F. M., Sdepanian, V. L., Pisa, I. T., & de Fátima Marin, H. (2011). Artificial intelligence techniques applied to the development of a decision–support system for diagnosing celiac disease. *International journal of medical informatics, 80*(11), 793-802.

Tereshchenkova, V. F., Goptar, I. A., Zhuzhikov, D. P., Belozersky, M. A., Dunaevsky, Y. E., Oppert, B., ... Elpidina, E. N. (2017). Prolidase is a critical enzyme for complete gliadin digestion in Tenebrio molitor larvae. *Archives of Insect Biochemistry and Physiology, 95*(4), e21395.

Than, T. D., Alici, G., Zhou, H., & Li, W. (2012). A review of localization systems for robotic endoscopic capsules. *IEEE transactions on biomedical engineering, 59*(9), 2387-2399.

Theodoridis, X., Grammatikopoulou, M. G., Petalidou, A., Patelida, M., Gkiouras, K., Klonizakis, M., ... Bogdanos, D. P. (2019). Dietary management of celiac disease: revisiting the guidelines. *Nutrition, 66*, 70-77.

Théophile, H., David, X. R., Miremont-Salamé, G., & Haramburu, F. (2014). Five cases of sprue -like enteropathy in patients treated by olmesartan. *Digestive and Liver Disease, 46*(5), 465-469.

Theron, M., Bentley, D., Nagel, S., Manchester, M., Gerg, M., Schindler, T., ... Perret, C. (2017). Pharmacodynamic monitoring of RO5459072, a small molecule inhibitor of cathepsin S. *Frontiers in immunology, 8*, 806.

Thomason, K., West, J., Logan, R., Coupland, C., & Holmes, G. (2003). Fracture experience of patients with coeliac disease: a population based survey. *Gut, 52*(4), 518-522.

Thompson, T. (2004). Gluten contamination of commercial oat products in the United States. *New England Journal of Medicine, 351*(19), 2021-2022.

Tian, N., Wei, G., Schuppan, D., & Helmerhorst, E. J. (2014). Effect of Rothia mucilaginosa enzymes on gliadin (gluten) structure, deamidation, and immunogenic epitopes relevant to celiac disease. *American Journal of Physiology-Gastrointestinal and Liver Physiology, 307*(8), G769-G776.

Tietge, U., Schmidt, H., & Manns, M. (1997). Neurological complications in celiac disease. *The American journal of gastroenterology, 92*(3), 540.

Ting, Y. T., Dahal-Koirala, S., Kim, H. S. K., Qiao, S. W., Neumann, R. S., Lundin, K. E., ... Rossjohn, J. (2020). A molecular basis for the T cell response in HLA-DQ2. 2 mediated celiac disease. *Proceedings of the National Academy of Sciences, 117*(6), 3063-3073.

Tollefsen, S., Arentz-Hansen, H., Fleckenstein, B., Molberg, Ø., Ráki, M., Kwok, W. W., ... Sollid, L. M. (2006). HLA-DQ2 and-DQ8 signatures of gluten T cell epitopes in celiac disease. *The Journal of clinical investigation, 116*(8), 2226-2236.

Toti, P., Balestri, P., Cano, M., Galluzzi, P., Megha, T., Farnetani, M., ... Fois, A. (1996). Celiac disease with cerebral calcium and silica deposits: X-ray spectroscopic findings, an autopsy study. *Neurology, 46*(4), 1088-1092.

Toufeili, I., Dagher, S., Shadarevian, S., Noureddine, A., Sarakbi, M., & Farran, M. T. (1994). Formulation of gluten -free pocket-type flat breads: Optimization of methylcellulose, gum arabic, and egg albumen levels by response surface methodology. *Cereal Chemistry, 71*(6), 594-600.

Tran, M. T., Faridi, P., Lim, J. J., Ting, Y. T., Onwukwe, G., Bhattacharjee, P., ... La Gruta, N. L. (2021). T cell receptor recognition of hybrid insulin peptides bound to HLA-DQ8. *Nature Communications, 12*(1), 5110.

Tran, T. H., & Li, H. (2014). Olmesartan and drug-induced enteropathy. *Pharmacy and Therapeutics, 39*(1), 47.

Troncone, R., & Ferguson, A. (1991). Animal model of gluten induced enteropathy in mice. *Gut, 32*(8), 871-875.

Trynka, G., Wijmenga, C., & van Heel, D. A. (2010). A genetic perspective on coeliac disease. *Trends in molecular medicine, 16*(11), 537-550.

Tufaro, D., Bassoli, A., & Cappa, C. (2022). Okra (Abelmoschus esculentus) powder production and application in gluten -free bread: Effect of particle size. *Food and Bioprocess Technology, 15*(4), 904-914.

Turner, S. J., Doherty, P. C., McCluskey, J., & Rossjohn, J. (2006). Structural determinants of T-cell receptor bias in immunity. *Nature Reviews Immunology, 6*(12), 883-894.

Tursi, A., Giorgetti, G. M., Iani, C., Arciprete, F., Brandimarte, G., Capria, A., & Fontana, L. (2006). Peripheral neurological disturbances, autonomic dysfunction, and antineuronal antibodies in adult celiac disease before and after a gluten -free diet. *Digestive diseases and sciences, 51*, 1869-1874.

Tye-Din, J. (2018). Interpreting tests for coeliac disease. *Australian journal of general practice, 47*(1/2), 28-33.

Tye-Din, J. A., Stewart, J. A., Dromey, J. A., Beissbarth, T., van Heel, D. A., Tatham, A., ... Jewell, D. P. (2010). Comprehensive, quantitative mapping of T cell epitopes in gluten in celiac disease. *Science translational medicine, 2*(41), 41ra51-41ra51.

Uhde, M., Ajamian, M., Caio, G., De Giorgio, R., Indart, A., Green, P. H., ... Alaedini, A. (2016). Intestinal cell damage and systemic immune activation in individuals reporting sensitivity to wheat in the absence of coeliac disease. *Gut, 65*(12), 1930-1937.

Upadhyay, A. A., Kauffman, R. C., Wolabaugh, A. N., Cho, A., Patel, N. B., Reiss, S. M., ... Sanz, I. (2018). BALDR: a computational pipeline for paired heavy and light chain immunoglobulin reconstruction in single-cell RNA-seq data. *Genome medicine, 10*, 1-18.

USAI, P., Usai Satta, P., Lai, M., Corda, M., Piras, E., Calcara, C., ... Bassotti, G. (1997). Autonomic dysfunction and upper digestive functional disorders in untreated adult coeliac disease. *European journal of clinical investigation, 27*(12), 1009-1015.

Uusitalo, U., Andren Aronsson, C., Liu, X., Kurppa, K., Yang, J., Liu, E., ... Hagopian, W. A. (2019). Early probiotic supplementation and the risk of celiac disease in children at genetic risk. *Nutrients, 11*(8), 1790.

Vader, L. W., Stepniak, D. T., Bunnik, E. M., Kooy, Y. M., De Haan, W., Drijfhout, J. W., ... Koning, F. (2003). Characterization of cereal toxicity for celiac disease patients based on protein homology in grains. *Gastroenterology, 125*(4), 1105-1113.

Vader, W., Kooy, Y., Van Veelen, P., De Ru, A., Harris, D., Benckhuijsen, W., ... Koning, F. (2002). The gluten response in children with celiac disease is directed toward multiple gliadin and glutenin peptides. *Gastroenterology, 122*(7), 1729-1737.

Vakiani, E., Arguelles-Grande, C., Mansukhani, M. M., Lewis, S. K., Rotterdam, H., Green, P. H., & Bhagat, G. (2010). Collagenous sprue is not always associated with dismal outcomes: a clinicopathological study of 19 patients. *Modern Pathology, 23*(1), 12-26.

Valitutti, F., Cucchiara, S., & Fasano, A. (2019). Celiac disease and the microbiome. *Nutrients, 11*(10), 2403.

Valle, J., Morgado, J. M. T., Ruiz-Martín, J., Guardiola, A., Lopes-Nogueras, M., García-Vela, A., ... Sánchez-Muñoz, L. (2017). Flow cytometry of duodenal intraepithelial lymphocytes improves diagnosis of celiac disease in difficult cases. *United European gastroenterology journal, 5*(6), 819-826.

van Beurden, Y. H., van Gils, T., van Gils, N. A., Kassam, Z., Mulder, C. J., & Aparicio-Pagés, N. (2016). Serendipity in Refractory Celiac Disease : Full Recovery of Duodenal Villi and Clinical Symptoms after Fecal Microbiota Transfer. *Journal of Gastrointestinal & Liver Diseases, 25*(3).

Van Buiten, C. B., Lambert, J. D., & Elias, R. J. (2018). Green tea polyphenols mitigate gliadin-mediated inflammation and permeability *in vitro*. *Molecular nutrition & food research, 62*(12), 1700879.

Van Buiten, C. B., Lambert, J. D., Sae-tan, S., & Elias, R. J. (2017). Inhibition of gliadin digestion by green tea polyphenols and the potential implications for celiac disease. *The FASEB Journal, 31*, 974.923-974.923.

Van De Wal, Y., Kooy, Y. M., Van Veelen, P. A., Peña, S. A., Mearin, L. M., Molberg, Ø., ... Benckhuijsen, W. E. (1998). Small intestinal T cells of celiac disease patients recognize a natural pepsin fragment of gliadin. *Proceedings of the National Academy of Sciences, 95*(17), 10050-10054.

van de Wal, Y., Kooy, Y. M., van Veelen, P., Vader, W., August, S. A., Drijfhout, J. W., ... Koning, F. (1999). Glutenin is involved in the gluten -driven mucosal T cell response. *European journal of immunology, 29*(10), 3133-3139.

van den Broeck, H. C., van Herpen, T. W., Schuit, C., Salentijn, E. M., Dekking, L., Bosch, D., ... van der Meer, I. M. (2009). Removing celiac disease-related gluten proteins from bread wheat while retaining technological properties: a study with Chinese Spring deletion lines. *BMC plant biology, 9*, 1-12.

Van Heel, D. A., Franke, L., Hunt, K. A., Gwilliam, R., Zhernakova, A., Inouye, M., ... Holmes, G. K. (2007). A genome-wide association study for celiac disease identifies risk variants in the region harboring IL2 and IL21. *Nature genetics, 39*(7), 827-829.

Van Hul, M., Geurts, L., Plovier, H., Druart, C., Everard, A., Ståhlman, M., ... Delzenne, N. M. (2018). Reduced obesity, diabetes, and steatosis upon cinnamon and grape pomace are associated with changes in gut microbiota and markers of gut barrier. *American Journal of Physiology-Endocrinology and Metabolism, 314*(4), E334-E352.

van Konijnenburg, D. P. H., Reis, B. S., Pedicord, V. A., Farache, J., Victora, G. D., & Mucida, D. (2017). Intestinal epithelial and intraepithelial T cell crosstalk mediates a dynamic response to infection. *Cell, 171*(4), 783-794. e713.

Van Leeuwen, M., Lindenbergh-Kortleve, D., Raatgeep, H., De Ruiter, L., De Krijger, R., Groeneweg, M., ... Samsom, J. (2013). Increased production of interleukin-21, but not interleukin-17A, in the small intestine characterizes pediatric celiac disease. *Mucosal immunology, 6*(6), 1202-1213.

van Riemsdijk, L. E., van der Goot, A. J., Hamer, R. J., & Boom, R. M. (2011). Preparation of gluten -free bread using a meso-structured whey protein particle system. *Journal of cereal science, 53*(3), 355-361.

Van Unen, V., Li, N., Molendijk, I., Temurhan, M., Höllt, T., van der Meulen-de, A. E., ... van Bergen, J. (2016). Mass cytometry of the human mucosal immune system identifies tissue-and disease-associated immune subsets. *Immunity, 44*(5), 1227-1239.

Veeraraghavan, G., Leffler, D. A., Kaswala, D. H., & Mukherjee, R. (2015). Celiac disease 2015 update: new therapies. *Expert review of gastroenterology & hepatology, 9*(7), 913-927.

Venuta, F., & Rendina, E. A. (2008). Combined pulmonary artery and bronchial sleeve resection. *Operative Techniques in Thoracic and Cardiovascular Surgery, 13*(4), 260-273.

Verdu, E. F., & Danska, J. S. (2018). Common ground: shared risk factors for type 1 diabetes and celiac disease. *Nature immunology, 19*(7), 685-695.

Verdu, E. F., & Schuppan, D. (2021). Co-factors, microbes, and immunogenetics in celiac disease to guide novel approaches for diagnosis and treatment. *Gastroenterology, 161*(5), 1395-1411. e1394.

Verdu, E. F., Huang, X., Natividad, J., Lu, J., Blennerhassett, P. A., David, C. S., ... Murray, J. A. (2008). Gliadin-dependent neuromuscular and epithelial secretory responses in gluten -sensitive HLA-DQ8 transgenic mice. *American Journal of Physiology-Gastrointestinal and Liver Physiology, 294*(1), G217-G225.

Viebke, C., Al-Assaf, S., & Phillips, G. O. (2014). Food hydrocolloids and health claims. *Bioactive Carbohydrates and Dietary Fibre, 4*(2), 101-114.

Viitasalo, L., Iltanen, S., Huhtala, H., Saavalainen, P., Kaukinen, K., Lindfors, K., & Kurppa, K. (2020). First-degree Relatives of Celiac Disease patients have increased seroreactivity to serum microbial markers. *Nutrients, 12*(4), 1073.

Viitasalo, L., Kurppa, K., Ashorn, M., Saavalainen, P., Huhtala, H., Ashorn, S., ... Iltanen, S. (2018). Microbial biomarkers in patients with nonresponsive celiac disease. *Digestive diseases and sciences, 63*, 3434-3441.

Viitasalo, L., Niemi, L., Ashorn, M., Ashorn, S., Braun, J., Huhtala, H., ... Kurppa, K. (2014). Early microbial markers of celiac disease. *Journal of clinical gastroenterology, 48*(7), 620-624.

Villanacci, V., Ceppa, P., Tavani, E., Vindigni, C., & Volta, U. (2011). Coeliac disease: the histology report. *Digestive and Liver Disease, 43*, S385-S395.

Virta, L. J., Kaukinen, K., & Collin, P. (2009). Incidence and prevalence of diagnosed coeliac disease in Finland: results of effective case finding in adults. *Scandinavian journal of gastroenterology, 44*(8), 933-938.

Vitetta, L., Vitetta, G., & Hall, S. (2018). Immunological tolerance and function: associations between intestinal bacteria, probiotics, prebiotics, and phages. *Frontiers in immunology, 9*, 2240.

Volta, U., & Villanacci, V. (2011). Celiac disease: diagnostic criteria in progress. *Cellular & molecular immunology, 8*(2), 96-102.

von Tirpitz, C., & Reinshagen, M. (2003). Management of osteoporosis in patients with gastrointestinal diseases. *European journal of gastroenterology & hepatology, 15*(8), 869-876.

Vriezinga, S. L., Auricchio, R., Bravi, E., Castillejo, G., Chmielewska, A., Crespo Escobar, P., ... Mummert, E. (2014). Randomized feeding intervention in infants at high risk for celiac disease. *New england journal of medicine, 371*(14), 1304-1315.

Wacklin, P., Laurikka, P., Lindfors, K., Collin, P., Salmi, T., Lähdeaho, M. L., ... Kurppa, K. (2014). Altered duodenal microbiota composition in celiac disease patients suffering from persistent symptoms on a long-term gluten -free diet. *Official journal of the American College of Gastroenterology| ACG, 109*(12), 1933-1941.

Wagh, S. K., Gadge, P. P., & Padul, M. V. (2018). Significant hydrolysis of wheat gliadin by bacillus tequilensis (10bT/HQ223107): a Pilot Study. *Probiotics and Antimicrobial Proteins, 10*(4), 662-667.

Wagh, S. K., Lammers, K. M., Padul, M. V., Rodriguez-Herrera, A., & Dodero, V. I. (2022). Celiac Disease and Possible Dietary Interventions: From Enzymes and Probiotics to Postbiotics and Viruses. I*nternational Journal of Molecular Sciences, 23*(19), 11748.

Wahab, P. J., Meijer, J. W., & Mulder, C. J. (2002). Histologic follow-up of people with celiac disease on a gluten -free diet : slow and incomplete recovery. *American Journal of Clinical Pathology, 118*(3), 459-463.

Walker, M. D., Williams, J., Lewis, S. K., Bai, J. C., Lebwohl, B., & Green, P. H. (2020). Measurement of forearm bone density by dual energy x-ray absorptiometry increases the prevalence of osteoporosis in men with celiac disease. *Clinical gastroenterology and hepatology, 18*(1), 99-106.

Walter, T., Wieser, H., & Koehler, P. (2015). Degradation of gluten in rye sourdough products by means of a proline-specific peptidase. *European Food Research and Technology, 240*(3), 517-524.

Wang, H., Xue, Y., Zhang, H., Huang, Y., Yang, G., Du, M., & Zhu, M. J. (2013). Dietary grape seed extract ameliorates symptoms of inflammatory bowel disease in IL 10-deficient mice. *Molecular nutrition & food research, 57*(12), 2253-2257.

Wang, K., Jin, X., Chen, Y., Song, Z., Jiang, X., Hu, F., ... Topping, D. L. (2016). Polyphenol-rich propolis extracts strengthen intestinal barrier function by activating AMPK and ERK signaling. *Nutrients, 8*(5), 272.

Wang, P., Li, D., Ke, W., Liang, D., Hu, X., & Chen, F. (2020). Resveratrol-induced gut microbiota reduces obesity in high-fat diet-fed mice. *International Journal of Obesity, 44*(1), 213-225.

Wang, Q., Tang, Y., Yang, Y., Zhao, J., Zhang, Y., Li, L., ... Ming, J. (2020). Interaction between wheat gliadin and quercetin under different pH conditions analyzed by multi-spectroscopy methods. *Spectrochimica Acta Part A: Molecular and Biomolecular Spectroscopy, 229*, 117937.

Wang, X., Qian, H., Ciaccio, E. J., Lewis, S. K., Bhagat, G., Green, P. H., ... Liu, Y. (2020). Celiac disease diagnosis from videocapsule endoscopy images with residual learning and deep feature extraction. *Computer Methods and Programs in Biomedicine, 187*, 105236.

Washington, K., Stenzel, T. T., Buckley, R. H., & Gottfried, M. R. (1996). Gastrointestinal pathology in patients with common variable immunodeficiency and X-linked agammaglobulinemia. *The American journal of surgical pathology, 20*(10), 1240-1252.

Wei, G., Helmerhorst, E. J., Darwish, G., Blumenkranz, G., & Schuppan, D. (2020). Gluten degrading enzymes for treatment of celiac disease. *Nutrients, 12*(7), 2095.

Wei, G., Tian, N., Valery, A. C., Zhong, Y., Schuppan, D., & Helmerhorst, E. J. (2015). Identification of pseudolysin (lasB) as an aciduric gluten -degrading enzyme with high therapeutic potential for celiac disease. *The American journal of gastroenterology, 110*(6), 899.

Weijers, H., Lindquist, B., Anderson, C., Rey, J., Shmerling, D., Visakorpi, J., ... Grüttner, R. (1970). Diagnostic criteria in coeliac disease. *Acta Paediatr Scand, 59*, 461-463.

West, J., Logan, R. F., Card, T. R., Smith, C., & Hubbard, R. (2003). Fracture risk in people with celiac disease: a population-based cohort study. *Gastroenterology, 125*(2), 429-436.

Wieser, H. (2000). Comparative investigations of gluten proteins from different wheat species I. Qualitative and quantitative composition of gluten protein types. *European Food Research and Technology, 211*(4), 262-268.

Wieser, H. (2007). Chemistry of gluten proteins. *Food microbiology, 24*(2), 115-119.

Wijarnpreecha, K., Lou, S., Panjawatanan, P., Cheungpasitporn, W., Pungpapong, S., Lukens, F. J., & Ungprasert, P. (2018). Cigarette smoking and risk of celiac disease:

A systematic review and meta-analysis. *United European gastroenterology journal, 6*(9), 1285-1293.

Wilson, N. K., Kent, D. G., Buettner, F., Shehata, M., Macaulay, I. C., Calero-Nieto, F. J., ... Schulte, R. (2015). Combined single-cell functional and gene expression analysis resolves heterogeneity within stem cell populations. *Cell stem cell, 16*(6), 712-724.

Wolf, C., Siegel, J. B., Tinberg, C., Camarca, A., Gianfrani, C., Paski, S., ... Pultz, I. S. (2015). Engineering of Kuma030: a gliadin peptidase that rapidly degrades immunogenic gliadin peptides in gastric conditions. *Journal of the American Chemical Society, 137*(40), 13106-13113.

Wong, S. H., & Yu, J. (2019). Gut microbiota in colorectal cancer: mechanisms of action and clinical applications. *Nature Reviews Gastroenterology & Hepatology, 16*(11), 690-704.

Wrigley, C., Békés, F., & Bushuk, W. (2006). Gluten: A balance of gliadin and glutenin. *Gliadin and glutenin: The unique balance of wheat quality*, 3-32.

Wronkowska, M., Haros, M., & Soral-Śmietana, M. (2013). Effect of starch substitution by buckwheat flour on gluten -free bread quality. *Food and Bioprocess Technology, 6*, 1820-1827.

Wu, H., Luo, T., Li, Y., Gao, Z., Zhang, K., Song, J., ... Cao, Y. (2018). Granny Smith apple procyanidin extract upregulates tight junction protein expression and modulates oxidative stress and inflammation in lipopolysaccharide-induced Caco-2 cells. *Food & function, 9*(6), 3321-3329.

Xia, J., Bergseng, E., Fleckenstein, B., Siegel, M., Kim, C. Y., Khosla, C., & Sollid, L. M. (2007). Cyclic and dimeric gluten peptide analogues inhibiting DQ2 -mediated antigen presentation in celiac disease. *Bioorganic & medicinal chemistry, 15*(20), 6565-6573.

Xia, J., Siegel, M., Bergseng, E., Sollid, L. M., & Khosla, C. (2006). Inhibition of HLA-DQ2 -mediated antigen presentation by analogues of a high affinity 33-residue peptide from α2-gliadin. *Journal of the American Chemical Society, 128*(6), 1859-1867.

Xu, H., Feely, S. L., Wang, X., Liu, D. X., Borda, J. T., Dufour, J., ... Khosla, C. (2013). Gluten-sensitive enteropathy coincides with decreased capability of intestinal T cells to secrete IL-17 and IL-22 in a macaque model for celiac disease. *Clinical Immunology, 147*(1), 40-49.

Xu, J., Zhang, Y., Wang, W., & Li, Y. (2020). Advanced properties of gluten -free cookies, cakes, and crackers: A review. *Trends in Food Science & Technology, 103*, 200-213.

Yan, D., & Holt, P. R. (2009). Willem Dicke. Brilliant clinical observer and translational investigator. Discoverer of the toxic cause of celiac disease. *Clinical and Translational Science, 2*(6), 446-448.

Yang, G., Bibi, S., Du, M., Suzuki, T., & Zhu, M. J. (2017). Regulation of the intestinal tight junction by natural polyphenols: A mechanistic perspective. *Critical Reviews in food science and nutrition, 57*(18), 3830-3839.

Yang, W. H., Zheng, B., Wu, M. N., Zhu, S. J., Fei, F. Q., Weng, M., ... Lu, P. R. (2019). An evaluation system of fundus photograph-based intelligent diagnostic technology for diabetic retinopathy and applicability for research. *Diabetes Therapy, 10*, 1811-1822.

Yang, X., Li, A., Li, X., Sun, L., & Guo, Y. (2020). An overview of classifications, properties of food polysaccharides and their links to applications in improving food textures. *Trends in Food Science & Technology, 102*, 1-15.

Yemenicioglu, A., Farris, S., Turkyilmaz, M., & Gulec, S. (2020). Natural hydrocolloids in the food sector–Recent applications beyond conventional uses. *International Journal of Food Science & Technology, 55*(4), 1387-1388.

Yeo, S., Park, H., Seo, E., Kim, J., Kim, B. K., Choi, I. S., & Huh, C. S. (2020). Anti-inflammatory and gut microbiota modulatory effect of Lactobacillus rhamnosus strain LDTM 7511 in a dextran sulfate sodium -induced colitis murine model. *Microorganisms, 8*(6), 845.

Yildiz, Ö., & Dogan, I. S. (2014). Optimization of gluten -free cake prepared from chestnut flour and transglutaminase: response surface methodology approach. *International Journal of Food Engineering, 10*(4), 737-746.

Ylimaki, G., Hawrysh, Z., Hardin, R., & Thomson, A. (1991). Response surface methodology in the development of rice flour yeast breads: sensory evaluation. *Journal of Food Science, 56*(3), 751-755.

Yokoyama, S., Perera, P. Y., Waldmann, T. A., Hiroi, T., & Perera, L. P. (2013). Tofacitinib, a janus kinase inhibitor demonstrates efficacy in an IL-15 transgenic mouse model that recapitulates pathologic manifestations of celiac disease. *Journal of clinical immunology, 33*(3), 586-594.

Zali, M. R., Sima, H., Hekmatdoost, A., Ghaziani, T., & Mashayekh, A. (2003). Seroprevalence of celiac disease in autoimmune hepatitis and chronic hepatitis B. *The American journal of gastroenterology, 98*(s9), S87.

Zamakhchari, M., Wei, G., Dewhirst, F., Lee, J., Schuppan, D., Oppenheim, F. G., & Helmerhorst, E. J. (2011). Identification of Rothia bacteria as gluten -degrading natural colonizers of the upper gastro-intestinal tract. *PloS one, 6*(9), e24455.

Zanchetta, M. B., Costa, A. F., Longobardi, V., Mazure, R., Silveira, F., Temprano, M. P., ... Smecuol, E. (2018). Improved bone microarchitecture in patients with celiac disease after 3 years on a gluten -free diet. *Clin Gastroenterol Hepatol, 16*(5), 774-775.

Zanchetta, M. B., Costa, F., Longobardi, V., Longarini, G., Mazure, R. M., Moreno, M. L., ... Smecuol, E. (2015). Significant bone microarchitecture impairment in premenopausal women with active celiac disease. *Bone, 76*, 149-157.

Zanchetta, M. B., Longobardi, V., Costa, F., Longarini, G., Mazure, R. M., Moreno, M. L., ... Smecuol, E. (2017). Impaired bone microarchitecture improves after one year on gluten -free diet: a prospective longitudinal HRpQCT study in women with celiac disease. *Journal of Bone and Mineral Research, 32*(1), 135-142.

Zanini, B., Lanzarotto, F., Mora, A., Bertolazzi, S., Turini, D., Cesana, B., ... Vassallo, F. (2010). Five year time course of celiac disease serology during gluten free diet: results of a community based "CD-Watch" program. *Digestive and liver disease, 42*(12), 865-870.

Zareie, P., Szeto, C., Farenc, C., Gunasinghe, S. D., Kolawole, E. M., Nguyen, A., ... Jones, C. M. (2021). Canonical T cell receptor docking on peptide–MHC is essential for T cell signaling. *Science, 372*(6546), eabe9124.

Zelnik, N., Pacht, A., Obeid, R., & Lerner, A. (2004). Range of neurologic disorders in patients with celiac disease. *Pediatrics, 113*(6), 1672-1676.

Zevallos, V. F., Raker, V. K., Maxeiner, J., Scholtes, P., Steinbrink, K., & Schuppan, D. (2019). Dietary wheat amylase trypsin inhibitors exacerbate murine allergic airway inflammation. *European journal of nutritio, 58*, 1507-1514.

Zevallos, V. F., Raker, V., Tenzer, S., Jimenez-Calvente, C., Ashfaq-Khan, M., Rüssel, N., ... Schuppan, D. (2017). Nutritional wheat amylase-trypsin inhibitors promote intestinal inflammation via activation of myeloid cells. *Gastroenterology, 152*(5), 1100-1113. e1112.

Zhang, H., & Tsao, R. (2016). Dietary polyphenols, oxidative stress and antioxidant and anti-inflammatory effects. *Current Opinion in Food Science, 8*, 33-42.

Zhang, L., Gui, S., Wang, J., Chen, Q., Zeng, J., Liu, A., ... Lu, X. (2020). Oral administration of green tea polyphenols (TP) improves ileal injury and intestinal flora disorder in mice with Salmonella typhimurium infection via resisting inflammation, enhancing antioxidant action and preserving tight junction. *Journal of Functional Foods, 64*, 103654.

Zhang, Y., Liang, Z., Zong, Y., Wang, Y., Liu, J., Chen, K., ... Gao, C. (2016). Efficient and transgene-free genome editing in wheat through transient expression of CRISPR/Cas9 DNA or RNA. *Nature Communications, 7*(1), 12617.

Zhao, R., Long, X., Yang, J., Du, L., Zhang, X., Li, J., & Hou, C. (2019). Pomegranate peel polyphenols reduce chronic low-grade inflammatory responses by modulating gut microbiota and decreasing colonic tissue damage in rats fed a high-fat diet. *Food & function, 10*(12), 8273-8285.

Zhernakova, A., Withoff, S., & Wijmenga, C. (2013). Clinical implications of shared genetics and pathogenesis in autoimmune diseases. *Nature Reviews Endocrinology, 9*(11), 646-659.

Zhou, R., Wei, H., Sun, R., & Tian, Z. (2007). Recognition of double-stranded RNA by TLR3 induces severe small intestinal injury in mice. *The Journal of Immunology, 178*(7), 4548-4556.

Zhou, T., Han, G., Li, B. N., Lin, Z., Ciaccio, E. J., Green, P. H., & Qin, J. (2017). Quantitative analysis of patients with celiac disease by video capsule endoscopy: A deep learning method. *Computers in biology and medicine, 85*, 1-6.

Zoghi, A., Mirmahdi, R. S., & Mohammadi, M. (2021). The role of hydrocolloids in the development of gluten -free cereal-based products for coeliac patients: a review. *International Journal of Food Science & Technology, 56*(7), 3138-3147.

Zou, N. N. H., & Hobbs, J. E. (2010). *The Role Of Labelling In Consumers'functional Food Choices.*

Zugna, D., Richiardi, L., Akre, O., Stephansson, O., & Ludvigsson, J. F. (2010). A nationwide population-based study to determine whether coeliac disease is associated with infertility. *Gut, 59*(11), 1471-1475.

Zühlke, S., Risnes, L. F., Dahal-Koirala, S., Christophersen, A., Sollid, L. M., & Lundin, K. E. (2019). CD38 expression on gluten -specific T cells is a robust marker of gluten re-exposure in coeliac disease. *United European gastroenterology journal, 7*(10), 1337-1344.

Zylberberg, H. M., Lebwohl, B., RoyChoudhury, A., Walker, M. D., & Green, P. H. (2018). Predictors of improvement in bone mineral density after celiac disease diagnosis. *Endocrine, 59*, 311-318.

About the Authors

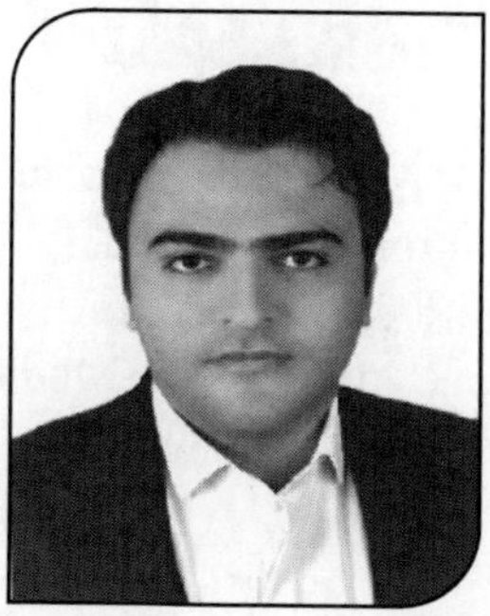

Dr. Amin Abbasi
Department of Food Science and Technology, Faculty of Nutrition and Food Sciences, Tabriz University of Medical Sciences, Tabriz, Iran
abbasia@sbmu.ac.ir; abasi@tbzmed.ac.ir

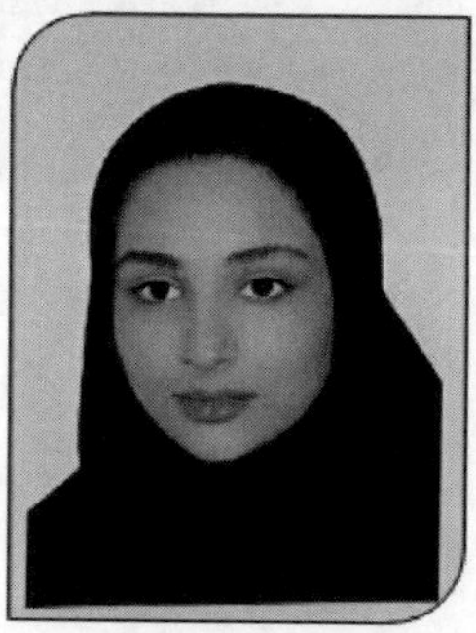

Sara Arshadi
Department of clinical Nutrition and Dietetics, National Nutrition and Food Technology Research Institute, Faculty of Nutrition Science and Food Technology, Shahid Beheshti University of Medical Sciences, Tehran, Iran
saraharshadii81@gmail.com

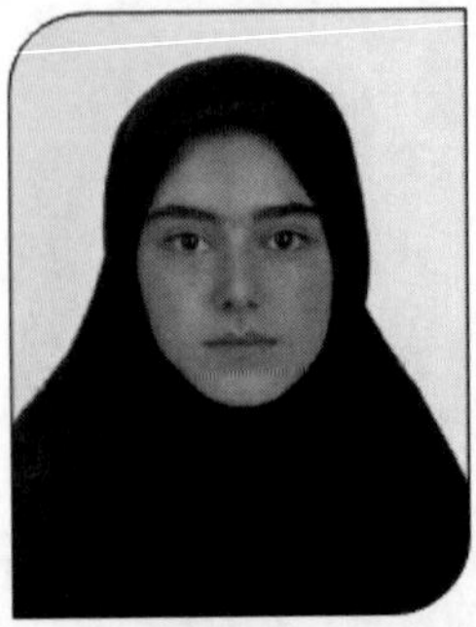

Negin Lohrasbi
Department of clinical Nutrition and Dietetics, National Nutrition and Food Technology Research Institute, Faculty of Nutrition Science and Food Technology, Shahid Beheshti University of Medical Sciences, Tehran, Iran
negin.lohrasbi250@gmail.com

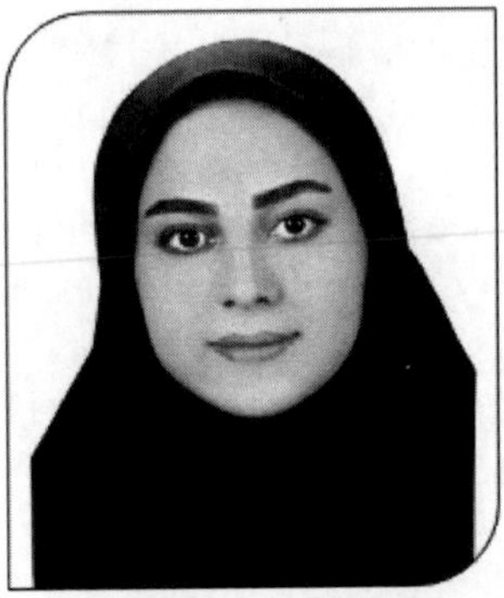

Faezeh Tejareh
Department of Nutrition, Science and Research Branch, Islamic Azad University, Tehran, Iran
faezehtejareh135@gmail.com

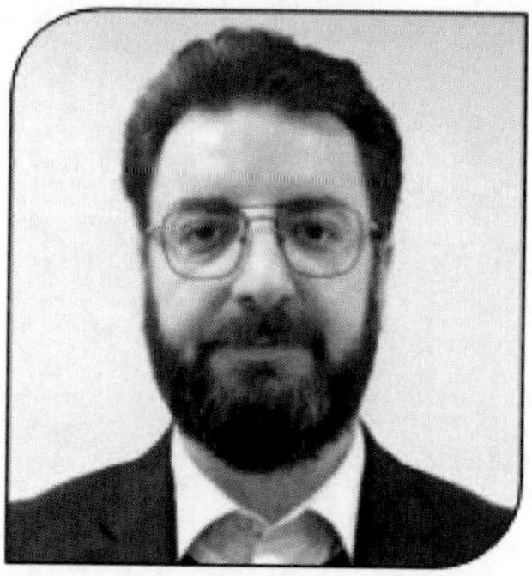

Dr. Mohammad Hashemi
Department of Nutrition, Faculty of Medicine, Mashhad University of Medical Sciences, Mashhad, Iran
mo_hashemi@hotmail.com.

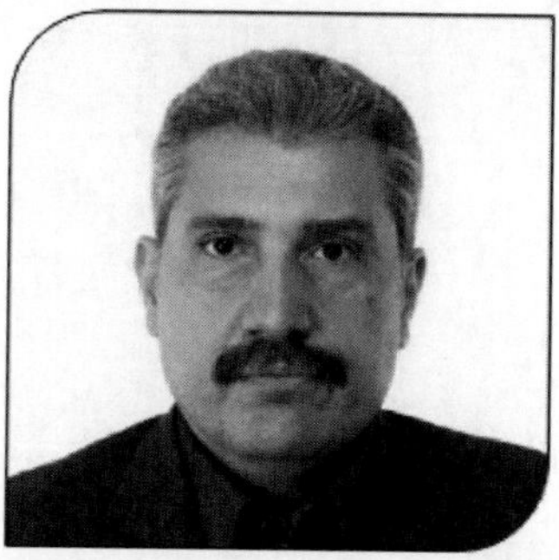

Prof. Hedayat Hosseini
Department of Food Science and Technology, National Nutrition and Food Technology Research Institute, Faculty of Nutrition Science and Food Technology, Shahid Beheshti University of Medical Sciences, Tehran, Iran
hedayat@sbmu.ac.ir

Index

Q

R

S

T

U

V

W

Z